RECENT CONCEPTS IN SARCOMA TREATMENT

DEVELOPMENTS IN ONCOLOGY

Recent volumes

M.P. Hacker, E.B. Double and I. Krakoff, eds., Platinum Coordination Complexes in Cancer Chemotherapy. ISBN 0-89838-619-5

M.J. van Zwieten, The Rat as Animal Model in Breast Cancer Research: A Histopathological Study of Radiation- and Hormone-Induced Rat Mammary Tumors. ISBN 0-89838-624-1

B. Löwenberg and A. Hagenbeek, eds., Minimal Residual Disease in Acute Leukemia. ISBN 0-89838-630-6

I. van der Waal and G.B. Snow, eds., Oral Oncology. ISBN 0-89838-631-4

B.W. Hancock and A.H. Ward, eds., Immunological Aspects of Cancer. ISBN 0-89838-664-0

K.V. Honn and B.F. Sloane, Hemostatic Mechanisms and Metastasis. ISBN 0-89838-667-5

K.R. Harrap, W. Davis and A.H. Calvert, eds., Cancer Chemotherapy and Selective Drug Development. ISBN 0-89838-673-X

C.J.H. van de Velde and P.H. Sugarbaker, eds., Liver Metastasis. ISBN 0-89838-648-5

D.J. Ruiter, K. Welvaart and S. Ferrone, eds., Cutaneous Melanoma and Precursor Lesions. ISBN 0-89838-689-6

S.B. Howell, ed., Intra-arterial and Intracavitary Cancer Chemotherapy. ISBN 0-89838-691-8

D.L. Kisner and J.F. Smyth, eds., Interferon Alpha-2: Pre-Clinical and Clinical Evaluation. ISBN 0-89838-701-9

P. Furmanski, J.C. Hager and M.A. Rich, eds., RNA Tumor Viruses, Oncogenes, Human Cancer and Aids: On the Frontiers of Understanding. ISBN 0-89838-703-5

J. Talmadge, I.J. Fidler and R.K. Oldham, Screening for Biological Response Modifiers: Methods and Rationale. ISBN 0-89838-712-4

J.C. Bottino, R.W. Opfell and F.M. Muggia, eds., Liver Cancer. ISBN 0-89838-713-2

P.K. Pattengale, R.J. Lukes and C.R. Taylor, Lymphoproliferative Diseases: Pathogenesis, Diagnosis, Therapy. ISBN 0-89838-725-6

F. Cavalli, G. Bonadonna and M. Rozencweig, eds., Malignant Lymphomas and Hodgkin's Disease: Experimental and Therapeutic Advances. ISBN 0-89838-727-2

L. Baker, F. Valeriote and V. Ratanatharathorn, eds., Biology and Therapy of Acute Leukemia. ISBN 0-89838-728-0

J. Russo, ed., Immunocytochemistry in Tumor Diagnosis. ISBN 0-89838-737-X

R.L. Ceriani, ed., Monoclonal Antibodies and Breast Cancer. ISBN 0-89838-739-6

D.E. Peterson, G.E. Elias and S.T. Sonis, eds., Head and Neck Management of the Cancer Patient. ISBN 0-89838-747-7

D.M. Green, Diagnosis and Management of Malignant Solid Tumors in Infants and Children. ISBN 0-89838-750-7

K.A. Foon and A.C. Morgan, Jr., eds., Monoclonal Antibody Therapy of Human Cancer. ISBN 0-89838-754-X

J.G. McVie, W. Bakker, Sj.Sc. Wagenaar and D. Carney, eds., Clinical and Experimental Pathology of Lung Cancer. ISBN 0-89838-764-7

K.V. Honn, W.E. Powers and B.F. Sloane, eds., Mechanisms of Cancer Metastasis. ISBN 0-89838-765-5

K. Lapis, L.A. Liotta and A.S. Rabson, eds., Biochemistry and Molecular Genetics of Cancer Metastasis. ISBN 0-89838-785-X

A.J. Mastromarino, ed., Biology and Treatment of Colorectal Cancer Metastasis. ISBN 0-89838-786-8

M.A. Rich, J.C. Hager and J. Taylor-Papadimitriou, eds., Breast Cancer: Origins, Detection and Treatment. ISBN 0-89838-792-2

D.G. Poplack, L. Massimo and P. Cornaglia-Ferraris, eds., The Role of Pharmacology in Pediatric Oncology. ISBN 0-89838-795-7

A. Hagenbeek and B. Löwenberg, eds., Minimal Residual Disease in Acute Leukemia 1986. ISBN 0-89838-799-X

F.M. Muggia and M. Rozencweig, eds., Clinical Evaluations of Anti-Tumor Therapy. ISBN 0-89838-803-1

F.A. Valeriote and L. Baker, eds., Biochemical Modulation of Anticancer Agents: Experimental and Clinical Approaches. ISBN 0-89838-827-9

B.A. Stoll, ed., Pointers to Cancer Prognosis. ISBN 0-89838-841-4

K.H. Hollmann and J.M. Verley, eds., New Frontiers in Mammary Pathology 1986. ISBN 0-89838-852-X

D.J. Ruiter, G.J. Fleuren and S.O. Warnaar, eds., Application of Monoclonal Antibodies in Tumor Pathology. ISBN 0-89838-853-8

M. Chatel, F. Darcel and J. Pecker, eds., Brain Oncology. ISBN 0-89838-954-2

J.R. Ryan and L.O. Baker, eds., Recent Concepts in Sarcoma Treatment. ISBN 0-89838-376-5

Recent Concepts in Sarcoma Treatment

Proceedings of the International Symposium on Sarcomas, Tarpon Springs, Florida, October 8–10, 1987

edited by

James R. Ryan MD
Associate Professor, Department of Orthopedic Surgery,
Chief Orthopedic Oncology,
Wayne State University School of Medicine, Detroit, Michigan 48201, USA

Laurence O. Baker D.O.
Professor, Department of Internal Medicine,
Director, Division of Hematology-Oncology,
Wayne State University School of Medicine, Detroit, Michigan 48201, USA

KLUWER ACADEMIC PUBLISHERS
DORDRECHT / BOSTON / LONDON

Library of Congress Cataloging in Publication Data

International Symposium on Sarcomas (1987 : Tarpon Springs, Fla.)
    Recent concepts in sarcoma treatment : proceedings of the
  International Symposium on Sarcomas, Tarpon Springs, Florida,
  October 8-10, 1987 / edited by James R. Ryan, Laurence H. Baker.
        p.   cm. -- (Developments in oncology)
    International Symposium on Sarcomas organized under the auspices
  of the Intergroup Sarcoma Committee of the National Cancer
  Institute.
    ISBN 0-89838-376-5
    1. Sarcoma--Treatment--Congresses.   I. Ryan, James R. (James
  Raymond), 1936-   . II. Baker, Laurence H. III. National Cancer
  Institute (U.S.). Intergroup Sarcoma Committee. IV. Title.
  V. Series.
    [DNLM: 1. Sarcoma--diagnosis--congresses. 2. Sarcoma--therapy-
  -congresses.   W1 DE998N / QZ 266 I61065r 1987]
  RC270.8.I53 1987
  616.99'4--dc19
  DNLM/DLC
  for Library of Congress   88-8976
                                                                  CIP

ISBN 0-89838-376-5

Published by Kluwer Academic Publishers,
P.O. Box 17, 3300 AA Dordrecht, The Netherlands.

Kluwer Academic Publishers incorporates
the publishing programmes of
D. Reidel, Martinus Nijhoff, Dr W. Junk and MTP Press.

Sold and distributed in the U.S.A. and Canada
by Kluwer Academic Publishers,
101 Philip Drive, Norwell, MA 02061, U.S.A.

In all other countries, sold and distributed
by Kluwer Academic Publishers Group,
P.O. Box 322, 3300 AH Dordrecht, The Netherlands.

PREFACE

There have been significant advances in the treatment of sarcomas in the past several years. Further, different clinical treatment programs are being advocated in different areas including surgery alone, surgery with preoperative or postoperative chemotherapy, surgery with different radiotherapy modalities, with each investigator espousing his own treatment program. On the other side, there is the question of whether these treatment programs are offering better results or whether the natural history of sarcomas has changed.

The International Symposium on Sarcomas was held at Innisbrook Resort, Tarpon Springs, Florida, October 8-10, 1987. This was the first international symposium to date involving all of the disciplines treating sarcomas including pathologists, orthopaedic surgeons, general surgeons, medical oncologists, pediatric oncologists, and radiation oncologists. The Symposium brought together a number of specialists working in the clinical field of sarcomas for a presentation of their specific treatment programs and their results. The presentations were followed by panel discussions to stimulate educational debate as to the different forms of treatment for sarcomas and to formulate some conformity in control of disease, control of spread, and ultimate function for the patient.

James R. Ryan, M.D.
December 1987

ACKNOWLEDGMENTS

I would like to thank everyone involved in the organization of the International Symposium on Sarcomas, under the auspices of the Intergroup Sarcoma Committee of the National Cancer Institute; Mrs. Gwen MacKenzie and her staff, Division of Hematology-Oncology, Wayne State University, for financial administration; and Mrs. Carol Grzesik for her help in organizing the Symposium and preparation of the manuscript.

Supported in part by PHS Grant Number 1 R13 CA45130-01 awarded by the National Cancer Institute, DHHS. Support also received from Bristol-Myers Laboratories.

TABLE OF CONTENTS

GRADING OF SOFT-TISSUE SARCOMAS

David C. Dahlin, M.D.*

The concept of the grading of malignant tumors was introduced by Broders in 1920 (1), who had studied 537 squamous cell carcinomas of the lip. Such tumors tended to be much more advanced at the time of his study, which was before 1920, than they are currently. Broders' study was actually the practical application of the Hansemann principle (2). Hansemann concluded, in the nineteenth century, that the most malignant tumors of various types metastasized the earliest and the most widely. Broders graded the tumors from 1 to 4 and showed that the grade 4 lesions, the most undifferentiated, had the poorest prognosis.

Reszel and co-workers (3) gave us information in 1966 that a numerical system of grading liposarcomas provided information on the likelihood of five- and ten-year survival, with the grade 4 lesions having the poorest prognosis. Kindbloom and co-workers (4), in 1975, also found that poorer differentiation correlated with poorer prognosis of liposarcomas. Russell and co-workers (5), in a study of a variety of soft-tissue sarcomas in 1977, reported that grade is a necessary requirement in the structuring of any staging system for soft-tissue sarcoma. Markhede, Angervall and Stener (6), who studied 97 patients with soft-tissue tumors, found that the likelihood of survival was related to the adequacy of the surgical removal and to the histologic grade of malignancy. Evans (7) in 1979, reported that dedifferentiated lipo-sarcomas, those with highly anaplastic areas, had a significantly poorer prognosis than the myxoid and well-differentiated types. Enzinger and Weiss (8), in their book on Soft-Tissue Tumors, in 1983, indicated the significance of grade of malignancy for many soft-tissue tumors. Orson and co-workers, in 1987 (9), studied 211 cases of liposarcoma and stated that "significant variation in survival time was related to histologic grade, Enneking's stage, tumor size and histologic type." Costa (10), in 1985, emphasized the value of grading both soft-tissue and bone sarcomas. Unni and Dahlin (11), in 1984, stated that grading is especially useful in chondrosarcoma, angiosarcoma of bone and in certain types of osteosarcoma.

At the Mayo Clinic, we have found that grading affords

----

*Professor Emeritus of Pathology, Mayo Clinic, Rochester, MN 55905.

1

J. R. Ryan and L. O. Baker (eds.), Recent Concepts in Sarcoma Treatment, 1–6.
© 1988 by Kluwer Academic Publishers.

important prognostic information for many soft-tissue sarcomas such as the following:

Fibrosarcoma
Liposarcoma
Malignant fibrous histiocytoma
Leiomyosarcoma
Hemangiopericytoma
Neurofibrosarcoma

A subjective element makes it difficult to state exactly what constitutes a specific grade of tumor. The general criteria for the elements of grading are the degree of cellularity, the degree of cellular anaplasia, mitotic activity (including abnormal mitoses) and necrosis. Attention must be given the overall pattern of the lesion. Mitotic activity may be great in the cellular central portion of florid myositis ossificans, but the peripheral maturation to osteoid and trabeculae of obviously benign bone afford the diagnostic clue that the lesion is a benign and non-neoplastic reparative process. Similarly, other benign processes may be recognized by their general morphology; mitoses must be ignored in them.

Fibrosarcoma, the first soft-tissue lesion on the list, can be graded from 1 to 4. It is necessary to exclude lesions now recognized such as malignant fibrous histiocytoma and monomorphic synovial sarcoma. After appropriate exclusion, the five-year survival for grade 1 and 2 fibrosarcoma has been 55 percent, for grade 3 it has been 34 percent and for grade 4 only 21 percent. These survival figures are similar to those of the earlier fibrosarcoma series in which variants had been included. This suggests that grade can help predict survival regardless of the exact histologic diagnosis.

Liposarcoma can be graded, and the numbers are of prognostic significance. Evans (7) has provided information that those liposarcomas that dedifferentiate into a higher grade have a poorer prognosis. The other sarcomas in the list of those that can be graded, malignant fibrous histiocytoma, leiomyosarcoma, hemangiopericytoma and neurofibrosarcoma, can be assessed as to cellularity, anaplasia, mitotic activity and necrosis. These features can provide a numerical system of grading that affords prognostic significance and allows the surgeon to select a more aggressive surgical removal for the lesions of higher grade.

Sarcomas of soft-tissue origin that we have found it impractical to grade to provide significant information concerning prognosis usually have little variation from case to case. They are:

Synovial sarcoma
Clear-cell sarcoma
Epithelioid sarcoma
Angiosarcoma
Lymphangiosarcoma
Alveolar soft parts sarcoma
Mesenchymal chondrosarcoma
Myxoid chondrosarcoma

The final list is of small-cell sarcomas. Members of this group are usually grade 4 malignant, so it is impractical to grade them. They are:

Rhabdomyosarcoma
Extraosseous Ewing's sarcoma
Undifferentiated small-cell sarcoma
Neuroblastoma

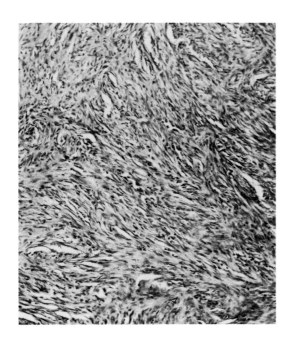

FIGURE 1A: Grade 1 fibrosarcoma. There are relatively few nuclei and minimal anaplasia. H&E x 160.

4

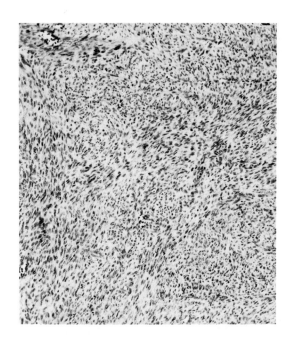

FIGURE 1B: Grade 2 fibrosarcoma with some increased cellularity and slight anaplasia. H&E x 160.

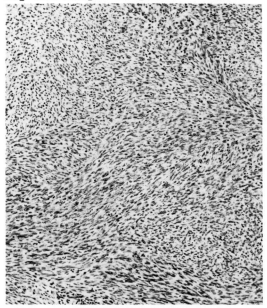

FIGURE 1C: Grade 3 fibrosarcoma. There is more cellularity
and anaplasia. H&E x 160.

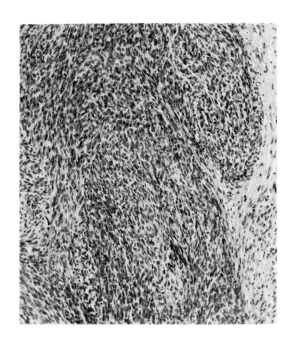

FIGURE 1D: Grade 4 fibrosarcoma. Note marked cellularity.
Mitotic figures were numerous.

REFERENCES

1. Broders AC: Squamous cell epithelioma of the lip. A study of 537 cases. JAMA 74:656-664, 1920.
2. Broders AC: The microscopic grading of cancer. In Pack GT, Livingston EM (eds.): Treatment of Cancer and Allied Diseases, Vol. 1, New York: Paul B. Hoeker Inc, pp 19-41, 1946.
3. Reszel PA, Soule EH, Coventry MB: Liposarcoma of the extremities and limb girdles. A study of 222 cases. J. Bone and Joint Surg 48-A(2):229-244, 1966.
4. Kindbloom LG, Angervall L, Svendsen P: Liposarcoma. A clinicopathologic, radiographic and prognostic study. Acta Pathol et Microbiol Scand. Section A, pp 1-71, Suppl no 253, 1975.
5. Russell WO, Cohen J, Enzinger F, Hajdu SI, Heise H, Martin RG, Meissner W, Miller WT, Schmitz RL, Suit HD: A clinical and pathological staging system for soft-tissue sarcomas. Cancer 40:1562-1570, 1977.
6. Markhede G, Angervall L, Stener B: A multivariate analysis of the prognosis after surgical treatment of malignant soft-tissue tumors. Cancer 49:1721-1733, 1982.
7. Evans HL: Liposarcoma. A study of 55 cases with a reassessment of its classification. Am J Surg Pathol 3:507-523, Dec 1979.

8. Enzinger FM, Weiss SW: Soft-Tissue Tumors. St. Louis: The CV Mosby Company, 1983.
9. Orson GG, Sim FH, Reiman HR, Taylor WF: Liposarcoma of the musculoskeletal system. In Press (submitted to Cancer Jan 30, 1987).
10. Costa J: Histologic classification and grading of sarcomas. Cancer Treat Symp 3:27-28, 1985.
11. Unni KK, Dahlin DC: Grading of bone tumors. Seminars in Diagn Pathol 1:165-172, 1984.

GRADING OF SOFT TISSUE SARCOMAS: EXPERIENCE OF THE EORTC SOFT TISSUE AND BONE SARCOMA GROUP

J.A.M. van Unnik[1,9], J.M. Coindre[2], G. Contesso[3],
Ch.E. Albus-Lutter[4], T. Schiodt[5], T. Garcia Miralles[6],
R. Sylvester[7], D. Thomas[7], and V. Bramwell[8]

In oncology, the best possible information about prognosis is of paramount importance. This holds true particularly for clinical trials but also for determining the most appropriate treatment in general. Regarding soft tissue sarcomas (STS), it is well known that some types of these malignancies have a favorable prognosis, e.g. myxoid liposarcoma, others such as rhabdomyosarcomas are generally related to a poor outcome. On the other hand, every worker in this field is familiar with the great variability in histopathology and clinical behavior of e.g. the fibro- and leiomatous tumors.

Many studies regarding clinico-pathological correlations in STS have been based on a combination of typing and grading of these malignancies in which a certain grade was automatically assigned to a certain tumor, e.g. highly differentiated liposarcoma - grade 1, rhabdomyosarcoma - grade 3, and other sarcomas were graded according to the number of mitoses, pleomorphism, etc. (1-4). In these studies, these parameters were generally only described in general terms and the way in which the authors arrived at a definite grade was not given in detail. One may suspect that the grading largely rested on experience and intuition. However, by applying analytic statistical methods, it was shown that some general parameters were highly correlated with prognosis, e.g. mitoses (5) and necrosis (6).

For several years, a group of pathologists in France and in Holland independently worked on a grading system. These pathologists were members of the pathology subcommittee of the EORTC soft tissue and bone sarcoma group or worked in close connection with the members of this subcommittee. In these studies, the significance of a great number of

----

1) Institute of Pathology Utrecht, Pasteurstraat 2, 3511 HX
   Utrecht, The Netherlands
2) Fondation Bergonie, Bordeaux, France
3) Institut Gustave-Roussy, Villejuif, France
4) Netherlands Cancer Institute, Amsterdam, The Netherlands
5) Department of Pathology, Rigshospitalet, Copenhagen,
   Denmark
6) Hospital General de Asturias, Oviedo, Spain
7) EORTC Data Center in Brussels, Belgium
8) Ontario Cancer Foundation, London, Ontario, Canada
9) To whom correspondence should be addressed

J. R. Ryan and L. O. Baker (eds.), Recent Concepts in Sarcoma Treatment, 7–13.
© 1988 by Kluwer Academic Publishers.

parameters was tested. The parameters used by one or both groups were: the degree of nuclear pleomorphism, the presence of giant cells, of vascular emboli, myxoid areas, the degree of cellularity, tumor differentiation, necrosis and mitotic rate. In order to enhance reproducibility, these parameters were defined as exactly as possible. Afterwards, a multivariate analysis was applied to determine minimum subsets of variables required to retain the prognostic information. These criteria were (semi) quantitatively used in a scoring system. The study of the group of Trojani et al.(7), comprising 155 patients of the French cancer centers, showed that tumor differentiation, mitotic rate and tumor necrosis were the three histological factors which provided the maximum prognostic information. A simple histopathologic grading system, applicable to all types of STS, was elaborated. This grading was strongly correlated with survival and the advent of metastases. Reproducibility of this grading among pathologists has been tested: agreement was 75% for the tumor grade and only 51% for the diagnosis of histologic types. The Dutch study of Albus-Lutter (8), making use of 400 patients of the Netherlands Cancer Institute in Amsterdam, came up with six factors, i.e. mitotic rate, myxoid component, differentiation, tumor necrosis and also the size of the tumor and the localization (superficial versus deep) as minimal criteria to predict the clinical course. In both studies, the type of sarcoma was not taken into consideration because of the marked alterations and differences in interpretation of existing classifications (9, 10) and the preponderance of grading over typing as prognostic indicator in these types of malignancies. However, in the study of Albus-Lutter, the number of patients was sufficient to apply an adapted grading system to some large diagnostic groups.

With the experience gained by these studies, a comparable study was undertaken on the 169 patients with STS of EORTC Trial 62771 (adjuvant cyvadic versus no chemotherapy) for whom we were able to carry out an external review of the slides. The chemotherapy in this trial did not influence the survival. The median age of the patients was 41 years with a range from 16-70 years. If after local surgery (local resection in 80% or amputation in 20%) microscopic tumor was left behind, radiotherapy was applied in 54%. Local recurrences at entry in the trial were observed in 17%. The diagnostic groups of STS were MFH 23%, fibrosarcoma 6%, liposarcoma 20%, leiomyosarcoma 8%, rhabdomyosarcoma 3%, angiosarcoma 2%, synoviosarcoma 18%, neurogenic sarcoma 7%, miscellaneous 7%, undifferentiated 6%.

The histopathologic parameters studied were: differentiation of the tumor, necrosis, myxoid areas and mitotic rate. Later on, the size of the tumor and type of surgical intervention (local resection versus amputation) were added.

In contrast to the foregoing studies, the quantitative parameters studied were not a priori grouped (mitotic rate <10<, or <20<, and diameter of the tumor <5<cm), but ob-

jectively divided into the most discriminating categories, which appeared to be for size <8<cm) and mitotic rate <3/10 HPF (high power fields), 3-20/10 HPF and >20/10 HPF (10 HPF is approximately 1,5 mm^2).

Results

All histological parameters examined were correlated with the duration of survival, but after multivariate analysis only the mitotic rate and the presence of necrosis retained their significance, of which the mitotic rate was by far the most important. Differences in the amount of necrosis (<10% necrosis versus 10-50% necrotic areas) were of no influence. The following score function was obtained:

Score A = 7.7745 x necrosis + 11.747 x mitoses
 Where necrosis is 0 if no necrosis and 1 if some
 necrosis, and mitoses is 0 if <3 mitoses/10 HPF,
 mitoses is 1 if 3-20 mitoses/10 HPF, and mitoses is
 2 if >20 mitoses/10 HPF.

Survival curves I, II and III are illustrated in Figure 1 and obtained as follows:

Curve I   if 0 <score <9 (number of patients 30)
Curve II if 10 <score <29 (number of patients 107)
Curve III if   score >30 (number of patients 28)

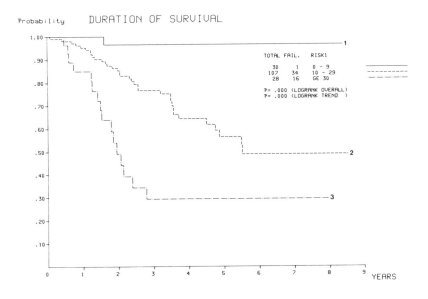

FIGURE 1: Overall survival curves, calculated according to score A, in which presence of necrosis and number of mitoses are involved.

In a simplified form, the same curves can be defined as follows:

TABLE 1:	Mitotic score	Necrosis score	Curve
	0	0	I
	0	1	I
	1	0	II
	1	1	II
	2	0	II
	2	1	III

The subordinate importance of necrosis is illustrated in Table I where the presence of necrosis only influences the grading in mitotic score 2.

If the tumor diameter is also used, then the score function becomes:

Score B = 8.3696 x necrosis + 13.438 x mitoses + 11.551 x tumor diameter in which the score for tumor size is 0 if diameter <8 cm and 1 if diameter $\geq$8 cm.

In Figure 2, the curves I, II and III are defined as:

I   if   0 $\leq$score $\leq$19 (number of patients 36)
II   if 20 $\leq$score $\leq$29 (number of patients 59)
III if   score $\geq$30 (number of patients 48)

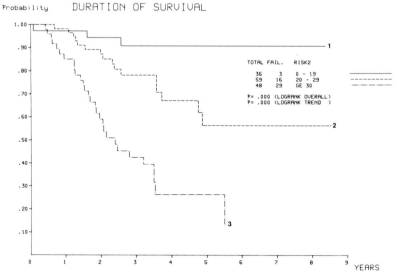

FIGURE 2: Overall survival curves, calculated according to score B, in which presence of necrosis, number of mitoses and tumor site are involved.

For the appearance of distant metastases, the diameter of the tumor is not significant. Based on mitotic rate and necrosis score A can be modified based on the following

formula:
    9.5835 x necrosis + 10.298 x mitoses in which necrosis
    and mitotic rate are defined as before (Figure 3).

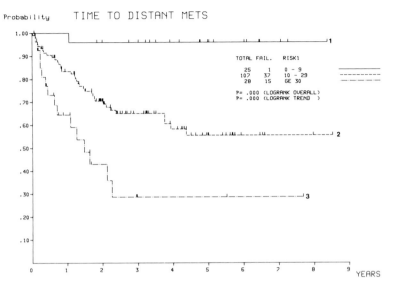

FIGURE 3: Appearance of distant metastasis is illustrated.
The various curves are calculated according to
score A (presence of necrosis and number of
mitoses).

    Using also the surgical procedure as a variable, an even
more accurate score function for survival may be obtained
as:
    Score C = 10.968 x surgical procedure + 14.219 x mitotic
    rate + 10.171 x tumor diameter + 7.1836 x necrosis.
    In this formula, the surgical procedure is given as 0 if
local resection and as 1 if amputation.
    The survival curves in Figure 4, I-IV based on these
parameters are defined as:
    I   if 0 $\leq$ score $\leq$ 20 (number of patients 37)
    II   if 21 $\leq$ score $\leq$ 30 (number of patients 44)
    III if 31 $\leq$ score $\leq$ 40 (number of patients 38)
    IV   if 41 $\leq$ score $\leq$ 60 (number of patients 23)

12

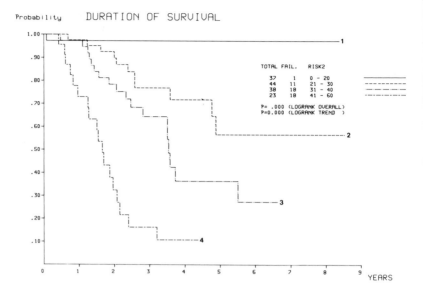

FIGURE 4: Overall survival curves calculated according to
score C, in which presence of necrosis, number of
mitoses, tumor size and surgical procedure are
involved.

In this way, depending on the available data, a rather
accurate prognostic indication can be given in this group of
malignancies.

REFERENCES

1. Russell WO, Cohen J, Enzinger F, et al: A Clinical and
    Pathological Staging System for Soft Tissue Sarcomas.
    Cancer 40:1562-1570, 1977.
2. Markhede G, Angervall L, Stener B: A Multivariate Analy-
    sis of the Prognosis After Surgical Treatment of Malig-
    nant Soft Tissue Tumors. Cancer 49:1721-1733, 1982.
3. Myhre-Jensen O, Kaae S, Hjollund-Maasen E, et al:
    Histopathological Grading in Soft Tissue Tumors. Rela-
    tion to Survival in 261 Surgically Treated Patients.
    Acta Pathol Microbiol Immunol Scand Sec 91, 145-150,
    1983.
4. Suit HD, Russell WO, Martin RG: Sarcoma of Soft Tissue:
    Clinical and Histopathological Parameters and Response
    to Treatment. Cancer 35:1478-1483, 1975.
5. Van de Werf-Messing B, Van Unnik JAM: Fibrosarcoma of
    the Soft Tissues. Cancer 18:1113-1123, 1965.
6. Costa J, Wesley RA, Glatstein E, Rosenberg SA: The
    Grading of Soft Tissue Sarcomas. Results of a Clinico-
    pathologic Correlation in a Series of 163 Cases. Cancer
    53:530-541, 1984.

7. Trojani M, Contesso G, Coindre JM, et al: Soft Tissue
    Sarcomas in Adults: Study of Pathological Prognostic
    Variables and Definition of a Histopathological Grading
    System. Int J Cancer 33:37-42, 1984.
8. Albus-Lutter Ch.E: Het Wekedelen Sarcoom, een Onderzoek
    Naar Klinisch-Pathologische Correlaties. Thesis,
    Utrecht, 1987.
9. Presant CA, Russell WO, Alexander RW, Fu YS: Soft Tissue
    and Bone Sarcoma Histopathology Peer Review: The Fre-
    quency of Disagreement in Diagnosis and the Need for
    Second Pathology Opinions. The Southeastern Cancer Study
    Group Experience. J. Clin Oncol 4:1658-1661, 1986.
10. Coindre JM, Trojani M, Contesso G, et al: Reproducibil-
    ity of a Histopathologic Grading System for Adult Soft
    Tissue Sarcomas. Cancer 58:306-309, 1986.

GRADING OF BONE TUMORS

Andrew G. Huvos, M.D.[*]

The modern clinicopathologic study of osseous neoplasms, both benign and malignant, emphasizes a variety of biologic techniques, among which, grading of tumors, DNA-related analyses encompassing cytogenetics, flow cytometric methods, cell kinetics, and restriction enzyme endonuclease mapping are the most prominently mentioned. These biologic methods have been found to be, individually or in combination with each other, useful in predicting prognosis in bone and soft tissue neoplasms.

There are contrary opinions on the feasibility of grading giant cell tumors of bone and reliably predicting subsequent clinical behavior. Some maintain that the histologic makeup does not consistently and reliably parallel the biologic potential of a given lesion. Neither local recurrence rate nor distant metastases can be predicted - they believe and state - by histologic appearance.(1,2) Others feel, however, that microscopic features should be buttressed with other parameters, such as erosion of cortex and extension to soft tissues, to provide a more predictive evaluation for prognostication.(3) And, there are those who believe the histologic features of a giant cell tumor reliably mirror subsequent clinical behavior and are of considerable help in predicting prognosis while providing valuable guidance in the required treatment.(4,5) A reasonably reproducible scheme in grading giant cell tumors of bone establishes three histologic grades. In Grade I, also referred to as conventional giant cell tumor, the stroma is inconspicuous and low profile as compared to the large numbers of giant cells that dominate the histologic picture. In Grade II, sometimes referred to as "borderline" lesions, the stroma is significantly more prominent and the number of giant cells is diminished in relation to the stromal component. The proliferating stromal cells are spindle shaped and elongated, featuring cellular atypia and moderate number of mitotic figures. In the malignant giant cell tumor, also known as Grade III giant cell tumor of bone, the spindly stroma is definitely sarcomatous, clearly predominates the giant cells, the latter becoming

---

[*]Attending Pathologist, Memorial Hospital for Cancer and Allied Diseases of the Memorial Sloan-Kettering Cancer Center, 1275 York Avenue, New York, NY 10021; Professor of Pathology, Cornell University Medical College, New York, NY.

14

J. R. Ryan and L. O. Baker (eds.), Recent Concepts in Sarcoma Treatment, 14–17.

scarcc. An overt sarcoma is diagnosable with relative ease here.(6)

The light-microscopic grading of osteogenic sarcoma remains a contested and unsettled problem. Several not inconsequential difficulties limit its uniform application for assessing prognosis for either single or a group of patients; Broder's original grading system, conceived in 1939, was meant only for fibrosarcomas. (7) In addition, most sarcomas are not homogenous microscopically. Samples of tissues taken from the periphery and from the central region may provide varying impressions as to its grade of malignancy. Small pieces of tissues obtained at biopsy, especially if it is a needle biopsy, is quite inaccurate. Evaluation of the proliferative activity of the lesional tissue is dependent on prompt and good fixation for the preservation of mitotic figures. Sarcomas of identical pattern and grade may vary in their clinical behavior according to their location in the bone.(5)

A case in point is the parosteal (juxtacortical) osteogenic sarcoma.(8,9) This distinctive type of heavily sclerotic sarcoma originates on the external surface of a bone, specifically in relation to the periosteum or the immediate parosteal connective tissues, or both. Microscopic examination, including careful histologic grading of malignancy, is absolutely essential not only for proper diagnosis but for assessing prognosis and required treatment. The majority of these sarcomas are of the classic low-grade, well differentiated, osteogenic sarcoma type. One should be always aware that these low-grade malignant tumors appear to be innocuous, and their biologic potential is often underestimated. A readily reproducible scale of histologic grading ranging from low -, to intermediate to fully malignant osteogenic sarcoma, characterize the juxtacortical types. The importance for the pathologist as well as the clinician here is that by reliably identifying the exact grade of the sarcoma, the treatment and the prognosis can be determined.

High-grade osteogenic sarcoma of the juxtacortical (parosteal) variety, sometimes also referred to as high-grade surface osteogenic sarcoma, should be treated as fully malignant intramedullary osteogenic sarcoma, i.e. neoadjuvant chemotherapy, en bloc resection, and postoperative adjuvant chemotherapy.

Malignant fibrous histiocytoma of bone is also a distinct clinicopathologic entity where histologic grading of the tumor not only establishes the right diagnosis but the treatment and prognosis as well.(10,11) On histologic examination, malignant fibrous histiocytoma of bone, which is ten times less frequent than osteogenic sarcoma, may be predominantly fibrous, histiocytic or xanthomatous, or it may present as a malignant giant cell tumor of bone. Survival, however, is not dependent on the histologic subtype of the sarcoma, but is strongly affected by the histologic grade of malignancy. Assessing the histologic grade of malignancy in a malignant fibrous histiocytoma of bone is quite important since it impacts on treatment and materially influences prognosis. In histologically low-grade malignant tumors, thorough curettage coupled with cryosurgery can provide an effective alternative to a more aggressive surgical intervention. In high-grade malignant fibrous histiocytoma of bone, preoperative, neoadjuvant chemotherapy should be followed by an en bloc, limb-sparing surgical excision in addition to postoperative adjuvant chemotherapy.(12) The meticulous evaluation of the exact grade of malignancy of these sarcomas places the surgical pathologist at the "cutting edge" of bone tumor treatment.

These data indicate that the histologic grade of a given tumor is an important predictor of prognosis. Unfortunately, the histologic grading of musculoskeletal tumors is, by the very nature of the process, subjective. Abnormal DNA content of a tumor, as gauged by flow cytometric analysis, in determining aneuploidy or other variation in the DNA histogram appears to indicate that the majority of the high-grade osteogenic sarcoma is aneuploid.(13,14) It is of importance to establish whether the subjective grading of sarcomas correlates with the proliferative index of the tumor and with the ultimate prognosis of the patient.

REFERENCES

1. Dahlin DC, Unni KK: Bone Tumors. General Aspects and Data on 8,542 Cases. 4th Edition. Springfield, Illinois, Charles C. Thomas Publ, p.134, 1986.
2. Unni KK, Dahlin DC: Grading of bone tumors. Semin Diagn Pathol 1:165-172, 1984.
3. Campanacci M, Giunti A, Olmi R: Giant-cell tumours of bone: A study of 209 cases with long-term follow-up in 130. Ital J Orthop Traumatol 1:249-277, 1975.
4. Hutter RVP, Worcester JN Jr, Francis KC, Foote FW Jr, Stewart F: Benign and malignant giant cell tumors of bone. A clinicopathological analysis of the natural history of the disease. Cancer 15:653-690, 1962.
5. Huvos AG: Bone Tumors: Diagnosis, Treatment and Prognosis. First Edition. Philadelphia, WB Saunders Co, 1979.
6. Nascimento AG, Huvos AG, Marcove RC: Primary malignant giant cell tumor of bone. A study of eight cases and review of the literature. Cancer 44:1393-1402, 1979.
7. Broders AC, Hargrave R, Meyerding HW: Pathological features of soft tissue fibrosarcoma. With special reference to the grading of its malignancy. Surg Gynecol Obstet 69:267-280, 1939.
8. Farr GH, Huvos AG: Juxtacortical osteogenic sarcoma. An analysis of fourteen cases. J Bone Joint Surg 54A:1205-1216, 1972.
9. Ahuja SC, Villacin AB, Smith J, Bullough PG, Huvos AG: Juxta-cortical (parosteal) osteogenic sarcoma. Histological grading and prognosis. J Bone Joint Surg 59A:632-647, 1977.
10. Huvos AG, Heilweil M, Bretsky SS: The pathology of malignant fibrous histiocytoma of bone. A study of 130

patients. Am J Surg Pathol 9:853-871, 1985.

11. Huvos AG, Woodard HQ, Heilweil M: Postradiation malignant fibrous histiocytoma of bone. A clinicopathologic study of 20 patients. Am J Surg Pathol 10:9-18, 1986.

12. Urban C, Rosen G, Huvos AG, Caparros B, Cacavio A, Nirenberg A: Chemotherapy of malignant fibrous histiocytoma. A report of five cases. Cancer 51:795-802, 1983.

13. Kreicbergs A, Brostrom LA, Cewrien G, Einhorn S: Cellular DNA content in human osteosarcoma. Aspects on diagnosis and prognosis. Cancer 50:2476-2481, 1982.

14. Mankin HJ, Connor JF, Schiller AL, Perlmutter N, Alho A, McGuire M: Grading of bone tumors by analysis of nuclear DNA content using flow cytometry. J Bone Joint Surg 67A:404-413, 1985.

THE PATHOLOGICAL STAGING OF SARCOMAS

José Costa, M.D.[1], and Serge Leyvraz, M.D.[1]

Staging systems are designed to group patients according to prognosis. They are important for patient's stratification in clinical trials and they are also useful in providing guidelines for the utilization of different therapeutic strategies. Staging systems are thus based on prognostic factors, the latter being defined as characteristics of the disease (lesion) or the patients which are of value in forecasting the natural history of the disease or its response to specific therapies.

Numerous staging systems have been designed (reviewed in 1) and each of them uses a variety of prognostic factors in different combinations (Table 1). One of the parameters - histological grade - is problematic because grading varies from center to center. This makes comparison of results difficult and as illustrated by Lindberg et al., the stage of 60% of patients in a series can be changed by simply altering the grading system (2).

TABLE 1

Staging Systems for STS

AJC	T (1-3 size+inv.); N; M; G (1-3)
MSK-Soc.	compt.; G (H-L); M
MSK-Hosp.	T (size); depth (S-D); G (H-L)
MGH	T (size, compt., inv.); G (1-3); N; M
SAKK	T (1-2 size); sympt.; G (1-3); N; M
IRS	local; region; metast.; unresected

AJC	- American Joint Committee
MSK-Soc.	- Musculo-Skeletal Society
MSK-Hosp.	- Memorial Sloan-Kettering Hospital
MGH	- Massachusetts General Hospital
SAKK	- Schweizerische Arbeitsgruppe fur Klinische Krebsforschung
IRS	- Intergroup Rhabdomyosarcoma Studies

---

[1]Institute of Pathology and Cancer Center, University of Lausanne, Lausanne, Switzerland.

J. R. Ryan and L. O. Baker (eds.), Recent Concepts in Sarcoma Treatment, 18–21.
© 1988 by Kluwer Academic Publishers.

Relatively few histopathological studies define with precision the grading systems they use (3,4,5,6,7) and fewer yet focus on the question of grading. It would be of interest and worthwhile to test the different grading systems using the same patient population. Perhaps a consensus in histological grading could be reached, as already stated (1), a number of differences between grading systems are likely to be more apparent than real.

Within the frame of a Swiss Multicentric Study, conducted under the auspices of the Swiss Group for Clinical and Epidemiological Cancer Research, we have modified the AJC staging for soft tissue sarcomas. The modification is based on our experience and that of Collin et al. (8), indicating that size, symptoms and grade are powerful independent variables determining the prognosis of patients with STS. The proposed modification of the AJC staging system (9) is summarized in Table 2. Although the number of groups is high when sufficient numbers of patients are available, it will be possible to test if some of the groups can be combined to give rise to a more limited number of stages.

TABLE 2

Modified AJC Staging for Soft Tissue Sarcomas

	Size	Sympt.	Grade	Node	Metastases
0	Tx	Sx	G1	NO	MO
1	T1	SA	G2	NO	MO
2	T1	SB	G2	NO	MO
3	T2	SA	G2	NO	MO
4	T2	SB	G2	NO	MO
5	T1	SA	G3	NO	MO
6	T1	SB	G3	NO	MO
7	T2	SA	G3	NO	MO
8	T2	SB	G3	NO	MO
9	Tx	Sx	G2-3	N1	MO
10	Tx	Sx	G2-3	Nx	M1

T1:	≤ 5 cm
T2:	>5 cm
SA:	no symptoms
SB:	symptoms
G1, G2, G3:	according to NCI grading
N1:	lymph nodes metastases
M1:	distant metastases

As emphasized by Suit (10), it is important to accumulate the data on each patient that will serve for a detailed clinco-pathological study of STS, staging being for these purposes inadequate. The features I believe essential to record in a prospective fashion are given in Table 3. Other features can be added to specifically address the problems of histopathological diagnosis grading and staging. A very important aspect of the pathological staging is the documentation of the local spread of the tumor. A careful mapping of the tissues involved by the tumor should be established. Close collaboration between the surgeon and the pathologist is needed to orient and localize the specimens and tissues sampled (Ref. 1, Fig. 5). If the pathologist collects the information outlined in Table 3, all staging systems can be used and again, like for grading, it would be of interest to test the performance of the different staging systems on a well-characterized patient population. This, of course, requires that a grading be agreed upon.

TABLE 3

Location	Local extension
Size	Metastases (L & H)
Histotype and Grade	Margins of resection
Necrosis	Invasion of adj. struct.
Mitotic rate	Cellularity
Matrix	Pleomorphism
Differentiation	Immunohistology
Electron microscopy	

As difficult, but perhaps less controversial, the diagnosis, grading and staging of bone sarcomas is best exemplified by osteosarcoma. Some comparative aspects of both staging of soft tissue and osteosarcoma are given in Table 4. The evaluation of the tumor response to the preoperative chemotherapy has become extremely important in osteosarcoma and it is possible that the same will be true for soft tissue sarcomas as intra-arterial or systemic preoperative chemotherapy is already being used in selected centers.

TABLE 4

Pathology of Sarcomas

	Soft Tissue	Bone
Diagnosis	"clin-histol. ent."	"historadiol. ent."
Location	axial/periph. depth	axial/periph. ep./meta/diaph. med./cort./periost.
Histotype	LM, Imm, EM	LM, X-ray
Grade	linked to histotype	linked to histo-radiol type and cytology
Local ext.	compart. adj. structures	soft tissue joint space
Metastases	hematogenous lymphatic	hematogenous skip
Path."preop Rx"	?	evaluation of response

REFERENCES

1. Costa J: The Grading and Staging of Soft Tissue Sarco-
    mas. In Pathology of Soft Tissue Tumors. Edited by
    Fletcher and McKee. In Press.
2. Lindberg R: Treatment of Localized Soft Tissue Sarcomas
    in Adults at M.D. Anderson Hospital and Tumor Institute.
    Cancer Treatment Symposia 3:51-65, 1985.
3. Costa J, Wesley RA, Glatstein E et al.: The Grading of
    Soft Tissue Sarcomas. Results of a Clinicopathological
    Correlation in a Series of 163 Cases. Cancer 53:530-541,
    1984.
4. Markhede G, Angervall L. and Stener B: A Multivariate
    Analysis of the Prognosis After Surgical Treatment of
    Soft Tissue Tumors. Cancer 49:1721-1733, 1982.
5. Rydholm A, Berg NO, Gullberg B et al.: Epidemiology of
    Soft Tissue Sarcomas in the Locomotor System. Acta Path
    Microbiol et Immunol Scand A 92:363-374, 1984.
6. Trojani M, Contesso G, Coindre JM et al.: Soft Tissue
    Sarcomas of Adults: Study of Pathological and Prognostic
    Variables and Definition of a Grading System. Int J
    Cancer 33:37-42, 1984.
7. Hajdu SI: Pathology of Soft Tissue Tumors. Edited by Lea
    and Febiger, Philadelphia.
8. Collin Ch., Godbold J, Hajdu SI, Brennan M: Localized
    Extremity Soft Tissue Sarcoma: An Analysis of Factors
    Affecting Survival. J Clin Oncol 5:601-612, 1987.
9. Leyvraz S, Costa J: The Multidisciplinary Approach to
    Soft Tissue Sarcoma. In press in Der Orthopade, 1987.
10. Suit HD, Mankin HJ, Shiller A et al.: Staging Systems
    for Sarcoma of Soft Tissue and Sarcoma of Bone. Cancer
    Treatment Symposia 3:29-36, 1985.

THE DIAGNOSIS OF SOFT TISSUE TUMORS. THE GÖTEBORG EXPERIENCE

Lennart Angervall, M.D., Ph.D.*, and
Lars-Gunnar Kindblom, M.D., Ph.D.*

Soft tissue tumors are classified on a histogenetic basis. Such a classification, with 15 main histogenetic groups, was established by WHO (1969) under the leadership of Dr. Franz Enzinger. An updated classification has been presented by Enzinger and Weiss in their textbook of soft tissue tumors. This classification comprises some 150 tumors and tumor-like lesions, of which, 30 are malignant soft tissue sarcomas. The subclassification of sarcomas is not based on the degree of cell and tissue differentiation or the histologic grade of malignancy, but is based on differences in histologic structure, age, clinical presentation and localization. For histologic malignancy grading we use a system with 4 grades, basically like the one developed and used at the Mayo Clinic. The grading of soft tissue sarcomas is based mainly on cellularity, cell atypia and the degree of anaplasia, mitotic activity and cell and tissue differentiation, and also on the manner of growth, necrosis and hemorrhage. Soft tissue sarcomas of various types with the same malignancy grade do not necessarily display identical clinical behavior. The usefulness of 4 grades of malignancy has been proven by our multivariate and hazard function prognostic analysis and studies of both single entities, namely liposarcoma and myxofibrosarcoma, and series of various types of soft tissue sarcomas. The distinction between benign and malignant tumors can not always be maintained. There are soft tissue tumors of intermediate, borderline, or uncertain malignancy, and these have been summarized in a tentative classification presented in our survey article in the Seminars in Diagnostic Pathology, vol. 3, November 1986.

There is a large group of tumors and tumor-like lesions, so-called pseudosarcomas, which may be mistaken for malignancy. A tentative classification comprising almost 40 lesions has been given in our survey article. The importance of being aware of, and having knowledge of pseudosarcomas can be illustrated by the finding that some 10% of 800 reviewed tumors reported to the Swedish Cancer Registry between 1958 and 1963 as soft tissue sarcomas were found to be benign tumors and tumor-like lesions. The most common were found to be nodular fasciitis, spindle cell and pleomorphic lipoma,

---

*Department of Pathology, Gothenburg University, Sahlgren Hospital, S-413 45 Göteborg, Sweden.

J. R. Ryan and L. O. Baker (eds.), Recent Concepts in Sarcoma Treatment, 22–26.
© 1988 by Kluwer Academic Publishers.

intravascular papillary endothelial hyperplasia, pigmented villonodular synovitis and ancient neurilemoma.

The yearly incidence of genuine soft tissue sarcomas in Sweden, which has a population of 8 million, is about 250 cases. This figure does not include mesothelioma, tumors from supporting tissues of parenchymal organs, and neuroectodermal organ tumors such as neuroblastoma and pheocromocytoma. It has been estimated that benign soft tissue tumors outnumber sarcomas more than 100 times.

In Göteborg, we generally omit incisional biopsy in the preoperative investigation of a soft tissue lesion. If a careful physical examination and various radiographic studies all agree on the diagnosis of malignancy, and the location of the tumor allows its complete removal with slight or no loss of function, preoperative biopsy is omitted. When additional information about the nature of the lesion is needed, fine needle aspiration cytology is the first choice. If the operation could result in serious functional disability, the diagnosis should generally be settled by incisional biopsy. We have shown in long-term follow-up studies that local function-preserving surgery based on the clinical diagnosis alone has resulted in a low local recurrence rate, even for high-grade malignant tumors. This, the so-called Stener principle, has also led to a very low amputation frequency. In a consecutive series of soft tissue sarcomas of the extremities treated according to this principle, the surgical treatment was based on the clinical and radiographic diagnosis alone in some 65%, also including fine needle aspiration in some 25% and including open biopsy in some 10%. The incidence of local recurrence was 3, 19, 30% for these 3 groups, respectively.

Angiography has long been an important tool in the preoperative investigation and remains so even after the introduction of computed tomography. We have developed a microangiographic technique which makes it possible to fill even the finest vessels with contrast medium, i.e., vessels with a diameter of 3-5 microns. By correlating microangiographic, angiographic and histologic studies, we have analyzed the vascularization of several types of soft tissue lesion and from these studies we have postulated that the vascularity of a soft tissue tumor is related to the degree of malignancy and to the tissue of origin. Important exceptions to the general rule that high vascularity indicates malignancy are hibernoma, hemangiopericytoma, deep hemangiomas, particularly intramuscular hemangiomas of the small vessel type, and muscle rupture in organization and other lesions with granulation tissue. The reason why hibernoma is highly vascular in spite of being a benign tumor may be that brown fat - its assumed tissue of origin - is rich in vessels.

At our laboratory, we have many years of experience in fine needle aspiration in the preoperative investigation of soft tissue and bone tumors. The technique has been found to be of value in distinguishing benign from malignant tumors, metastases from primary sarcomas and, in some cases, the histogenetic type can also be strongly suggested and the degree of malignancy indicated. We have developed an embedding technique for fine needle aspirates which permits a combined light and electron-microscopic examination, and we have also recently started to apply immunohistochemistry in the cytologic diagnosis of soft tissue lesions. Combined ultrastructural and immunohistochemical examinations in the cytologic diagnosis have been found to be of particular value for the diagnosis of rhabdomyosarcoma. Our experience from ultrastructural studies of the preoperative cytologic diagnosis of soft tissue tumors has been summarized in a separate article in Seminars in Diagnostic Pathology, November 1986.

In the diagnosis of all kinds of tumors, we use hematoxylin and eosin and the van Gieson trichrome as routine stainings. The van Gieson trichrome staining is of particular value in the diagnosis of leiomyomatous tumors because of the bright yellow, picrinophilic stain it gives to the cytoplasm of leiomyomatous tumors, which helps to distinguish them from other spindle cell tumors. In Table 1, there is a list of cell and tissue products which can be demonstrated by special stainings and histochemical methods of interest in the diagnosis of selected cases of soft tissue lesions. We have paid special attention to the characterization of glycosaminoglycans in soft tissue tumors as well as bone tumors. The histochemical separation of sulphated and non-sulphated glycosaminoglycans, in the first place, has been performed by the use of basic dyes applied at controlled pH's and by the so-called Scott technique (staining with Alcian blue at varying electrolyte concentrations). These methods are of value for the distinction of chondromatous tumors from other lesions.

TABLE 1

HISTOCHEMISTRY

Mucosubstances
Glycogen
Fibrillary proteins (collagen, reticulin, elastin)
Lipids
Hemosiderins
Reducing pigments

For 20 years we have been applying electron microscopy in our research on soft tissue tumors, and also in the diagnostic work involved in selected cases. So far, we have experience of more than 1,000 soft tissue lesions. Generally, ultrastructural examination is of the most benefit when light microscopy has restricted the diagnostic possibilities to a very few. In the diagnosis of soft tissue tumors, we

TABLE 2

COMBINED EM AND IMMUNOHISTOCHEMISTRY IN THE DIAGNOSIS OF SOFT TISSUE SARCOMAS

	Immunohisto-chemistry	EM
SMALL AND ROUND CELL TUMORS		
Rhabdomyosarcoma	desmin, myoglobin	myofilaments, Z-lines
Extraskeletal Ewing's sarcoma	vimentin	undifferentiated cells, glycogen
Malignant hemangiopericytoma	laminin, collagen IV	pericyte-like, external lamina
Neuroblastoma Neuroepithelioma	NSE, neurofilament	neurosecretory granules
Malignant lymphoma	LC	uncharacteristic
SPINDLE CELL TUMORS		
Leiomyosarcoma	desmin	myofilaments, actin bundles
Malignant schwannoma	S-100 protein	external lamina long-spaced collagen
Malignant fibrous histiocytoma, spindle cell type	A1AT,A1ACT, FER	fibroblastic and histiocytic features
Malignant mesothelioma	cytokeratin, EMA CEA	microvilli, cell junctions, intermediate cytofilaments
Synovial sarcoma	vimentin, cytokeratin	luminal spaces, external lamina, cell junctions
EPITHELIOID TUMORS		
Epithelioid hemangio-endothelioma, angiosarcoma	F VIII RAG, laminin, collagen IV	endothelial features, vascular differentiation
Malignant granular cell tumor	S-100 protein	lysosomes, autophagic vacuoles
Alveolar soft part sarcoma	vimentin, desmin	crystalline structures
Epithelioid sarcoma	cytokeratin, vimentin, EMA, actin	epithelium-like features
Clear cell sarcoma	S-100 protein	large nucleoli, glycogen, occasional melanosomes
Metastases Carcinoma	cytokeratin, EMA	epithelial features
Malignant melanoma	S-100 protein	melanosomes
PLEOMORPHIC TUMORS		
Malignant fibrous histiocytoma, pleomorphic type	vimentin, A1AT, A1ACT, FER	fibroblastic and histiocytic features
Pleomorphic carcinoma	cytokeratin, EMA, CEA	epithelial features
MYXOID TUMORS		
Myxoid liposarcoma, Myxofibrosarcoma	vimentin	lipoblastic and fibroblastic-myofibroblastic-histiocytic features, respectively
Extraskeletal myxoid chondrosarcoma	S-100 protein, vimentin	chondroblastic features
Chordoma	cytokeratin, EMA, vimentin, S-100 protein	notochord-like cells

have found electron microscopy to be of special value: 1) to show leiomyoblastic and Schwann cell differentiation in spindle cell tumors, 2) to show rhabdomyoblastic and nerve cell differentiation in round cell malignancies, 3) to prove vascular differentiation in endothelial and pericytic neoplasms, 4) to distinguish sarcoma from carcinoma, especially small cell carcinoma from rhabdomyosarcoma, Ewing's sarcoma and malignant lymphoma, and pleomorphic carcinoma from the pleomorphic type of malignant fibrous histiocytoma, and 5) to identify poorly-differentiated metastases of malignant melanoma.

During the last 8 years, immunohistochemical techniques have been used increasingly at our laboratory, both in research and routine diagnostic work on soft tissue tumors. Our experience of combined electron microscopic and immunohistochemical analysis in the study of small and round cell, spindle cell, epithelioid, pleomorphic and myxoid soft tissue tumors is summarized in Table 2.

The special morphologic techniques have contributed to a better understanding of the histogenesis and cell differentiation of soft tissue tumors. It should be emphasized, however, that in most cases of soft tissue lesions, the diagnosis is arrived at by the light microscopy of routine stainings whilst taking the clinical presentation into consideration. In cases presenting diagnostic problems, the diagnosis can often be based on the combined clinical, gross, light and electron microscopic and immunohistochemical findings.

Our experience in the diagnosis and prognosis of soft tissue tumors is given in more detail, as well as references to our most important works in this field, in our survey article.

REFERENCE

1. Seminars in Diagnostic Pathology (Editor, Daniel J. Santa Cruz, M.D). Soft Tissue Tumors (Guest Editor, Lennart Angervall, M.D.). Vol 3, No 4, Grune & Stratton, Harcourt Brace Jovanovich, Inc, 1986.

THE ROLE OF THE PATHOLOGIST IN THE TREATMENT OF OSTEOSARCOMA*

P. Picci[1], G. Bacci, R. Capanna, M. Avella, N. Baldini,
P. Ruggieri, R. Biagini, G. Pignatti

The role of the pathologist has changed in the modern treatment of osteosarcoma. Not only must the correct diagnosis be made, but also:
1. an evaluation of necrosis and
2. an evaluation of surgical margins must be given.

The method of study is very important and has to be standardized in each case to obtain as much information as possible. The method we employ is a careful macroscopic examination of the specimen, and any site where we find some suspect area for viable tumor or for marginal or intralesional margin is colored with china ink. In detecting these areas, the collaboration of the surgeon is of paramount importance. Tetracyclin is also useful to evaluate the extension of the tumor. X-rays of the specimen are also used to see the exact extension and to identify particular or unsafe sites to be closely studied. From each case, two entire sections of the tumor were obtained and photographed on a normal Polaroid camera. These sections were divided in blocks and a map was used to design and to number these blocks. From 5 to 26 blocks were obtained from each specimen.

The first point is the evaluation of necrosis, and particularly we have to evaluate the amount and the distribution of this necrosis. The amount of necrosis is important because it is the most reliable prognostic factor at this moment and determines further treatments. We decided to use a very simple grading system for necrosis: "good" greater than 90%, "fair" between 60-90%, "poor" lower than 60%. A confirmation of the importance of necrosis as a prognostic factor is shown by our results (Table 1)

Another important study is the distribution of necrosis. We do that to obtain more information regarding staging, surgery and prognosis. Each section is photographed and a map is reconstructed. Areas with persisting viable tumor are

---

[1]Universita di Bologna, Cattedra di Clinica Ortopedica 1,
 Istituto Ortopedico Rizzoli, Via Codivilla 9, Bologna,
 Italy

---

*Supported in part by a grant from National Council for
 Research, project Oncology n. 88.0267944, and by a grant
 from Regione Emilia Romagna, law n. 1970 of May 13th, 1986.

27

J. R. Ryan and L. O. Baker (eds.), Recent Concepts in Sarcoma Treatment, 27–29.
© 1988 by Kluwer Academic Publishers.

TABLE 1:   Disease-Free Survival in Terms
of Necrosis

GOOD	42/51	82%
FAIR	21/45	47%
POOR	5/15	33%

identified; areas of peritumoral hemorrhage are also identified.

Table 2 summarizes our experience in 97 patients and we
saw that soft tissue invasion was present in 90 cases and in
70% of these cases we found viable tumor. The cortex was
invaded in 94 cases and in 50% we found viable tumor. The
subcortical marrow was involved in all of our cases and in
58% we found viable tumor. Again, areas in contact with
cartilage were involved in 65 patients and in 65% of these we
found viable tumor. Lacunae were present in 45 cases and in
64% of these cases the lacunae were surrounded by viable
tumor, and the ligaments were involved in 16 cases and 62%
had viable tumor. Peritumoral hemorrhage was present in 40%
of our cases. What conclusions do we draw from this
distribution? First of all, we got some indications for
staging.

1. We think it is better to avoid, as much as
possible, open biopsies because they may cause lacunae. We
found these lacunae mostly in areas where an open biopsy had
been performed. Probably, open surgery may alter the vascularization of the surgical bed and therefore impede drugs to
permeate the surrounding tumor. Needle biopsies are therefore
preferred.

TABLE 2:   Preferential Sites of Viable Tumor After
Chemotherapy

	Present in (no of cases)	Viable Tumor
Soft tissue invasion	90	63 (70%)
Tumor in the cortex	94	47 (50%)
Tumor in the subcortical marrow	97	56 (58%)
Pericartilaginous tumor	65	42 (65%)
Lacunae	45	29 (64%)
Tumor in the ligaments	16	10 (62%)

Peritumoral hemorrhage was present in 40% of the cases
(39/97)

2. Staging needle biopsies to evaluate necrosis before surgery (we do not use them, but a lot of people do) have to be aimed where viable tumor most likely persists. In other words, it is useless to perform a staging needle biopsy in the center of the medullary canal because it will be negative in most cases.

3. Pay attention to peritumoral hemorrhage because this may alter the CT scan giving false positive results and lead to greater surgery than necessary.

Then there are some indications for surgery.

1. Wide margins remain absolutely necessary because we have seen that viable tumor remains at the periphery of the tumor, in the soft tissue and in the cortex.

2. When ligaments are involved, extra-articular resection is mandatory. A new role of the pathologist is also in the evaluation of surgical margins. Using china ink on the specimen areas we suspected to be marginal or intralesional can be exactly evaluated on histological examination. In this way, in fact, a black line on the slide accurately marks the tissues where the lancet passed through.

Regarding the effect of preoperative chemotherapy, we noted on the classic standard x-ray that in some cases there was a delimitation of the tumor and an improvement in calcification of the tumor. Sometimes it appeared very well demarcated with respect to the surrounding tissue. Therefore, more than a reduction in size, we noted an increase in sclerosis and the appearance of a radiopaque shell. With angiograms, again, we noted a marked reduction of the vessels and again, in some cases, a clear demarcation with a shell. This is confirmed by the CT scan. We saw the same things macroscopically when the specimen arrived in the laboratory; particularly we noted that the muscles over the tumor were movable. In other words, there was no infiltration of the tumor in the soft tissues. This is more evident cutting the specimen when you see that muscles fall down and are not attached to the tumor.

Histologically, we noticed that in good responders, combined with necrosis, abundant osteoid is present signifying that tumoral cells before dying produced this characteristic and well-differentiated stroma.

Our conclusions are: probably the effect of preoperative chemotherapy is not only in necrosis, but in differentiation too. This differentiation we saw is evident radiographically, macroscopically, microscopically, and results in a delimitation of the tumor from surrounding tissues. In other words, a good response to chemotherapy can probably modify the relationship of the tumor with the surrounding tissue, giving it a new intracompartmentability.

MUSCULOSKELETAL TUMOR STAGING - 1987 UPDATE

William F. Enneking, M.D.[*]

Since 1960, prospective primary observational data has been gathered and stored on primary benign and malignant neoplasms of the musculoskeletal system in the W. Thaxton Springfield Study Center at the University of Florida. In 1974, based upon analysis of this data, a staging system for primary malignant tumors of connective tissue histogenesis was constructed together with definitions of oncologic surgical margins and oncologic surgical procedures. By 1979, 258 cases had been staged and enough time had passed to evaluate the system. At that time, the Musculoskeletal Tumor Society (MTS) contributed an additional 139 cases from thirteen member institutions to form an initial study group of 397 cases.

After analysis of the data, the system was modified to the form first published in 1980 (5). Because of the emphasis placed on correlating the system with surgical margins and procedures, it was termed a Surgical Staging System. The System was based on three factors: Grade (G), Anatomic Site (T), and Metastases (M).

Grade was subdivided into low (G_1) or high grade (G_2) on a combination of histologic and radiographic criteria. Before selecting this two grade system, both three and four grade systems were considered.

The four grade system described by Broders et al. for soft tissue fibrosarcomas was based on histologic criteria originally applied to carcinomas, and many of the criteria were not widely applicable to sarcomas of both bone and soft tissue.

A three grade system described by Evans et al. (7) and Sanerkin (11) for chondrosarcomas, and by Enzinger et al. (6) for soft tissue sarcomas, was also examined. The criteria for bone and soft tissue lesions were quite disparate, did not facilitate the principal objective of the system -- surgical planning. In the nomenclature of surgical margins (intracapsular, marginal, wide, and radical) used to stratify surgical procedures -- both limb-salvage resections and amputations -- the data indicated that there were only two margins that obtained adequate local control -- wide and radical. Both

----

[*]Department of Orthopedic Surgery, University of Florida College of Medicine, Box J-246, JHM Health Center, Gainesville, FL 32610.

J. R. Ryan and L. O. Baker (eds.), Recent Concepts in Sarcoma Treatment, 30–39.

intracapsular and marginal margins resulted in unacceptably high recurrence rates. As there was no intermediate surgical margin to correlate with an intermediate grade lesion, a three grade system was discarded in favor of a two grade system with both histologic and radiographic criteria.

Anatomic site was subdivided into intracompartmental (A) or extracompartmental (B) location based upon radiographic and surgical criteria that demonstrated whether or not the lesion was confined within well-defined anatomic compartments (bone, joint, intramuscular compartments), bounded by the natural barriers to tumor extension (cortical bone, articular cartilage, joint capsule, major fascial septae). Although size was recognized as a significant variable of the anatomic site, it was not included as a criteria because it did not form a basis for surgical planning. The determinant surgical criteria of the anatomic site was the involvement of the major neurovascular structures. This was best accounted for by compartmentalization and virtually ignored by size.

On the other hand, the prognostic significance of size was accounted for in the system by the close correlation between size and compartmentalization -- i.e., the great preponderance of small lesions were intracompartmental and the large lesions were virtually all extracompartmental.

The third factor, metastasis, was expressed as clinically present (M_1) or absent (M_0). The data demonstrated there was no difference in the prognosis in those cases in which there was regional lymph node metastasis (N) and those in which distant metastases were present (M). Thus, both were combined into a single criteria.

The fine details of the system were published (5) and are summarized in Table 1.

TABLE 1

SURGICAL STAGING SYSTEM - 1980

| G_1-Low Grade Malignant | T_1-Intracompartmental | M_0-No Metastasis |
| G_2-High Grade Malignant | T_2-Extracompartmental | M_1-Metastasis |

I
  A - G_1 T_1 M_0

  B - G_1 T_2 M_0

II
  A - G_2 T_1 M_0

  B - G_2 T_2 M_0

III
  A - G_{1-2} T_1 M_1

  B - G_{1-2} T_2 M_1

Analysis of the data in 1980 showed that there was a stepwise difference in prognosis for each progression in the system. These differences were the same whether the lesions were staged intramurally or extramurally, or whether the lesions had originated in bone or soft tissue. At this point in time, the Musculoskeletal Tumor Society adopted the system for its institutional protocols and studies. It has been widely adopted in the literature for staging both bone and soft tissue lesions and has been used as the staging system for the 1983, 1985, and 1987 International Symposia on limb-salvage. (4,9)

In 1986, after greater experience with the system, the criteria for compartmentalization were clarified and an extension of the system to allow staging of benign lesions was presented. (3) In this extension, grade was further subdivided into G_0 (benign), G_1 (low grade malignant), and G_2 (high grade malignant). The criteria for anatomic site was similarly extended into T_0 (intracapsular), T_1 (extracapsular, intracompartmental), and T_2 (extracapsular, extracompartmental). In addition, the term "intracapsular" was substituted for "intralesional" as a surgical margin. This format represents the current Surgical Staging System of the MTS and is summarized as Table 2.

TABLE 2

SURGICAL STAGING SYSTEM - 1986

G_0-Benign	T_0-Intracapsular	M_0-No Metastasis
G_1-Low Grade Malignant	T_1-Extracapsular, Intracompartmental	M_1-Metastasis
G_2-High Grade Malignant	T_2-Extracapsular, Extracompartmental	

BENIGN	MALIGNANT
1 - G_0 T_0 M_0	I
	A - G_1 T_1 M_0
2 - G_0 T_1 M_0	B - G_1 T_2 M_0
3 - G_0 T_2 M_{0-1}	
	II
	A - G_2 T_1 M_0
	B - G_2 T_2 M_0
	III
	A - G_{1-2} T_1 M_1
	B - G_{1-2} T_2 M_1

At about the same time that the MTS Surgical System was developing, the American Joint Commission for Cancer Staging and End Results Reporting (AJC) had formed two independent Task Forces charged with the responsibility for developing separate staging systems for bone and soft tissue sarcomas.

The Task Force on Bone reported in 1977 that they had failed to devise a satisfactory system and recommended that "institutions with access to large numbers of patients, consistency in management, and long-term follow-up undertake this task." (2) This was what was done at the University of

Florida and evolved into the MTS System. The next report of
the AJC-Bone Task Force in 1985 was the recommendation that
the AJC adopt the criteria for G, T, and M of the MTS System,
but in order to conform to the four stage format, the AJC
modified the numbering of the stages. (8) In this modification, Stage I and II remained synonymous with those of the
MTS, Stage III was left undefined, and Stage IV of the AJC-
Bone System was the same as Stage III of the MTS System
(Table 3). Thus, although the criteria and stratification
were the same in both systems, the nomenclature was different. The other minor difference was that the MTS System,
being confined to lesions of connective tissue histogenesis,
excluded Ewing's Sarcoma, while the AJC-Bone System specifically included it. Since 1985 the AJC-Bone System has not
been widely used in the literature.

TABLE 3

AJC SURGICAL STAGING SYSTEM - BONE - 1985

G_1-Low Grade Malignant	T_1-Intracompartmental	M_0-No Metastasis
G_2-High Grade Malignant	T_2-Extracompartmental	M_1-Metastasis

I

   A - G_1 T_1 M_0

   B - G_1 T_2 M_0

II

   A - G_2 T_1 M_0

   B - G_2 T_2 M_0

III

   A - G_{1-2} T_1 M_1

   B - G_{1-2} T_2 M_1

The AJC-Soft Tissue Task Force in 1977 published a
proposed system for staging soft tissue lesions. (10) This
system was markedly different from either the AJC-Bone or the
combined MTS Systems. It was a four stage system based upon
histologic grade (G), size and/or invasion of bone, artery,
or nerve (T), nodal metastases (N), and distant metastases
(M).

Grade was subdivided into three grades; low grade (G),
moderate grade (G2), and high grade (G3). In addition, certain histogenic types (synovial sarcoma, angiosarcoma, and
rhabdomyosarcoma) were arbitrarily assigned to the high grade
group irrespective of the histologic criteria as if those
lesions never were of low or intermediate grade.

T was subdivided by two criteria, by size in the lower
stages and by whether or not the lesion invaded bone, artery,
or nerve in the higher grades. T_1 was assigned to lesions
under five centimeters, and T_2 to lesions greater in size
than five centimeters. T_3 was assigned to lesions that
invaded bone, artery, or nerve. Metastasis was subdivided

by regional node involvement (N) or distant Metastasis (M).
N_O signified no node involvement, and N_1 signified metastatic
node involvement. Similarly, M_O and M_1 signified the absence
or presence of distant metastasis.

These criteria were used to construct the four stage
system shown in Table 4. The first three stages were stratified by histologic grade and subdivided on the basis of size
alone. In stage three, a third subdivision was added for
lesions with nodal metastasis. Stage four was subdivided into
two groups, the first with invasion of bone, artery, or
nerve, and the second on the basis of distant metastasis.
Analysis of the data from 423 verified cases showed there was
a stepwise progression in prognosis for each stage, but that
there was no difference between the subdivisions in the
stages based on size, and that those lesions placed in Stage
III on the basis of node metastasis had a worse prognosis
than those placed in Stage IV on the basis of bone, artery,
or nerve invasion.

	TABLE 4		
	AJC - SOFT TISSUE SARCOMA - 1977		
G_1-Low Grade Malignant	T_1- <5 cm	N_O-No Node Metastasis	M_O-No Distant Metastasis
G_2-Moderate Grade Malignant	T_2- >5 cm	N_1-Node Metastasis	M_1-Distant Metastasis
G_3-High Grade Malignant	T_3- Involves Bone, Artery, Nerve		

I				III			
a - G_1 T_1 N_O M_O				a - G_3 T_1 N_O M_O			
b - G_1 T_2 N_O M_O				b - G_3 T_2 N_O M_O			
				c - G_{1-3} T_{1-2} N_1 M_O			
II				IV			
a - G_2 T_1 N_O M_O				a - G_{1-3} T_3 N_{0-1} M_O			
b - G_2 T_2 N_O M_O				b - G_{1-3} T_{1-3} N_{0-1} M_1			

The system has not been widely used in the ensuing
decade. The principal reason for its lack of utilization
appeared to be its complexity leading to poor compliance, its
inconsistencies, and the difficulties in correlating the
stages with surgical planning.

Some examples of inconsistencies; assigning a higher
stage to a small, superficial low grade synovial sarcoma
(Stage IIIa) than to a large, deep moderate grade liposarcoma
(Stage IIb), or assigning a higher stage to a small low grade
fibrosarcoma invading bone (Stage IVa) than to a large high
grade malignant fibrous histiocytoma with lymph node metastasis (Stage IIIc).

Recognizing these shortcomings, the AJC-Soft Tissue Task
Force has recently recommended several modifications to the
system. (12) The recommendation, as yet unpublished, re-

moves bone, artery, and nerve invasion as a criteria for T, removes histogenic type as a criteria for G, and places both node and distant metastasis in the same stage. Stages I, II, and III are determined by grade and subdivided by size, while Stage IV represents metastasis subdivided by node and distant metastasis (Table 5). The modifications make this system less complex and remove the majority of the inconsistencies from the original version.

TABLE 5

AJC SOFT TISSUE SARCOMA - MODIFIED - 1987

G_1-Low Grade Malignant	T_1- <5 cm	N_0-No Node Metastasis	M_0-No Distant Metastasis
G_2-Moderate Grade Malignant	T_2- >5 cm	N_1-Node Metastasis	M_1-Distant Metastasis
G_3-High Grade Malignant			

I				III				
A - G_1	T_1	N_0	M_0	A - G_3	T_1	N_0	M_0	
B - G_1	T_2	N_0	M_0	B - G_3	T_2	N_0	M_0	
II								
A - G_2	T_1	N_0	M_0	A - G_{1-3}	T_{1-2}	N_1	M_0	
B - G_2	T_2	N_0	M_0	B - G_{1-3}	T_{1-2}	N_{0-1}	M_1	

Discussion

At the present moment, there are three different staging systems for bone and soft tissue sarcomas:
1. The MTS System for both bone and soft tissue sarcomas,
2. The AJC-Bone System, and
3. The modified AJC-Soft Tissue System.

The MTS System has the advantages of simplicity, a high degree of compliance, wide understanding and international usage, ease of correlation with surgical planning, and the same criteria for both bone and soft tissue lesions.

The AJC-Bone System is virtually the same as the MTS System. It has not been widely publicized and is virtually unknown outside of the AJC-Task Force. The inconsistency of assigning metastatic disease to Stage IV in one system and to Stage III in another system leads to confusion. On the other hand, there is value to uniformity in formulating the various staging systems for different classes of malignancy wherein Stage IV always represents distant metastasis.

The AJC-Soft Tissue System, as originally proposed, differed markedly from the other two systems. The modifications simplifying the system and removing the inconsistencies brings it into closer alignment with the other two systems.

In view of the recent modifications of both the AJC-Bone and AJC-Soft Tissue systems, this would seem to be a propitious moment to consider combining the three into a unified whole by examining the differences in criteria for each of the factors and attempting to reconcile the differences.

G - All systems utilize histologic grade. Both systems for bone use a two grade system for malignant lesions, while the AJC-Soft Tissue System uses a three grade system. The two grade system places the clearly low and high grade lesions in two separate stages and requires the selection of one or the other stages for lesions with intermediate histologic characteristics. This selection is enhanced by data from clinical, radiographic, and specialized imaging techniques that are considered along with the histologic criteria. (3) In the era in which it was devised, when surgery alone was the usual method of treatment, the two grade format correlated well with surgical planning. Low grade lesions were well managed with procedures obtaining wide margins and the selection between resection and amputation correlated well with whether the lesion was situated intra- or extracompartmentally. High grade lesions required procedures that obtained radical margins and, again, the selection of resection versus amputation to obtain a radical margin correlated well the anatomic setting of the lesion.

The three grade system also allows the clearly low and high grade lesions to be placed in separate stages, but adds another stage for intermediate grade lesions. While the criteria for the gradation are purely histologic and do not take into account radiographic or specialized imaging data, criteria for the three grade system have been published for both some bone lesions, notably chondrosarcoma (7,11), and soft tissue sarcomas. (6) These criteria are widely understood and applied by pathologists. Of considerable significance is the potential for flow cytometry and similar techniques to increase the accuracy of histologic grading.

Correlation between a three grade system and surgical planning offers a wider range of surgical options than the two grade system. In this era of combining marginal, wide, and occasionally radical margins with pre- and postoperative adjuvant modalities, a three grade system appears to offer potentially better therapeutic correlations than a two grade system.

Both Systems have shown significant differences in prognosis between the stages based on either the two or three grade system.

In sum, there does not appear to be a clear cut advantage of one system over the other. Those whose perspective is primarily surgical appear to prefer the two grade system and those whose perspective is primarily pathologic favor the three grade system.

T - site and/or size is determined by different criteria in the MTS and AJC-Soft Tissue Systems, while they are the same between the MTS and AJC-Bone Systems. In the MTS and AJC-Bone Systems, T is used to designate the anatomic site and is subdivided into intracompartmentally (T_1) and extracompartmentally (T_2) situated lesions. In the modified AJC-Soft Tissue System, T is stratified by size less (T_1) or greater (T_2) than five centimeters. There are cogent reasons

for favoring compartmentalization over size as the criteria
for subdividing T. The anatomic setting of a lesion is the
key determinant in surgical planning, while size per se is
not. Compartmentalization has both anatomic and functional
implications, while size does not. With current imaging
techniques, compartmentalization can be precisely determined
and is recorded for reproducibility. Size changes from a wet
to dry specimen, from the radiographic image to the operating
room, and from the operating room to the pathology suite.
Compartmentalization takes into account size, while size
alone does not take into account compartmentalization. While
in the original AJC-Soft Tissue System compartmentalization
was indirectly accounted for, albeit somewhat awkwardly, in
the modified system it is ignored in favor of size alone.
While it is true that size is related to prognosis, it is
almost a linear progression until twenty centimeters. Thus,
although lesions greater than five centimeters have a worse
prognosis than lesions less than five centimeters, the same
can be said for eight, ten, twelve, or fifteen centimeters as
the dividing line. This, in all likelihood, accounts for why
there is little prognostic significance to a two step division in T on the basis of any one size..

In sum, there is a clear cut advantage to using the
concept of compartmentalization over that of size as the
criteria for T.

M - metastasis is treated the same by the AJC-Bone and
the MTS Systems by combining nodal and distant metastasis
into a single M. However, the AJC-Bone System calls this
Stage IV and leaves Stage III unnamed because in other AJC
systems, stage is reserved for metastatic disease. In the
modified AJC-Soft Tissue System, metastasis is subdivided
into nodal (N) and distant (M) and placed as subdivisions of
Stage IV. In their 1977 report, the AJC-Soft Tissue Task
Force had nodal metastasis as Stage III,c and distant metastasis as Stage IV,b. There was no difference in prognosis
between these two stages. Be that as it may, there does not
seem to be a compelling reason to favor separating or combining nodal and distant metastasis. Combining them, as in the
AJC Bone and MTS Systems is simpler, while separating them as
in the AJC-Soft Tissue System may, with more cases, provide a
significant stratification to Stage IV. It is evident that
having a single system for both bone and soft tissue lesions
would be better than the current multiple systems. The
alternatives are to universally adopt the three stage combined MTS System, reconcile the differences into a combined
four stage system, or continue with the current situation.
The latter alternative is the least desirable. Any reconcil-
iation should logically be based upon the most useful criteria for G, T, and M.

As to grade, the three step system appears preferable.
Grading into low, moderate, and high grades is widely practiced by pathologists and a three step system will, in all
likelihood, accommodate better to future diagnostic and
therapeutic developments.

Clearly, the anatomic localization of the lesion is the

preferable criteria for subdividing T. The rapid advances in radiography and specialized imaging techniques continue to increase the resolution by which compartmentalization can be determined.

The presence of metastasis should be expressed in a single stage and it would seem preferable to designate both regional and distant metastases as subsets.

For the advantages of uniformity, a four stage, three grade format in which T is determined by compartmentalization and M is subdivided into N and M combines the better features of the three systems. This format is shown in Table 6.

TABLE 6

A UNIFIED SYSTEM - 1987

G_1- Low Grade Malignant T_1- Intracompartmental N_0-No Node Metastasis M_0-No Distant Metastasis

G_2- Moderate Grade Malignant T_2- Extracompartmental N_1-Node Metastasis M_1-Distant Metastasis

G_3- High Grade Malignant

I
   A - G_1 T_1 N_0 M_0

   B - G_1 T_2 N_0 M_0

III
   A - G_3 T_1 N_0 M_0

   B - G_3 T_2 N_0 M_0

II
   A - G_2 T_1 N_0 M_0

   B - G_2 T_2 N_0 M_0

IV
   A - G_{1-3} T_{1-2} N_1 M_0

   B - G_{1-3} T_{1-2} N_{0-1} M_1

There is no doubt that conversion from either the current widely used three stage MTS System or the AJC Systems to a four stage unified system would cause serious burdens to those individuals, institutions, and inter-institutional groups whose protocols and data storage is based on one of the current systems. Whether or not conversion to a unified (modified combined) four stage system is worth the price of these burdens is the heart of the matter. However, there is no question that universal adoption of one or the other of these systems would be a significant step forward in musculo-skeletal oncology.

REFERENCES

1. Broders AC, Hargrave R, Myerding HW: Pathologic Features of Soft Tissue Fibrosarcoma. Surg Gynecol Obstet 69:267-280, 1939.
2. Copeland MM, Robbins GF, Myers MN: Development of a Clinical Staging System for Primary Malignant Tumors of Bone: A Progress Report. In Management of Primary Bone and Soft Tissue Tumors. Chicago, Year Book Medical Publishers, Inc., p. 35, 1977.
3. Enneking WF: A System of Staging Musculoskeletal Neo-plasms. Clin Orthop Rel Res 204:9-24, March 1986.
4. Enneking WF (ed.): Limb Salvage in Musculoskeletal

Oncology. New York, Churchill Livingston, 1987.

5. Enneking WF, Spanier SS, Goodman MA: A System for the Surgical Staging of Musculoskeletal Sarcoma. Clin Orthop Rel Res 153:106-120, December 1980.

6. Enzinger FM, Lattes R, Tartoni H: Histologic Typing of Soft Tissue Tumors. World Health Organization, Geneva, 1969.

7. Evans HL, Ayala AG, Romsdahl MM: Prognostic Factors in Chondrosarcoma of Bone: A Clinico-pathologic Analysis with Emphasis on Histologic Grading. Cancer, 40:818, 1977.

8. Hutter R, Bears O, Henson D, Myers M: Manual for Staging of Cancer, 3rd edition, Philadelphia, Lippincott, 1985.

9. Kotz R (ed.): Proceedings of the 2nd International Meeting on the Design and Application of Tumor Pros-thesis for Bone and Joint Reconstruction. Vienna, Egermann Druckereigesellschaft, 1983.

10. Russell WW, Cohen J, Enzinger F, Hajdu, SI, Heise H, Martin RG, Meissner W, Miller WT, Schmitz RL, Suit HD: A Clinical and Pathologic Staging System for Soft Tissue Sarcomas. Cancer 40:1562, 1977.

11. Sanerkin NG: The Diagnosis and Grading of Chondrosarcoma of Bone. Cancer 45:582, 1980.

ELECTRON MICROSCOPY OF SARCOMAS

Bruce Mackay, M.D., Ph.D.*

The ability of the pathologist to classify malignant
neoplasms has improved dramatically in the past two decades
with the expanded application of immunocytochemical staining
procedures and electron microscopy to the study of tumors.
The roles of these techniques in the evaluation of neoplasms
that can not be classified by conventional light microscopy
is in part determined by the general category into which a
particular tumor falls. Most bone sarcomas can be identified
without difficulty from their radiologic appearance and
histopathology as seen in paraffin sections. Many soft
tissue sarcomas are in contrast difficult to classify by
light microscopy alone. The significance to the clinician and
his patient of precision in the subclassification of a soft
tissue sarcoma is somewhat limited at the present time because there are not many clear-cut differences in behavior
among the various subtypes. Accurate designations are nevertheless necessary to improve our understanding of the biologic behavior and response to therapy of the tumors; and with
the increasing complexity of multi-modality therapy, it is
reasonable to hope that closer correlations between sarcoma
type and management will emerge.
   The designations applied to most bone tumors are fairly
precise. The number of different cell types is small and each
tends to have distinctive appearances, and the nature of the
tumor matrix is often helpful. Consequently, the contribu-
tions of ultrastructural studies on bone neoplasms are to a
large extent academic. Small cell tumors are an exception,
and electron microscopy is useful to distinguish Ewing's
sarcoma from small cell osteosarcoma. The soft tissue sarcomas are in contrast unique among human tumors for the
degree to which their component cells can lack distinctive
morphologic features that would serve to indicate the subtype. The degree of overlap by light microscopy among different forms of soft tissue sarcomas is considerable. In many
instances, however, examination of the fine structure of the
cells with the electron microscope will reveal the sarcoma
type. (1)
   The pathologist approaches the study of a problem tumor

---

*Professor of Pathology, The University of Texas System
Cancer Center, M.D. Anderson Hospital and Tumor Institute,
1515 Holcombe Blvd., Houston, TX 77030.

J. R. Ryan and L. O. Baker (eds.), Recent Concepts in Sarcoma Treatment, 40–47.
© 1988 by Kluwer Academic Publishers.

(2) by examining hematoxylin and eosin-stained paraffin sections with the light microscope. At least two thirds of soft tissue sarcomas can be confidently categorized in this way, and the clinical and radiologic findings will often aid in determining whether a particular tumor is primary within bone or soft tissues, and if it is benign or malignant. When the light microscopy is not diagnostic, histochemical stains for glycogen and other substances may be used, but they are of limited value. Immunostaining methods are more selective, though only a few are directly applicable to the subtyping of soft tissue tumors. Not all tumors suspected by light microscopy to be sarcomas are in fact mesenchymal, and stains for cytokeratins, S-100 protein and leucocyte common antigen stains are useful screening procedures to determine if a particular tumor falls into the soft tissue group. Immunostaining methods have an advantage over electron microscopy as diagnostic aids in that they are available to every pathologist through commercial kits, and can therefore be performed and evaluated in any laboratory. However, good controls are essential, and the findings must be assessed in the context of the clinical and light microscopic findings since certain sarcomas are cytokeratin (3) or S-100 (4) positive.

Electron microscopy is used sparingly for diagnostic purposes, and the reasons include the limited number of conveniently available facilities and the cost of maintaining them, the expense of the ultrastructural diagnostic procedure, and a shortage of experienced pathologists who are familiar with the ultrastructural spectrum that can be encountered in human tumors. In the case of the sarcomas, relatively small numbers of specimens of most of the subtypes have been studied at the ultrastructural level and much information has yet to be garnered, but the data is slowly accumulating in spite of the fact that its practical application is limited. If there were clearer indications that the findings would help in the selection of treatment, electron microscopy would be more widely employed.

Some Practical Points.

Effective procedures for procuring and preparing tissue for electron microscopy are vitally important because any distortion in the tissue specimen is immediately apparent at the ultrastructural level. Crushing and drying artifacts can not be tolerated, and prompt immersion of small pieces of a solid tumor in buffered glutaraldehyde is mandatory. One advantage of electron microscopy is the small amount of tissue that is required, and needle biopsies and fine needle aspirates (5) are adequate provided they are representative and are processed correctly. A disadvantage of these small specimens is their limited ability to reveal architectural patterns of the cells that are readily apparent in larger specimens, but in spite of this shortcoming, low magnification electron micrographs can be highly informative and reveal details of the organization of a tumor and the relationships between cells and stroma that are not apparent by routine light microscopy.

The ultrastructural examination of a problem tumor

should be carried out by a pathologist who is familiar with the clinical situation and has examined the paraffin sections and compared them with light microscopic sections of the plastic-embedded tissue for electron microscopy. Usually the structure of a soft tissue sarcoma is fairly uniform throughout the tumor, but sampling of a heterogeneous neoplasm can influence the appearances seen at the ultrastructural level. Correlation of the light and electron microscopy is therefore essential.

Examples:

It is not possible in the limited space available to review the broad field of bone and soft tissue sarcomas. The following four illustrative cases provide an indication of the detailed information on sarcoma cell structure that can be obtained by transmission electron microscopy.

Case 1. (See Figure 1.) Fibrosarcoma involving the femur and adjacent soft tissues of the thigh of a 21-year-old female. Parts of three tumor cells are shown. They are characterized by the presence of abundant endoplasmic reticulum occupying most of the cytoplasm. The cells are connected to one another by primitive cell junctions. The magnification is x 13,000.

FIGURE 1

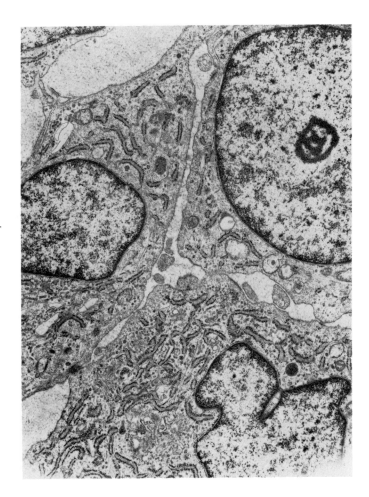

44

Case 2. (See Figure 2.) Malignant fibrous histiocytoma from the thigh of a 60-year-old male. The cells in this area of the tumor were round to ovoid. Compared with the fibrosarcoma cells in the previous illustration, they contain relatively little endoplasmic reticulum, but small cell junctions are again present. Magnification x 7,000.

FIGURE 2

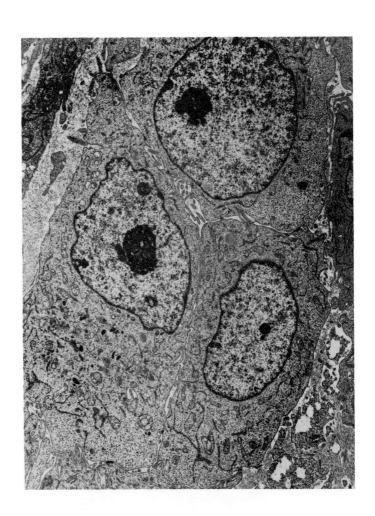

Case 3. (See Figure 3.) Rhabdomyosarcoma of the bladder in a 2-year-old girl. A small area of the cytoplasm of a tumor cell is shown. Thick and thin (myosin and actin) myofilaments are organized into fragments of myofibrils. Magnification x 40,000.

FIGURE 3

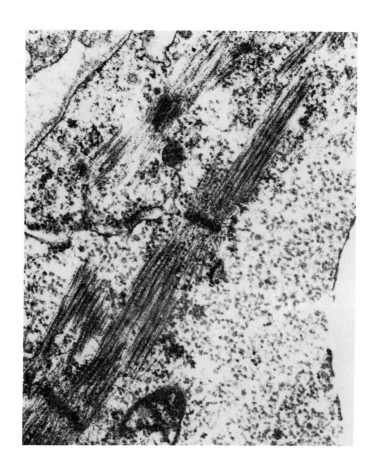

Case 4. (See Figure 4.) Extraskeletal myxoid chondro-sarcoma of the thigh from a 70-year-old woman. Arrays of microtubules were present in the cisternae of the endoplasmic reticulum. In this illustration, the microtubules are mostly cut in cross section. Magnification x 61,000.

FIGURE 4

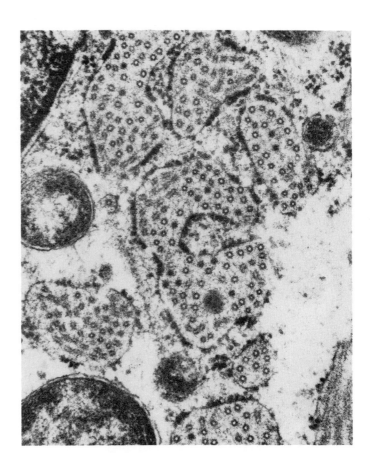

REFERENCES

1. Troncoso P, Ordonez NG, Mackay B: Soft tissue tumors. Clin Lab Med 7:249-260, 1987.
2. Mackay B, Ordonez NG: The role of the pathologist in the evaluation of poorly differentiated tumors and metastatic tumors of unknown origin. In Poorly Differentiated Neoplasms and Tumors of Unknown Origin. Fer MF, Greco FA, Oldham RK (eds.), Florida, Grune and Stratton, pp 3-74, 1986.

3. Meis JM, Mackay B, Ordonez NG: Epithelioid sarcoma: An immunohistochemical and ultrastructural study. Surg Pathol (in press).
4. Benson JD, Kraemer BB, Mackay B: Malignant melanoma of soft parts: An ultrastructural study of four cases. Ultrastruct Pathol 8:57-70, 1985.
5. Mackay B, Fanning T, Bruner JM, Steglich MC: Diagnostic electron microscopy using fine needle aspiration biopsies. Ultrastruct Pathol 11:659-672, 1987.

IMMUNOHISTOCHEMISTRY IN SARCOMAS

John J. Brooks, M.D.*

Introduction

The usefulness of immunohistochemistry in the diagnosis of sarcomas has certainly blossomed in recent years. Here, its overall importance in the diagnosis of soft tissue tumors will be documented and related to the clinical importance of proper sarcoma diagnosis. Secondly, specific markers will be briefly outlined and their limitations underscored. Last, new directions and approaches for the future using this technology will be proposed.

As one can see from the schematic diagram (Figure 1), the diagnosis of a sarcoma is fraught with difficulty. One may confuse such tumors histologically with carcinomas, melanomas, lymphoma, and also a host of benign tumors and pseudosarcomas. Any methodology which helps us through this treacherous territory is certainly welcome. Over the years, methodologic sensitivity in immunohistochemistry has improved dramatically (Table 1).

Why has immunohistochemistry been so useful in the diagnosis of sarcomas? In this overview, a number of facts are immediately apparent. First of all, most non-sarcomas can be excluded through the use of various markers. Secondly, most sarcoma types do have a specific and reliable marker. Third, most paraffin embedded tissues will contain the required immunoreactivity; and fourth, new and evermore useful markers and fine adjustments are continually forthcoming in this field.

In the partial listing within Table 2, it is apparent that there is a helpful or diagnostic immunohistochemical marker for nearly every soft tissue phenotype. The overall sensitivity and specificity for many of these markers is approximately 75% and 100%, respectively. Among spindle cell sarcomas for example, desmin immunoreactivity is conclusive in demonstrating a smooth muscle origin. Likewise, S-100 immunoreactivity is extremely helpful in delineating a soft tissue tumor as a malignant Schwannoma (or more properly, a

---

*Associate Professor of Pathology and Laboratory Medicine, Hospital of the University of Pennsylvania, 34th & Spruce Sts., Philadelphia, PA 19104.
Member, Soft Tissue Pathology Committee of the Eastern Cooperative Oncology Group (Grant NCI CA 15488).

J. R. Ryan and L. O. Baker (eds.), Recent Concepts in Sarcoma Treatment, 48–58.
© *1988 by Kluwer Academic Publishers.*

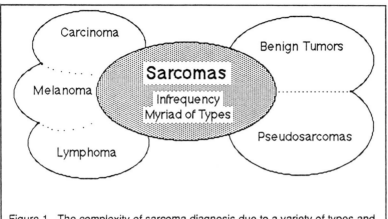

Figure 1. The complexity of sarcoma diagnosis due to a variety of types and
subtypes together with numerous mimicks.

Table 1. IMMUNOHISTOCHEMISTRY: Advances in Sensitivity

Method	Relative Value
Immunofluorescence	1
Direct (1 step)	10
Indirect (2 step)	100
PAP (3 step)	1000
ABC (3 step)	10,000

malignant peripheral nerve sheath tumor). More recently, new
antibodies have been helpful in the diagnosis of
rhabdomyosarcoma; for example, a monoclonal antibody to
muscle specific actin (so-called HHF35) has been developed by
Dr. Gown of Seattle. Likewise, immunoreactive cytokeratin is
characteristically found in monophasic synovial sarcoma,
rescuing this more frequently diagnosed entity from the ranks
of the diminishing group of sarcomas of uncertain histogenesis.

Specific Markers

Vimentin has been hailed as the intermediate filament
for mesenchymal tissues, and indeed it is found within essentially all normal mesenchymal tissue elements. However,
vimentin immunoreactivity is not that informative from a
diagnostic viewpoint, as a great variety of tumors, including
many carcinomas and melanoma, express vimentin. Non-muscle
specific myosins and actins can be found in many cells and,
like collagens, have not been diagnostically useful. Immuno-

Table 2. IMMUNOHISTOCHEMISTRY IN SARCOMAS: Phenotypic Markers: Sensitivity & Specificity

Phenotype	Marker	Sens.	Spec.
1. Muscle (skeletal)	Desmin	>90%	100%
2. Muscle (smooth)	Desmin	70%*	100%
3. Endothelium	Factor VIII	>90%	100%
4. Neural (neuronal)	Neurofilament	>90%	100%
5. Neural (n. sheath)	S100	70%	(-)
6. Neural (CCS[a])	S100	75%	(-)
7. Cartiliginous	S100	>90%	(-)
8. Fatty	S100	0-100%	(-)
9. "Synovial"	Cytokeratin	75%	100%
10. Other "Epithelial[b]"	Cytokeratin	75%	100%
11. Fibrohistiocytic	A-chymotrypsin	80%	(low)
12. Fibrous	--	--	--

*Site dependent; a = clear cell sarcoma; b = epithelioid & rhabdoid sarcomas.

reactive laminin may be helpful in distinguishing between tumors lacking laminin (fibroblastic) and tumors containing laminin (Schwannian and smooth muscle lesions).

Endothelial Markers

One of the most specific markers for a soft tissue phenotype is Factor VIII related antigen. This large protein, produced by endothelial cells, has been detected in numerous benign and malignant endothelial lesions with high degree of sensitivity and specificity. For optimum results, trypsinization is commonly used to detect it. Although essentially all angiosarcomas (even poorly differentiated types) are positive, this marker is found only focally in Kaposi's sarcoma. Ulex lectin may also be observed in endothelial cells and vascular tumors, but it is not specific for endothelium: caution must be used if carcinoma is a diagnostic possibility. Blood group antigens also appear on endothelial cells and, within mesenchymal lesions, are found only on tumors of endothelial origin.

Muscle Markers

The intermediate filament desmin is apparently the most sensitive and specific marker for muscle lesions. This protein can be found in tumors of both smooth and skeletal muscle origin. Within rhabdomyosarcomas, over 90% of cases will be positive including those of very poor differentiation. In a number of comparative studies, desmin has proved superior to other muscle markers for the identification of rhabdomyosarcoma. In smooth muscle tumors, immunoreactivity for desmin is quite variable and particularly dependent upon tumor site. It is likely that desmin is affected adversely by formalin fixation. Since desmin has thus far been extremely specific, a positive result in a spindle cell sarcoma should be interpreted as presumptive evidence for a smooth muscle origin. Rare cases of desmin positive malignant fibrous histiocytoma could conceivably represent pleomorphic or dedifferentiated leiomyosarcoma.

Myoglobin is another muscle marker found exclusively in skeletal muscle and lesions thereof. Although quite specific for rhabdomyosarcoma, its sensitivity is definitely less than that of desmin. Thus, while the overall sensitivity has been reported to range from 50-90% in RMS, comparative studies have always shown desmin immunoreactivity to be superior. Recently, monoclonal antibodies to muscle-specific myosins have been described and the results reported appear extremely promising.

Neural Markers

Neurofilament, the intermediate filament of neurons, is highly specific and important in identifying peripheral tumors of neural origin such as neuroblastoma, ganglioneuro-blastoma, and paraganglioma. Importantly, it will not react with other non-neuronal lesions such as those of nerve sheath origin. In its original description, the so-called neuron specific enolase (NSE) was considered to be fairly specific for neuronal lesions as well as selected other tumors. However, this has turned out not to be the case and a vast array of human tumors contain immunoreactive NSE; its usefulness has drastically decreased.

Despite the fact that S-100 antigen is found in a wide variety of tissues and cell types, S-100 antigen is nonetheless quite usual in diagnostic immunohistochemistry. In mesenchymal cell types, S-100 immunoreactivity is found within chondrocytes, adipocytes, and lesions of Schwannian origin. Due to the fact that the differential diagnosis of a problematic soft tissue lesion rarely involves more than one of these three phenotypes, S-100 immunoreactivity in a soft tissue lesion has real meaning. Within malignant peripheral nerve sheath tumors, sensitivity has been reported from between 50-75%. Indeed, a positive S-100 test in a spindle cell sarcoma, particularly if floridly positive, can be taken as supportive information for a tumor of Schwannian derivation, given the appropriate histopathology. It is true that there are occasional cases of leiomyosarcoma which exhibit some S-100 immunoreactivity. Usually this is to a mild degree and is likely due to the less specific alpha subunit of S-100. Clear cell sarcoma is another S-100 positive tumor. The immunoreactivity seen in chondrosarcomatous areas can be quite helpful in answering questions concerning the presence of cartilaginous foci. Although some authors have obtained nearly 100% sensitivity of S-100 within liposarcomas, other authors have not had such success. It can be helpful in distinguishing myxoid liposarcoma from myxoid malignant fibrous histiocytoma. Lastly, myelin basic protein and Leu 7 have been identified in many lesions and do not appear to be useful.

Epithelial Markers

The two classic types of sarcomas which display epithelial markers are synovial sarcoma and epithelioid sarcoma. Briefly, biphasic synovial sarcomas are nearly always positive for cytokeratin and epithelial membrane antigen, whereas monophasic tumors will exhibit the same immunoreactivity in approximately 3/4ths of cases. Other tumors, such as the newly described rhabdoid sarcoma of soft tissue and chordoma, also exhibit cytokeratin immunoreactivity. Aside from this group of tumors, cytokeratin is, as a general rule, not found in other sarcomas. The occasional reports of cytokeratin immunoreactivity in malignant fibrous histiocytomas or in leiomyosarcomas are somewhat suspect due to shared epitopes and regions of homology between cytokeratin and other intermediate filament proteins. For the time being, a cytokeratin positive spindle cell lesion resembling fibrosarcoma or hemangiopericytoma is considered a monophasic synovial sarcoma. Unfortunately, epithelial membrane antigen does not exhibit the complete specificity that cytokeratin does, but it is still a useful adjunct if used with caution.

Fibrohistiocytic Markers

Specific markers for the fibrohistiocytic phenotype have been hard to come by. The major markers discussed in the literature for this group of lesions have been alpha 1-anti-chymotrypsin and its relative alpha 1-anti-trypsin. However, long ago it was recognized that both of these markers may be identified in carcinomas and melanomas. While it is true that a large percentage of malignant fibrous histiocytomas express these two antigens, the specificity of these reactions has lately been questioned. It is clear that this marker may be found in other phenotypes, particularly smooth muscle. Further, routine "histiocytic markers" such as lysozyme and ferritin have been far less sensitive. Thus, it is unfortunate that the most common adult sarcoma (MFH) does not have an associated specific marker, but future developments may change this.

A panel approach is commonly performed now in the immunohistochemical approach to a difficult lesion. Using such a panel, characteristic immunoreactive profiles of each soft tissue tumor type will become apparent (Table 3). Such a panel approach also decreases the possibility of over interpretation of equivocal results, since other markers act as important controls. There are also a number of unstated rules for interpretation. For example, the rule of antigen precedence (so-called) states that, given a series of positive markers, the most specific and reliable marker takes precedence over all others and forms the basis for any further interpretation. That is just one example amongst many, the fibrohistiocytic lesion can only be diagnosed after a series of other markers in a panel have been shown to be negative.

What about the relationship between immunohistochemistry and other diagnostic techniques for sarcomas? Electron microscopic examination is unquestionably quite helpful in a large number of sarcomas. However, it is also clear that not all sarcomas will have the characteristic ultrastructural findings; for example, not all rhabdomyosarcomas will contain z-bands. However, it is emphasized here that, while the ultrastructure of sarcomas is quite important, the basic

Table 3. IMMUNOHISTOCHEMISTRY IN SARCOMAS:
Phenotypic Prolifes Using Panel Approach

Rhabdomyosarcoma	CK-,	S100-,	**DES+**
Nerve sheath tumors	CK-,	**S100+,**	DES-
Synovial sarcoma	**CK+,**	S100-,	DES-

CK = cytokeratin; DES = desmin.

principle behind immunohistochemistry is <u>cellular biochem-istry</u>, detecting products of the cell machinery. This bio-chemistry truly characterizes a specific phenotype and its products are probably expressed more frequently than specific structural markers. In other words, when it comes to cell identification, "by their deeds you shall know them". This methodology is also cheaper and more available than electron microscopy.

Clinical Importance

What is the importance of immunohistochemistry in terms of diagnosis and therapy? There are definite therapeutic advantages which result from a proper diagnosis in turn based upon this remarkable methodology. First of all, the patient does receive proper therapy having been placed in the proper category (Table 4). Second, one can only assess the

Table 4. IMMUNOHISTOCHEMISTRY IN SARCOMAS: Clinical.
Importance of Histogenesis for Diagnosis and Therapy

1. Proper Placement for Proper Therapy
   - Three Categories: Round cell
                        Spindle cell
                        Other types*

2. Assessment of Therapeutic Effectiveness
   - Uniform Groups of Cases

*In contrast to common belief, there are a group of unusual sarcomas with peculiar natural histories, such as Epithelioid & Clear cell sarcoma, Alveolar soft part sarcoma, Rhabdoid sarcoma, Angiosarcoma, Kaposi's sarcoma, and Liposarcoma; these do not fit well in the other two groups.

effectiveness of new chemotherapeutic agents on a completely uniform group of cases, and the uniformity is now provided by specific immunoreactivity. Misdiagnosed cases have been excluded through the use of immunohistochemistry, and changes in diagnosis occur with regularity. As can be seen in Table 5, experience with immunohistochemistry in the soft tissue

Table 5.   IMMUNOHISTOCHEMISTRY IN SARCOMAS. Changes in Diagnosis:
Eastern Cooperative Oncology Group Sarcoma Experience

Major:	1.	Sarcoma to non-sarcoma.	8/108 (7%)
	2.	One type to another with Rx implications (e.g. rhabdomyosarcoma change).	4/108 (4%)
	3.	Sarcoma to reactive lesion.	1/108 (1%)
Minor:	1.	Other changes, no impact on Rx (e.g. one spindle cell type to another).	33/108 (31%)
Total			46/108 (46%)

committee of the Eastern Cooperative Oncology Group has resulted in a significant percentage of diagnostic changes, some of which are quite important clinically. Major changes in diagnosis (meaning either that the "sarcoma" had been reclassified as a non-sarcoma or reactive lesion, or that the type was changed to one with therapeutic implications [e.g. rhabdomyosarcoma]) occurred in 12% of all cases. Obviously, minor changes in diagnosis are less important and have no impact on therapy (as an example, the change of one spindle cell sarcoma to another type). However, they do affect analysis of therapeutic effectiveness on specific sarcoma types.

Future Developments

In the future, immunohistochemistry could well be used to understand more theoretical aspects of sarcomas (Table 6). For example, one can use this technology to analyze the phenomenon of dedifferentiation (antigenic shift from one phenotype to another) and its clinical importance. Similarly,

Table 6. IMMUNOHISTOCHEMISTRY IN SARCOMAS:
New Approaches & Future Applications:

1. Proliferation markers - for Grading
2. Biologic markers
        e.g. Growth factors, receptors
        e.g. Enzymes associated with
        aggressive behavior
3. Cell surface markers for immunotherapy

one can use immunohistochemistry to analyze the autocrine growth hypothesis, reported to be the major mechanism for sarcoma growth. For example, in a recent study, we found that a number of sarcomas co-expressed growth factors and growth factor receptors, confirming self stimulation of growth. Future applications may also include the analysis of proliferation markers, aiding in the exact and objective grading of sarcomas, one of the major predictors of ultimate survival. Enzymes associated with aggressive behavior could be detected. Finally, cell surface antigen analysis may be critical for immunotherapy or the use of biologic response modifiers.

In summary, the clinical importance of immunohisto-chemistry resides in its use as a critical adjunct for proper diagnosis which, in turn, leads to proper therapy. It has been extremely powerful in this role and its full potential has not yet been reached.

REFERENCES

1. Taylor CR: Immunomicroscopy: A Diagnostic Tool for the Surgical Pathologist. Philadelphia, WB Saunders Co, 1986.
2. Rohol PJM, deJong ASH, Ramaekers FCS: Application of markers in the diagnosis of soft tissue tumors. Histo-pathology 9:1019-1035, 1985.
3. Battifora H: Monoclonal antibodies in the histologic diagnosis of cancer. Lab Management pp.38-53, May 1985.
4. Hsu S, Raine L, Fanger H: Use of avidin-biotin-peroxi-dase complex (ABC) in immunoperoxidase techniques. A comparison between ABC and unlabelled antibody (PAP) procedures. J. Histochem Cytochem 29:577-80, 1981.
5. Gown A, Vogel A: Monoclonal antibodies to human inter-mediate filament proteins. Distribution of filament proteins in normal human tissues. Am J Pathol 114:309-321, 1984.
6. Miettinen M, Hehto V, Badley R, Virtanen I: Expression of intermediate filaments in soft tissue sarcomas. Int J Cancer 30:541-546, 1982.
7. Mukai K, Stollmeyer, Rosai J: Immunohistochemical local-ization of actin: Applications in surgical pathology. Am J Surg Pathol 5:91-97, 1981.
8. Tsukada T, McNutt M, Ross R, Gown A: HHF35, a muscle actin-specific monoclonal antibody II. Reactivity in normal, reactive, and neoplastic human tissue. Am J Pathol 127:389-402, 1987.
9. Eusebi V, Ceccarelli C, Gorza L, Schiaffino S, Bussolati G: Immunocytochemistry of rhabdomyosarcoma: The use of four different markers. Am J Surg Pathol 10:293-299, 1986.
10. Ogawa K, Oguchi M, Yamabe H, Nakashima Y, Hamashima Y: Distribution of collagen type IV in soft tissue tumors. An immunohistochemical study. Cancer 58:269-277, 1986.
11. Miettinen M, Foidart J, Ekblom P: Immunohistochemical demonstration of laminin, the major glycoprotein of basement membranes, as an aid in the diagnosis of soft tissue tumors. Am J Clin Pathol 79:306-311, 1983.
12. Corson J, Weiss L, Banks-Schlegel S, Pinkus G: Keratin proteins and carcinoembryonic antigen in synovial sar-coma: an immunohistochemical study of 24 cases. Hum Pathol 15:615-621, 1984.

13. Mukai K, Rosai J, Burgdorf W: Localization of factor VIII-related antigen in vascular endothelial cells using an immunoperoxidase method. Am J Surg Pathol 4:273-276, 1980.

14. Guarda L, Ordonez N, Smith J, Hanssen G: Immunoperoxidase localization of factor VIII in angiosarcomas. Arch Pathol Lab Med 106:515-516, 1982.

15. Guarda L, Silva E, Ordonez N, Smith J: Factor VIII in Kaposi's sarcoma. Am J Clin Pathol 76:197-200, 1976.

16. Auerbach H, Brooks JJ: Kaposi's sarcoma: Observations and a hypothesis. Lab Invest 52:4A, 1985.

17. Miettinen M, Holthofer H, Lehto V, Miettinen A, Virtanen I: Ulex Europaeus 1 lectin as a marker for tumors derived from endothelial cells. Am J Clin Pathol 79:32-36, 1983.

18. Wick M, Manivel J: Epithelioid sarcoma and epithelioid hemangioendothelioma: an immunohistochemical and lectin-histochemical comparison. Virchows Arch Pathol Anat 87:319-326, 1987.

19. Miester P, Methras W: Immunohistochemical markers of histiocytic tumors. Hum Pathol 11:300-301, 1980.

20. duBoulay C.: Demonstration of alpha 1 antitrypsin and alpha 1 anti-chymotrypsin in fibrous histiocytomas using the immunoperoxidase technique. Am J Surg Pathol 6:559-564, 1982.

21. Kindblom L, Jacobson G, Jacobsen M: Immunohistochemical investigations of tumors of supposed fibro-histiocytic origin. Hum Pathol 13:834-840, 1982.

22. Miettinen M, Lehto V, Badley R, Virtanen I: Alveolar rhabdomyosarcoma: demonstration of the muscle type of intermediate filament protein, desmin and a diagnostic aide. Am J Pathol 108:426-251, 1982.

23. Altmannsberger M, Osborn M, Treuner J, Holscher A, Weber K, Chaeuer A: Diagnosis of human childhood rhabdomyosarcoma by antibodies to desmin. The structural protein of muscle specific intermediate filaments. Virchows Arch (Cell Pathol) 39:203-215, 1982.

24. Hashimoto H, Daimaru Y, Tsuneyoshi M, Enjoji M: Leiomyosarcoma of the external soft tissues. A clinicopathologic, immunohistochemical and electron microscopic study. Cancer 57:2077-2088, 1986.

25. Saul SH, Rast M, Brooks JJ: The immunohistochemistry of gastrointestinal stromal tumors: evidence supporting an origin from smooth muscle. Am J Surg Pathol 11:464-473, 1987.

26. Altmannsberger M, Osborn M, Schauer A, Weber K: Antibodies to different intermediate filament proteins. Cell type-specific markers on paraffin-embedded human tissues. Lab Invest 45:427-434, 1981.

27. Corson J, Pinkus G: Intracellular myoglobin: a specific marker for skeletal muscle differentiation in soft tissue sarcomas. Am J Pathol 103:384-389, 1981.

28. Brooks J: Immunohistochemistry of soft tissue tumors. Myoglobin as a tumor marker for rhabdomyosarcoma. Cancer 50:1757-1763, 1982.

29. Kindblom L, Eidal T, Karlsson K: Immunohistochemical localization of myoglobin in human muscle tissue and embryonal and alveolar rhabdomyosarcoma. Acta Path Microbiol Immunol Scand Sect. A 90:167-174, 1982.
30. deJong ASH, van Raamsdonk W, van Kessel-van Vark M, Albus-Lutter CE: Skeletal muscle actin as tumor marker in the diagnosis of rhabdomyosarcoma in childhood. Am J Surg Pathol 9:467-474, 1986.
31. Trojanowski J, Lee V, Schlaepfer W: An immunohisto-chemical study of human central and peripheral nervous tumors using monoclonal antibodies against neurofila-ments and glial filaments. Hum Pathol 15:248-257, 1984.
32. Sasaki A, Ogawa A, Nakazato Y, Ishida Y: Distribution of neurofilament protein and neuron-specific enolase in peripheral neuronal tumors. Virchows Arch 407:33-4, 1985.
33. Mukai M, Torikata C, Iri H, Morikawa Y, Shimizu K, Shimoda T, Nukina N, Ihara Y, Kageyama K: Expression of neurofilament triplet proteins in human neural tumors. Am J Pathol 122:28-35, 1986.
34. Lloyd R, Warner T: Immunohistochemistry of Neuron-specific enolase. Chapter 7 In Advances in Immunohisto-chemistry. R. Delellis (ed.), New York, Masson Publish-ing USA, 1984.
35. Dranoff G, Bigner D: A word of caution in the use of neuron specific enolase expression in tumor diagnosis. Arch Pathol Lab Med 108:535, 1984.
36. Nakajima T, Watanabe S, Sato Y, Kameya T, Hirota T, Shimosato Y: An immunoperoxidase study of S100 protein distribution in normal and neoplastic tissues. Am J Surg Pathol 6:715-727, 1982.
37. Weiss S, Langloss J, Enzinger F: Value of S100 protein in the diagnosis of soft tissue tumors with particular reference to benign and malignant Schwann cell tumors. Lab Invest 49:299, 1983.
38. Daimuru Y, Hashimoto H, Enjoji M: Malignant periph-eral nerve-sheath tumors (malignant schwannomas). An immuno-histochemical study of 29 cases. Am J Surg Pathol 9:434-444, 1985.
39. Chung E, Enzinger F: Malignant melanoma of soft parts. A reassessment of clear cell sarcoma. Am J Surg Pathol 7:405-413, 1983.
40. Mukai M, Torikata C, Iri H, Mikata A, Kawai T, Hanaoka H, Yakumaru K, Kageyama K: Histogenesis of clear cell sarcoma of tendons and aponeuroses. Am J Pathol 114:264-272, 1984.
41. Cocchia D, Lauriola L, Stolfi V, Tallini G, Michetti F: S-100 antigen labels neoplastic cells in liposarcoma and cartilaginous tumours. Virchows Arch Pathol Anat 402:139-145, 1983.
42. Hashimoto H, Daimaru Y, Enjoji M: S100 protein distribu-tion in liposarcoma. An immunoperoxidase study with special reference to the distinction of liposarcoma from myxoid malignant fibrous histiocytoma. Virchows Arch Pathol Anat 405:1-10, 1984.

43. Wick M, Swanson P, Scheithauer B, Manivel J: Malignant peripheral nerve sheath tumor: an immunohistochemical study of 62 cases. Am J Clin Pathol 87:425-433, 1987.

44. Fisher C: Synovial sarcoma: ultrastructural and immuno-histochemical features of epithelial differentiation in immunohistochemical features of epithelial differentiation in monophasic and biphasic tumors. Hum Pathol 17:996-1008, 1986.

45. Abenoza P, Manivel JC, Swanson PE, Wick MR: Synovial sarcoma: ultrastructural study and immunohistochemical analysis by a combined peroxidase-antiperoxi-dase / avidin-biotin peroxidase complex procedure. Hum Pathol 17:1107-1115, 1986.

46. Chase D, Enzinger F, Weill S, Langloss J: Keratinin epithelioid sarcoma: an immunohistochemical study. Am J Surg Pathol 8:435-441, 1984.

47. Tsuneyoshi M, Daimaru Y, Hashimoto H, Enjoji M: Malignant soft tissue neoplasms with the histologic features of renal rhabdoid tumors: an ultrastructur-al and immunohistochemical study. Hum Pathol 16: 1235-1242, 1985.

48. Gusterson B: Is Keratin present in smooth muscle? Histopathol 11:549-552, 1987.

CELLULAR COMPOSITION OF SARCOMAS

Steven I. Hajdu, M.D.*

Benign, reactive, and neoplastic mesenchymal cells are pluripotential cells.(3,6,8,16) In the course of differentiation, maturation, they become specialized and may assume the cytologic characteristics of fibroblasts, myoblasts, lipoblasts, angioblasts, chondroblasts and osteoblasts.(3,4, 9) Further differentiation, maturation, may lead to the appearance of end-stage forms, e.g., fibrocytes, myocytes (muscle cells), lipocytes (adipocytes), endothelial cells and chondrocytes. The various phases in cell-cycle that may influence differentiation, or so-called dedifferentiation, of mesenchymal cells is poorly understood, but genetic coding of the neoplastic cells and local tissue conditions have been suggested to play important roles in the development of mature and immature cellular elements.(3,10,15)

Homogenous and inhomogenous appearance of sarcomas, as seen by surgeons and radiologists, is mostly due to admixture of diverse cellular elements at different stages of maturation. Although extracellular deposit of intracellular products, e.g., collagen, osteoid, mucopolysaccharides of neoplastic cells is a major contributor to the gross and microscopic appearance of the matrix of sarcomas, non-neoplastic cellular elements of the stroma, and that of local tissues and organs may also influence the consistency and overall histologic and cytologic composition of sarcomas.(6, 7,10,17,19)

The assembly of neoplastic cells (slender and plump spindle cells, granular and clear epithelioid cells, isomorphic and pleomorphic giant cells) and matrix cells with their corresponding products leads to the appearance of tissue patterns.(3,6,8) Although it is general knowledge that tumors are named after the dominant and most differentiated cellular elements, histologic diagnosis, to a large extend, depends on microscopic recognition of the dominant tissue pattern.(6,14) However, poorly differentiated sarcomas, e.g., certain types of malignant fibrous histiocytomas and

----

*Attending Pathologist, Surgical Pathology and Autopsy Services, Dept. of Pathology, Chief, Cytology Service, Memorial Sloan-Kettering Cancer Center, 1275 York Avenue, New York, NY 10021.
Professor of Pathology, Cornell University Medical College, New York, New York.

J. R. Ryan and L. O. Baker (eds.), Recent Concepts in Sarcoma Treatment, 59–64.
© 1988 by Kluwer Academic Publishers.

pleomorphic, high grade sarcomas, e.g., pleomorphic liposarcomas, myosarcomas and malignant peripheral nerve tumors,
are notorious for forming nonspecific tissue patterns.(3,6,8)
These sarcomas, and a number of other neoplasms, e.g., tendosynovial sarcoma, angiosarcoma and alveolar soft part
sarcoma, warrant careful scrutiny of intracytoplasmic
products by special histochemical, immunohistochemical or
ultrastructural techniques in order to ascertain the precise
identity of the sarcoma.(3,9)

In Table 1, 200 soft tissue sarcomas, studied after
consistent and serial tissue blocking, are listed according
to their gross (macroscopic) and microscopic appearance. The
sarcomas were primary tumors and, with four exceptions, were
bigger than 5 cm.; none were treated prior to surgical excision. It is noteworthy that macroscopically there were only
three consistently homogenous sarcomas: malignant fibroblastic fibrous histiocytoma (dermatofibrosarcoma protuber-
ans), desmoid fibrosarcoma and monophasic tendosynovial
sarcoma. The same three sarcomas, plus embryonal rhabdomyo-

TABLE 1

COMPARISON OF MACROSCOPIC AND MICROSCOPIC
APPEARANCE OF SARCOMAS*

SARCOMAS	TOTAL NO. OF SARCOMAS	NUMBER OF INHOMOGENOUS SARCOMAS MACROSCOPICALLY	MICROSCOPICALLY
Malignant fibroblastic fibrous histiocytoma	10	1	0
Malignant pleomorphic fibrous histiocytoma	10	10	10
Desmoid tumor	10	2	0
Fibrosarcoma	10	7	7
Biphasic tendosynovial sarcoma	10	7	5
Monophasic tendosynovial sarcoma	10	3	0
Epithelioid sarcoma	10	8	8
Well-differentiated liposarcoma	10	6	4
Myxoid liposarcoma	10	9	6
Lipoblastic liposarcoma	10	6	8
Pleomorphic liposarcoma	10	10	10
Leiomyosarcoma	10	7	7
Embryonal rhabdomyosarcoma	10	8	3
Pleomorphpic rhabdomyosarcoma	10	10	10
Hemangiopericytoma	10	5	3
Angiosarcoma	10	9	8
Malignant peripheral nerve tumor	10	10	10
Chondrosarcoma	10	8	3
Osteosarcoma	10	10	10
Alveolar soft part sarcoma	10	5	1
Total	200	141	118

*Modified from: Hajdu and Hajdu, Cytopathology of Soft Tissue and Bone Tumors, Karger,
Basel, 1988.

sarcomas and chondrosarcomas, were the ones that appeared microscopically homogenous, single cell type. However, despite homogenous histologic composition, cytologic samples, e.g., aspirates from such tumors without recognizable tissue patterns or laboratory demonstration of specific cellular products, may not permit definitive microscopic diagnosis. (11,12,13,14)

Table 2 shows composition of soft tissue sarcomas (listed in Table 1) according to histologic grade and presence of microscopically detectable benign neoplastic and reactive, non-neoplastic areas in the sarcomas. The high rate of low grade sarcomatous areas as seen, e.g., in malignant pleomorphic fibrous histiocytomas, lipoblastic and pleomorphic liposarcomas and malignant peripheral nerve tumors, should serve as warning to those who depend, in grading of soft tissue sarcomas, on limited biopsy samples. (9,14) The almost consistent finding of benign neoplastic areas in sarcomas, such as certain fibrous histiocytomas, liposarcomas, myosarcomas and malignant peripheral nerve tumors, call

TABLE 2

MICROSCOPIC COMPOSITION OF SARCOMAS

SARCOMAS	TOTAL NO. OF SARCOMAS	LOW GRADE SARCOMA	HIGH GRADE SARCOMA	LOW AND HIGH GR. SARCOMA	BENIGN NEOPLASMS	REACTIVE LESIONS
			NUMBER OF SARCOMAS WITH AREAS OF:			
Malignant fibroblastic fibrous histiocytoma	10	10	-	-	3	2
Malignant pleomorphic fibrous histiocytoma	10	1	2	7	9	8
Desmoid tumor	10	10	-	-	2	3
Fibrosarcoma	10	1	4	5	1	2
Biphasic tendosynovial sarcoma	10	1	9	-	1	2
Monophasic tendosynovial sarcoma	10	-	10	-	-	2
Epithelioid sarcoma	10	-	10	-	-	2
Well-differentiated liposarcoma	10	10	-	-	6	2
Myxoid Liposarcoma	10	10	-	-	4	3
Lipoblastic liposarcoma	10	-	4	6	2	1
Pleomorphic liposarcoma	10	-	3	7	1	4
Leiomyosarcoma	10	3	4	3	5	3
Embryonal rhabdomyosarcoma	10	1	6	3	-	2
Pleomorphic rhabdomyosarcoma	10	-	9	1	-	2
Hemangiopericytoma	10	2	4	4	1	2
Angiosarcoma	10	2	3	5	4	5
Malignant peripheral nerve tumor	10	2	1	7	8	6
Chondrosarcoma	10	8	1	1	5	2
Osteosarcoma	10	-	8	2	3	4
Alveolar soft part sarcoma	10	-	10	-	-	2
Total	200	61	88	51	55	65

for further caution in planning, or postponing, definitive therapy on the basis of small or less than adequate incisional biopsy. It is worth remembering that pathologists and clinicians assume a great responsibility when they advise radical therapy, but they assume a still greater responsibility when they advise against it.(1,2,14)

It is general knowledge that histologic grade of sarcomas is the single most important component on which the selection of the most appropriate modality of therapy, and ultimately the prognosis, depends.(3,5,6,18) There is no single rule or formula for accurate grading of sarcomas, but the more experienced the pathologist is, and the more adequate and representative the histologic sample is, the more accurate the label as to grade will be. In our experience, in nine of ten cases the histologic grade cannot be accurately assessed without knowing the histologic type of the sarcoma. (3,6,14)

TABLE 3

COMPARISON OF MACROSCOPIC AND MICROSCOPIC FEATURES OF SARCOMAS
IN ORDER OF DIAGNOSTIC IMPORTANCE*

SARCOMAS	MACROSCOPIC APPEARANCE	MICROSCOPIC APPEARANCE			
		PATTERN	CELLS	MATRIX	PRODUCTS
Malignant fibroblastic fibrous histiocytoma	3	1	2	4	5
Malignant pleomorphic fibrous histiocytoma	4	3	1	2	5
Desmoid tumor	4	2	1	3	5
Fibrosarcoma	5	1	2	3	4
Biphasic tendosynovial sarcoma	5	1	2	4	3
Monophasic tendosynovial sarcoma	5	1	2	3	4
Epithelioid sarcoma	4	1	2	5	3
Well-differentiated liposarcoma	5	2	1	4	3
Myxoid liposarcoma	5	1	2	3	4
Lipoblastic liposarcoma	5	3	1	2	4
Pleomorphic liposarcoma	5	4	1	2	3
Leiomyosarcoma	5	2	1	4	3
Embryonal rhabdomyosarcoma	5	3	1	4	2
Pleomorphic rhabdomyosarcoma	5	4	1	3	2
Hemangiopericytoma	4	1	2	3	5
Angiosarcoma	4	1	2	3	5
Malignant peripheral nerve tumor	3	2	1	4	5
Chondrosarcoma	4	3	1	2	5
Osteosarcoma	4	5	2	1	3
Alveolar soft part sarcoma	5	1	2	4	3

*one is most important and five is least important diagnostic feature

Table 3 shows the sarcomas (presented in Tables 1 and 2) according to pathologists' dependence on pattern of growth, cell morphology, appearance of the matrix and specific cellular products in histologic typing of sarcomas. It is apparent that the above components are interrelated and carry different weights in histologic typing of different sarcomas. But, accurate pattern recognition and identification of cellular elements seem to be the key to reproducible histologic labeling and grading of sarcomas. Over-dependence on any one of the four components (pattern, cells, matrix and products), with complete disregard of the others, undoubtedly leads to histologic misdiagnoses. Similarly, overemphasis of mitotic count and tumor necrosis in grading of soft tissue sarcomas, at the expense of differentiation, cellularity, vascularity and amount of matrix, is a sure guarantee of inaccurate assignment of histologic grade.(3,6,14)

In conclusion, the complex and inhomogenous composition of sarcomas warrant caution in interpretation of biopsy samples. Perhaps, it is also worth remembering that stromal elements may contribute substantially to the appearance of sarcomas and, on occasion, it cannot be determined whether the cells are from the sarcoma or from the stroma. Finally, there cannot be a shortcut to orderly pathologic processing and evaluating of surgical specimens from such diverse and inhomogenous malignant neoplasms as sarcomas without detrimental results.

REFERENCES

1. Brennan MF, Shiu MH, Collin C, Hilaris BS, Magill G, Lane J, Godbold J, Hajdu SI: Extremity soft tissue sarcomas. Cancer Treat Symposia 3:71-81, 1985.
2. Donohue JH, Collin C, Friedrich C, Godbold J, Hajdu SI, Brennan MF: Metastases from low grade extremity soft tissue sarcomas. Cancer (in press).
3. Hajdu SI: Pathology of Soft Tissue Tumors. Philadelphia, Lea & Febiger, 1979.
4. Hajdu SI: The paradox of sarcomas. Acta Cytol 24:373-383, 1980.
5. Hajdu SI: Soft tissue sarcomas: classification and natural history. Ca. 31:271-280, 1981.
6. Hajdu SI: Differential Diagnosis of Soft Tissue and Bone Tumors. Philadelphia, Lea & Febiger, 1986.
7. Hajdu SI, Bean MA, Fogh J, Hajdu EO, Ricci A: Papanicolaou smear of cultured human tumor cells. Acta Cytol 18:327-332, 1974.
8. Hajdu SI, Hajdu EO: Cytopathology of Sarcomas and Other Nonepithelial Malignant Tumors. Philadelphia, WB Saunders Company, 1976.
9. Hajdu SI and Hajdu EO: Cytopathology of Soft Tissue and Bone Tumors. Karger, Basel (in press).
10. Hajdu SI, Lemos LB, Kazakewich H, Helson L, Beattie EJ: Growth pattern and differentiation of human soft tissue sarcomas in nude mice. Cancer 47:90-98, 1981.
11. Hajdu SI, Melamed MR: Needle biopsy of primary malignant bone tumors. Surg Gynecol Obstet 133:829-832, 1971.
12. Hajdu SI, Melamed MR: The diagnostic value of aspiration

smears. Amer J Clin Pathol 59:350-356, 1973.
13. Hajdu SI, Melamed MR: Limitations of aspiration cytology in the diagnosis of primary neoplasms. Acta Cytol 28:337-345, 1984.
14. Hajdu SI, Shiu MH, Brennan MF: The role of the pathologist in the management of soft tissue sarcomas. World J Surg (in press).
15. Hartnack Federspiel B, Sobin LH, Helwig EB, Mikel UV, Bahr GF: Morphometry and cytophotometric assessment of DNA in smooth-muscle tumors (leiomyomas and leiomyosarcomas) of the gastrointestinal tract. Anal Quantit Cytol Histol 9:105-114, 1987.
16. Katenkamp D, Raikhlin NT: Stem cell concept and heterogeneity of malignant soft tissue tumor - a challenge to reconsider diagnostics and therapy. Exp Path 28:3-11, 1985.
17. Nachman J, Simon MA, Dean L, Shermeta D, Dawson P, Vogelzang NJ: Disparate histologic responses in simultaneously resected primary and metastatic osteosarcoma following intravenous neoadjuvant chemotherapy. J Clin Oncol 5:1185-1190, 1987.
18. Russell WO, Cohen J, Enzinger F, Hajdu SI, Heise R, Martin RG, Meissner W, Miller WT, Schmictz RL, Suit HD: A clinical and pathological staging system for soft tissue sarcomas. Cancer 40:1562-1570, 1977.
19. Sethi J, Hirshaut Y, DeHarven E, Hajdu SI: Growing human sarcomas in culture. Cancer 40:744-755, 1977.

PREOPERATIVE EVALUATION OF EXTREMITY SARCOMAS

James R. Ryan, M.D.*

The preoperative evaluation of extremity sarcomas is necessary to give the surgical oncologist the information necessary to surgically stage the lesion to plan his surgical procedure. Flow cytometry, tumor markers, etc. will not be discussed, rather, the rationale for surgical preoperative evaluation.

It may go without saying that the first step in evaluation of the patient is a detailed history, physical examination and then routine radiographs of the lesion. However, as has been published, and all surgical oncologists have seen, patients with extremity sarcomas have had arthrograms of the joint near the lesion or other specialized studies which were not indicated if an adequate history and physical examination were undertaken. It seems in this day of more sophisticated tests, that the physician is forgetting the importance of the history and physical examination. Probably 90-95% of the information needed by the surgeon can be garnered by these three examinations. After these have been completed, specialized examinations can be performed.

One of the earliest examinations advocated was angiography.(1-7) The earlier literature recommended it for diagnostic purposes to differentiate between malignancy and benign lesions, while the later literature also advocated it for surgical staging, feeling that it showed the relationship of the lesion to major vessels and could outline soft tissue extension. The problem with angiography is that it is an invasive procedure which is painful and, in children, usually requires a general anesthetic.

Scintigraphy became popular--gallium-67 citrate for soft tissue, and technetium, either 99 m-labelled hydroxyethylidene diphosphonate or methylene diphosphonate for bone. The literature on gallium for soft tissue lesions is divided.(8-13) Lepanto especially felt it was of little value in childhood tumors. More recent literature, however, feels that it is a reliable indicator of malignant disease and useful in the staging of soft tissue sarcomas. Another value of gallium scanning is that it is probably the most sensitive test in picking up metastatic soft tissue disease. The value of

----
*Associate Professor, Department of Orthopaedic Surgery, Wayne State University School of Medicine, 4201 St. Antoine (7C), Detroit, MI 48201.

J. R. Ryan and L. O. Baker (eds.), Recent Concepts in Sarcoma Treatment, 65–68.
© 1988 by Kluwer Academic Publishers.

technetium scanning has been widely reviewed in the literature, both for bony lesions and soft tissue lesions.(14-22)
Its major value in bony lesions is probably identification of
bony metastases which is the second most common site, second
to the lungs. In Goldstein's series, 16% of cases had bony
metastases prior to pulmonary metastases, while in the
McKillop series, 43% had bony metastases and the sensitivity
of the test was 100%. Technetium scanning has also been
advocated for soft tissue lesions. Blood pooled imaging has
been reported to be very sensitive for the diagnosis of
malignant disease. It is also felt by several authors that it
is the most reliable test to reveal periosteal invasion of a
soft tissue lesion either by the tumor, pseudocapsule, or
extensions secondary to previous surgery. Hudson and Enneking
have emphasized that accurate scintigraphy is necessary with
high resolution images and a tangential relationship with
multiple views to be of benefit, and that routine whole-body
scans are inadequate. Kirchner and Simon emphasized that the
combination of gallium scintigraphy with technetium scintigraphy, including blood pooled imaging for soft tissue tumors,
is extremely reliable in the diagnosis of malignancy. If all
three tests are negative, the lesion is definitely benign.

When computerized axial tomography became available
everyone was excited about its capabilities for extremity
sarcomas.(23-30) It was advocated for diagnosis, staging,
follow-up results of therapy, evaluation of disseminated
disease, and as a guide for biopsy. It was found to give a
better indication of tumor location, extent and relationships
than radiographs, tomograms, scintigraphy or clinical findings. It was found superior to other examinations in determining the intra- and extraosseous involvement of bony sarcomas. It is felt to be the most reliable indicator of pulmonary metastatic disease.

The evolution of magnetic resonance imaging has again
excited the medical community.(31-39) Its tremendous potential advantages are that it has no ionizing radiation, it is
not invasive, and it may be repeated. The recent literature
indicates that it is superior to all other modalities including computerized axial tomography, both in determining extent
of bone marrow involvement and soft tissue involvement, both
of bony and soft tissue lesions. Several authors also indicated its superiority in determining tissue planes in relationship to neurovascular structures, Sundaram going so far
as to indicate that it is almost 100% sensitive and 100%
specific. Unfortunately, as is true with most new tests, the
early literature tends to laud the test and later we find the
foibles and pitfalls of the examination.

Other examinations that have been advocated include
tomography, ultrasound and tomoscintigraphy, none of which
appear to give any more information than the examinations
already discussed.

Today, there is a great variation in the surgical treatment of both bony and soft tissue sarcomas, from those who
recommend radical resection to those with adjuvant chemo-
and/or irradiation therapy, recommending essentially excis-

ional biopsy. For those advocating the latter procedure, one could argue that all of these examinations are not necessary as all vital structures are going to be salvaged anyway. However, it is important that all patients be surgically staged so that we are comparing the same disease entities when we are publishing our results in the literature.

Consequently, at the present time, the preoperative evaluation of the potential sarcoma patient is a complete history and physical examination, routine radiographs of the lesion, bone and gallium scintigraphy, computerized axial tomography of the chest and lesion, and magnetic resonance imaging of the lesion. The same information can usually be obtained by enhanced computerized axial tomography and magnetic resonance imaging as angiography, and routine angiography is generally not necessary.

Hopefully, one noninvasive test such as magnetic resonance imaging may be the only specialized procedure necessary in the future. However, we are not at that stage today to know the full capabilities of magnetic resonance imaging. After these steps have been completed then, obviously, a biopsy is necessary to complete the surgical staging.

REFERENCES

1. Farinas PL: Radiology 29:29-32, 1937.
2. Dos Santos R: J Bone Joint Surg 32B:17-29, 1950.
3. Strickland B: Brit J Radiol 32:705-713, 1959.
4. Halpern M: Radiol Clin N Am 8:277-288, 1970.
5. Yaghmai I: Cancer 27:1134-1147, 1971.
6. Voegeli E: Skeletal Radiol 1:3-14, 1976.
7. Hudson TM: Diagnostic Radiol 138:283-292, 1981.
8. Lepanto PB: AJR 126:179-186, 1976.
9. Kaufman JH: Radiology 123:131-134, 1977.
10. Bitran JD: Cancer 42:1760-1765, 1978.
11. Chew FS: Sem Nucl Med 11:266-276, 1981.
12. Kirchner PT: J Bone Joint Surg 66A:319-327, 1984.
13. Finn HA: J Bone Joint Surg 69A:886-891, 1987.
14. Vera R: Radiology 101:125-132, 1971.
15. Sills M: Radiology 113:391-392, 1974.
16. Richman LS: AJR 124:577-586, 1975.
17. Blatt CJ: NY State J Med 77:2118-2119, 1977.
18. Goldstein H: Radiology 135:177-180, 1980.
19. Enneking WF: J Bone Joint Surg 63A:249-257, 1981.
20. McKillop JH: Cancer 48:1133-1138, 1981.
21. Hudson TM: J Bone Joint Surg 66A:1400-1407, 1984.
22. Kirchner PT: J Bone Joint Surg 66A:319-327, 1984.
23. Berger PE: Radiology 127:171-175, 1968.
24. DeSantos LA: Radiology 128:89-94, 1978.
25. Lukens JA: AJR 139:45-48, 1982.
26. Whelan MA: AJR 139:1191-1195, 1982.
27. Powers SK: J Neurosurg 59:131-136, 1983.
28. Vanel D: AJR 143:519-523, 1984.
29. Rosenthal DI: Orthop Clin N Am 16:461-470, 1985.
30. Shirkhoda A: AJR 144:95-99, 1985.
31. Brady TJ: Radiology 149:181-187, 1983.

32. Cohen MD: Radiology 151:715-718, 1984.
33. Hudson TM: Skel Radiol 13:134-146, 1985.
34. Pettersson H: Acta Radiol (Diagn) (Stockholm) 26:225-234, 1985.
35. Aisen AM: AJR 146:749-756, 1986.
36. Daffner RH: AJR 146:353-358, 1986.
37. Sundaram M: J Bone Joint Surg 68A:809-819, 1986.
38. Zimmer WD: Clin Orthop & Rel Res 208:289-299, 1986.
39. Boyko OB: AJR 148:317-322, 1987.

OPEN BIOPSY OF SARCOMAS

Marvin M. Romsdahl, M.D., Ph.D.*

While all aspects of the clinical management of patients with musculoskeletal neoplasms are important to obtain the most favorable outcome, establishing the correct pathological diagnosis by a biopsy procedure is of paramount importance. One must acknowledge, however, that evaluation of such patients includes other important considerations, with biopsy ideally following an orderly plan of clinical and diagnostic examinations.

Factors relative to biopsy have become more relevant in recent years as a result of certain evolving developments. First, and most significant, the optimal treatment of both bone and soft tissue tumors is accomplished by utilizing multidisciplinary modalities in a variety of combinations and sequences. Consequently, the proposed treatment plan may well indicate, or strongly suggest, the preferred type of biopsy for a certain clinical presentation.

Second, an awareness of tumor cell growth and kinetics, wound contamination, anatomical compartment containment, and tumor boundary relationships to normal tissue all serve to permit a more critical approach to both diagnosis and treatment. Third, recent technological developments have resulted in a number of new and/or improved radiographic tools that permit more precise assessment of the size, location, and even the character of the neoplasm.

Collectively, these features allow more precision in management decisions. Among these, the issue of biopsy is highly important because it should be done in a manner that permits accurate histological diagnosis and does not limit or unnecessarily alter subsequent evaluations or treatments.

The need for a carefully planned biopsy is emphasized in a study that showed an 18.2% incidence of major errors in diagnosis.(1) These errors were considered to misguide the implementation of treatment deemed correct for the corrected diagnosis. Similarly, 18.2% (60 of 329) of biopsies were deemed to alter the assumed optimal treatment plan. Four and one-half percent of the patients evaluated were judged to require an amputation that may have been avoided with a well

----

*Professor of Surgery, Department of General Surgery, The University of Texas System Cancer Center, M.D. Anderson Hospital and Tumor Institute, 1515 Holcombe Blvd., Box 106, Houston, TX 77030.

J. R. Ryan and L. O. Baker (eds.), Recent Concepts in Sarcoma Treatment, 69–75.

planned biopsy procedure. Finally, it was determined that the prognosis and outcome were worsened in 8.5% of patients because of flaws in the biopsy procedure. The authors found that 75% of biopsies that significantly altered treatment were performed in referring institutions instead of the treating center. In summary, these features lead to strong recommendations that diagnostic biopsies, establishing an accurate pathological diagnosis, and definitive treatment should all be done in the treating institution.

Accordingly, it is important to have a well-conceived plan to provide the patient who develops a musculoskeletal mass or pain, the most common initial symptoms, the best possible comprehensive management. Initially, it is prudent to stage systematically the patient's disease by performing examinations that bear on the size, extent, and location of the neoplasm. This process, together with knowledge concerning epidemiological factors including age and site prevalence, will usually narrow the list of neoplasms in the differential diagnosis.

Having a knowledge of the natural history of these tumors and an impression of the most effective treatment for each type, it is now proper to address the issue of biopsy to determine the pathological identity of the neoplasm. When the management team--which should comprise surgeons, medical oncologists, diagnostic radiologists, and radiotherapists-- agree on the histological diagnosis, the most effective treatment plan can be determined.

Pathology

The pathologist should be provided with clinical and diagnostic information before the biopsy is performed. The responsible clinician should consider the expertise in his institution concerning cytological, frozen-section, routine, and ultrastructural examinations. In some circumstances, surface markers using immunodiagnostic technology will prove useful. Since such tests may require fresh tissues, one should plan for this prior to the actual biopsy. Distinguishing among certain bone and soft tissue tumors can be a challenge to the most experienced pathologist. Consequently, it is not usually feasible to expect a final diagnosis based on frozen-section examination. However, with careful attention to staging and contemplation of diagnostic possibilities, one can often feel confident of the diagnosis made in this setting.

The pathologist should document pertinent details in his report relative to the specimen size, tumor size, and especially vital information concerning the surgical margins. Details important to the clinician include knowing if the lesion is predominantly expansile, infiltrative, whether a pseudocapsule is identified, and the dimension of "normal" tissue, if any, at the tumor boundary. Such information, most accurately obtained when surgical specimens are submitted, is very important in treatment planning and assessment of ultimate management results. Describing the precise histology is meritous; however, it does not provide all information that may affect treatment planning and use of different

modalities.
Rationale for Performance of Open Biopsy

Closed biopsy, whether done with a fine-gauge needle for cytological examinations or one of several specially designed needles that yield a small "core" of tissue, is being used with increased frequency.(2) It is especially applicable when complete staging strongly suggests the clinical presentation and expected pathological diagnosis. This applies equally to both bone and soft tissue tumors. However, certain circumstances may prevail which indicate a need for an open biopsy:

1. Open biopsy is required when the tissue secured by closed biopsy is not sufficient or adequate for diagnosis. The pathologist should be provided sufficient material, as well as representative and viable tissue, on which to base his histological interpretations.

2. Homogeneous tumors are generally most ideal for closed biopsy. However, certain lesions are typically heterogenous, such as cartilaginous tumors and malignant fibrous histiocytoma. Open biopsy may be required to interpret correctly the true nature of the tumor, and if grading of the neoplasms is to be done.

Technique for Open Biopsy

Having determined that open biopsy is indicated, the surgeon should be aware of circumstances that attend this type of biopsy and, accordingly, practice certain precautions.

Open biopsy, as opposed to closed biopsy, is associated with a larger number of wound complications, has greater risk for hematoma, tumor spillage into "normal" tissues, and infection; and for bone lesions, it has a greater chance of subsequent fracture.(3) Therefore, the surgeon should exercise great care in the operative procedure, utilizing measures that reduce chances for infection and maximally contain the tumor. To accomplish this goal, the decision regarding incisional or excisional biopsy needs to be addressed. General anesthesia should be utilized in either case to allow careful wound management and to avoid deviation from good operative principles of neoplasm surgery.

Incisional Biopsy

The indications for incisional biopsy, which is the type of biopsy most commonly employed, apply most convincingly to large neoplasms strongly suspect for being malignant. Tumors considered by preoperative staging to have close relationships to major nerves and vessels, bone, or tendinous insertions should have incisional biopsy, as opposed to excisional biopsy. One can then strongly consider the use of a nonsurgical modality before definitive surgical resection, and thereby expect to render the procedure more complete.

A sharp scalpel should always be used to prevent crushing and injury to tissues in the operative field. The incision should be as short as feasible, longitudinal to the axis of the extremity (Figure 1), and directed precisely toward

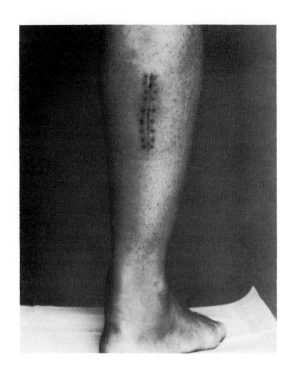

FIGURE 1A: Correctly placed longitudinal incision
of posterior calf region facilitated second
operation.

the neoplasm. In placement of the incision, it is important
to consider that the entire incision, with skin borders to
include suture penetrations, will be enveloped in a future
planned operation. In this respect, the entire operative
field including scar, adjacent skin, subcutaneous tissue, and
enveloping fascia,should be resected in contiguity with
biopsy tract and remaining neoplasm. This procedure has often
been referred to as "enveloping" the entire neoplastic
process since its goal is to remove tumor and any area
potentially contaminated by tumor cells in the previous
biopsy procedure. The biopsy incision site should consider
the worse possible outcome of management, this being the need
for an eventual major operative procedure such as amputation,
disarticulation, or hemipelvectomy--should treatment fail.
    Surgical biopsy principles, such as strict hemostasis,
maximum sterility, and least possible injury to normal tissues, should be practiced. The incision is directed straight
to the surface of the neoplasm without undermining skin,
subcutaneous tissue, or fascia. Muscles may be directly

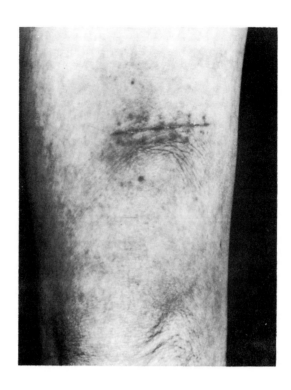

FIGURE 1B: Incorrectly placed transverse incision of anterior thigh complicated subsequent wide excision surgery.

incised as well, should they cover the neoplasm. The pseudo-capsule interphase should be included in a single specimen that also includes a section of neoplasm. Should a pseudo-capsule not be appreciated, it is prudent to perform a biopsy on the interface of normal tissue and neoplasm, even if the lesion should prove to be benign. In general, the periphery of the tumor is most viable and the central area is most often necrotic and does not contribute to histological diagnosis. Multiple biopsy samples should be avoided, with major emphasis being placed on the proper placement of the biopsy sample rather than the amount of material submitted. This decreases chances of tumor cell contamination and possible tumor growth in the operative wound. Strict hemostasis is obtained and the wound is vigorously irrigated with saline solution. Surgical instruments utilized at this point are discarded from the operative field, gloves are changed, and the wound closed meticulously in layers, without the placement of a drain.

    If there exists any doubt that the lesion biopsied

represents the presumed neoplasm, or whether sufficient tissue for diagnosis has been obtained, it is appropriate to request a frozen-section diagnosis. This helps ensure that the final diagnosis can be accurately made after more deliberate and complete histological examination of the specimen.

Principles regarding incisional biopsy of bone tumors are important to avoid complications and potential unfavorable alterations in management. First, a nonosseous soft tissue extension of the bone tumor should be the biopsy target instead of the bone cortex. This will reduce prospects for a pathological fracture and thereby possibly avoidance of an amputation. Second, if a biopsy of the bone must be performed, this should be accomplished by round or oval fenestrations, ideally made with a circular saw to avoid unnatural bone stress with its propensity to cause fracture. Rectangular and square bone holes should be avoided since they are at high risk for fracture.

Following bone biopsy, the "window" should be replaced if it is not necessary for pathological examination. Alternatively, the bone biopsy site may be sealed with methyl methacrylate to minimize wound contamination. It is recommended that tumor biopsy wounds not be drained; however, should the surgeon feel that drainage is mandatory, the drain should come through the incision or as close to the incision as feasible to localize any potential wound contamination.

Excisional Biopsy

Excisional biopsy may be the procedure of choice for musculoskeletal tumors that are 1) superficial, 2) under 5 cm in diameter, 3) judged to be benign or modestly aggressive by clinical presentation, or 4) can be widely excised without major impairment or alteration of anatomical structure. Should the experience of the physician indicate doubt concerning these characteristics, an incisional biopsy should clearly be done since it allows the widest range of options for future management.

In performing excisional biopsy, the general rules pertaining to direction of incisions is the same as for incisional biopsy. It is, however, important to limit the extent of the operative field if postoperative radiotherapy is to be considered. The goal of radiotherapy in this setting is to destroy "subclinical" or "microscopic" disease and, therefore, must include all areas disturbed by the surgical procedure. Using careful operative technique, one develops skin flaps, usually at the subcutaneous level, to beyond the margins of the neoplasm. At this point, and with careful palpation of the lesion, one incises enveloping fascia, muscle, and other structure about the mass to secure a 2-cm tissue margin. In the event the lesion approximates bone, it is practical to include periosteum with your specimen rather than have a "close" margin. The goals of excisional biopsy are to obtain a definitive diagnosis as well as complete surgical excision. When done with sufficient tumor margins, radiotherapy or chemotherapy as adjunctive treatment options can be employed without further surgery.

In practice, and where a malignant tumor is a distinct

possibility, it is generally beneficial to excise lesions extra widely than to err in the direction of a "close" or "positive" tumor margin. This will avoid wound tumor cell contamination and possibly the need for a subsequent operation to "envelope" the entire operative region, including the healed incision and surrounding operative field. Following meticulous hemostasis, the wound is irrigated with saline solution, surgical instruments and gloves are changed, and the wound is closed in anatomical layers, preferably without the use of a drain. However, it is prudent to use a drain when the operative field is extensive and fluid accumulation is expected to be of large amounts. Extremity immobilization and other factors relative to wound care are employed based on the experience of the surgeon. Wound care is an important aspect of surgery for musculoskeletal tumors, especially when skin is sacrificed at secondary operations or when skin is involved or adherent to the primary neoplasm. Wound dehiscence caused by tension is often an invitation to a second complication, namely, infection and scarring.

Summary
The physician responsible for management of the patient with a bone or soft tissue tumor must actively participate in analyzing all aspects of the staging process. Choosing the type of biopsy is a responsible issue, based on the different diagnoses possible, and a distinct treatment plan, based on documentation of the expected biopsy outcome. While multidisciplinary management is progressively being utilized to improve survival and local recurrence rates, it is highly beneficial that a responsible clinician bring those diagnostic and treatment modalities together in such a manner as to provide optimal management for the patient.

REFERENCES

1. Mankin HJ, Lange TA, Spanier SS: The hazards of biopsy in patients with malignant primary bone and soft tissue tumors. J Bone Joint Surg 64A(8):1121-1127, 1982.
2. Carrasco CH, Wallace S, Charnsangavej C, Richli W: Percutaneous skeletal biopsy. Seminars in Interventional Radiology 2(3):278-284, 1985.
3. Simon MA: Biopsy of musculoskeletal tumors. J Bone Joint Surg 64A(8):1253-1257, 1982.

FINE NEEDLE ASPIRATION CYTOLOGY IN DIAGNOSIS AND MANAGEMENT OF BONE AND SOFT TISSUE TUMORS

Harold J. Wanebo, M.D.[1], and Philip Feldman, M.D.

Fine needle aspiration (FNA) cytology (biopsy) has been utilized for tumors of soft tissue and bone since 1931 when the technique was first reported by Coley et al. in the diagnosis of bone tumors.(1) Although open biopsy is the established method of providing a tissue diagnosis of soft tissue and bone tumors, there is a role for FNA in the diagnosis and management of these tumors.(2-6) The main indications for FNA are to provide rapid diagnosis of soft tissue or bone lesions in which 1) the identity of the tumor is unknown (whether benign or malignant, primary or metastatic), and 2) to confirm the apparent diagnosis in cases where there is good clinical and radiologic evidence that the tumor is malignant or benign. There are several advantages of FNA:

1. It provides rapid diagnosis of most primary tumors as well as those which are present at multiple sites (lung, bone, soft tissue).

2. It permits early diagnosis of poorly accessible tumors such as intrathoracic or intra-abdominal (retroperitoneal), or pelvic tumors.

3. It may avoid the need for open biopsy (if metastatic), or accelerate the performance of the biopsy (if considered a primary tumor).

4. It is atraumatic and can minimize the psychic and financial costs associated with open biopsies in some patients.

5. FNA is useful in follow-up assessment of patients under therapy.

The limitations of FNA are as follows:

1. The technique is highly dependent on experience and expertise of the cytopathologist.

2. FNA is a complementary technique and requires correlation with clinical and radiologic information.

3. A nondiagnostic FNA or a `benign' FNA diagnosis of benign requires tissue diagnosis via open biopsy. An open biopsy is generally required to determine exact histology, tissue type, and grade of most bone and soft tissue sarcomas.

In selected patients, the FNA diagnosis coupled with the

----

[1]Chief of Surgery, Roger Williams General Hospital, 825 Chalkstone Avenue, Providence, RI 02908; Professor of Surgery, Brown University.

J. R. Ryan and L. O. Baker (eds.), Recent Concepts in Sarcoma Treatment, 76–80.
© 1988 by Kluwer Academic Publishers.

clinical and radiologic findings may permit adequate assessment of the tumor and obviate the need for an open biopsy. Thus, a large tumor within an extremity or in the pelvis or retroperitoneum which is clinically and radiologically aggressive may be adequately assessed by FNA diagnosis of `sarcoma' to permit initiation of treatment without need to obtain an open biopsy. In general, it may be easier to use FNA in diagnostic assessment and in treatment planning of selected primary tumors of soft tissue compared to bone tumors. FNA should be considered an excellent supplementary technique to clinical and radiologic assessment.

University of Virginia Experience

FNA was used to diagnose 22 primary tumors of soft tissue and bone, and 21 metastatic sarcomas to soft tissue and/or bone (Tables 1, 2 and 3). The primary tissue types are listed in Table 1. All but one of the primary sarcoma were diagnosed by FNA (21 of 22, 95% diagnostic rate), and the reading commonly given was `sarcoma' with further suggestion of probable type in most cases. An open biopsy was done prior to definitive surgery or preoperative therapy. The sarcoma tissue types essentially included the full range of types usually reported. Although only seven primary bone tumors were studied, these included Ewing's, osteosarcoma, chondrosarcoma, and giant cell tumor, all of which were diagnosed by FNA. Among the 21 metastatic sarcomas (all were diagnosed by FNA), there were also a variety of types involved (Table 2). Most were soft tissue origin, but it did include Ewing's (1), chordoma (2), and osteosarcoma (2). A variety of metastatic sites were assessed including head and neck (3), extremities (6), trunk and pelvis (11), and visceral (lung, intra-abdominal) (6).

TABLE 1: Fine Needle Aspiration Cytology of Bone and Soft Tissue Tumors

Primary	Total	+ FNA
Soft tissue tumors	15	14
Bone	7	7
	22	21 (95%)
Metastatic	21	21

Discussion

In general, this small series is representative of reports of larger series. (3-6) Among the primary tumors, all had a tissue diagnosis obtained by open biopsy. In retrospect, many of the extremity tumors were large, and were clinically and radiologically aggressive (i.e. filled a compartment or extended to or invaded nerve/vessel), or had marked vascularity by arteriography, and could have been

TABLE 2: **Primary Soft Tissue Tumors   Diagnosed by Fine Needle Aspiration Cytology**

Rhabdomyosarcoma	2/2
Synovial sarcoma	2/2
Malignant fibrous histiocytoma	5/5
Angiosarcoma	1/1
Epithelioid	1/1
Schwannoma	1/1
Liposarcoma	1/1
Hemangiopericytoma	0/1
Total diagnosed by FNA	13/14

Primary Bone Tumors Diagnosed by Fine Needle Aspiration Cytology

Ewing's	1
Osteosarcoma	4
Chondrosarcoma	1
Giant cell tumor	1
Total diagnosed by FNA	7/7

created by combined therapy with surgical resection without need for doing open biopsy. FNA was the major diagnostic measure used in 34 of 97 patients with extremity soft tissue sarcomas treated by Markhede et al. (mostly by limb-salvage resection). An amputation would generally not be done without open biopsy (unless there was obvious extensive disease).

Among the small number of primary bone tumors, the FNAC of vertebral (chondrosarcoma) and giant cell tumor were done followed by subsequent definitive surgery. Among the major bone lesions, osteosarcoma and chondrosarcoma, the FNA diagnosis was not definitive enough (in part because of sampling limitations) to adequately assess primary tissue type and grade to permit definitive therapy. Tissue diagnosis provides needed information regarding exact tissue types, mitotic rate, and tumor necrosis which are required by some.

The management of the metastatic or recurrent sarcomas was greatly facilitated by FNA. Open biopsy was not required and, in some cases, would have been difficult or imposed a major added burden on the patient who has metastases to clinically occult sites: pelvis, lung, retroperitoneal strictures. The current wedding of radiologic techniques, chest x-ray, fluoroscopy, ultrasound and CT permits exact needle placement for FNA.(6) Treatment with CT/RT or surgery can proceed on the basis of the diagnosis obtained.

Summary

FNA is a useful technique or preliminary assessment of most primary soft tissue and some bone tumors. In many of the

**TABLE 3: Fine Needle Aspiration Cytology
of Metastatic Sarcomas**

Metastatic sites - 21

Head and neck - 3
  Node - RMS - 1
  Antrum - Myosarcoma - 1
  Mandible - Ewing's - 1

Trunk - 5
  <u>Thoracic</u> - 2
    Chest wall - osteosarcoma - 1
    Breast - RMS - 1

  <u>Extra-abdominal</u> - 2
    Synovial sarcoma - 1
    Myxoliposarcoma - 1

Extremity - 5
  <u>Soft Tissue</u> - 2
    Knee - liposarcoma - 1
    Axilla - RMS - 1

  <u>Bone</u> - 3
    Leiomyosarcoma - 1
    Rhabdomyosarcoma - 2

Pelvis - 4
  <u>Soft Tissue/Bone</u>
    Chordoma - 2
    Rhabdomyosarcoma - 1
    Myeloma - 1

Visceral - 6
  <u>Lung</u> - 3
    MFH-1
    Osteosarcoma - 1
    Ewing's - 1

  <u>Intra-abdominal</u> - 3
    Pancreas - RMS - 1
    Adrenal - liposarcoma - 1
    Psoas - angiosarcoma - 1

cases with soft tissue tumors, the FNA diagnosis, when coupled with clinical and radiologic data, may be adequate to permit definitive combined therapy. Currently, most soft tissue tumors and accessible bone tumors will require confirmation and tissue diagnosis by open biopsy. For metastatic sarcomas, FNA is ideal. It permits a rapid, accurate, but inexpensive diagnosis, and facilitates therapy. Further advancements with immunologic and cytochemical stains should enhance FNA and permit its broader use in the diagnosis of tumors of soft tissue and bone.

REFERENCES

1. Coley BL, Sharp GS, Ellis EB: Diagnosis of bone tumors by aspiration. Am J Surg 13:215-224, 1931.
2. Hajdu SJ and Hajdu EO: Cytopathology of sarcomas and other non-epithelial malignant tumors. Philadelphia, WB Saunders, 1976.
3. Koss LG, Woyke S, Olszewski W: Tumors of soft tissue. In Aspiration Biopsy: Cytologic Interpretation and Histologic Bases. New York-Tokyo, Igaku-Shoin, pp.272-283, and The Bone (in same text), pp.422-441, 1984.
4. Willems JS: Aspiration biopsy cytology of soft tissue tumors. In Clinical Aspiration Cytology, Linsk JA and Franzen S (eds.) pp.319-347, Philadelphia, JB Lippincott, 1983.
5. Willems JS: Aspiration biopsy cytology of tumors and tumor-suspected lesions of bone. In Clinical Aspiration Cytology, pp.349-359, Philadelphia, JB Lippincott, 1983.
6. Murphy WA, Destovet JM, Gilula: Percutaneous skeletal biopsy 1981. A procedure for radiologists - results, review and recommendations. Radiology 139:545-549, 1981.
7. Markhede G, Angervall L, Stener B: A multivariate analysis of the prognosis after surgical treatment of malignant soft tissue tumors. Cancer 49:1721-1733, 1982.

THE ROLE OF FROZEN SECTIONS IN THE DIAGNOSIS AND MANAGEMENT OF BONE AND SOFT-TISSUE TUMORS

K. Krishnan Unni, M.B., B.S.*

Introduction

The frozen section, and the immediate rendering of a diagnosis, is used by pathologists worldwide. Most pathologists will not hesitate to recommend mastectomy on the basis of a frozen-section diagnosis of carcinoma. However, these same pathologists may be hesitant about recommending amputation on the basis of a frozen-section diagnosis of sarcoma. The reason for this difference is that breast cancer is relatively common and most pathologists have enough experience to gain confidence, whereas sarcomas are rare and most pathologists have not had much experience with them. With experience, the pathologist will find that the diagnosis of most sarcomas is no more difficult than that of breast cancer.

Historical Notes

Dr. Louis B. Wilson, working at the Mayo Clinic, is generally credited with developing the frozen-section technique into a valid and reliable diagnostic tool. However, pathologists probably attempted to prepare frozen sections even before that time, because in his first article on the subject (1), Dr. Wilson admitted to having shared the "common distrust" of frozen sections for microscopic diagnosis. Dr. William J. Mayo wrote a short segment on "The Story of the Fresh Frozen Section" for the staff meetings of the Mayo Clinic on September 11, 1929 (2). Mayo credited Dr. Wilson's training as a botanist to Wilson's success with the frozen-section method. In a letter written to a surgeon in an eastern university hospital (quoted by Dr. Mayo), Dr. Wilson also acknowledged using methods that he learned as a botanist. He noted that his first frozen sections were made "by putting the tissues outside the window when the weather was 20º F below zero in January 1905!"

Dr. Wilson published a second article in 1913 (3) and, by this time, was confident enough in his method to say that it was rarely necessary to defer the diagnosis until after paraffin sections were made.

Dr. Malcolm Dockerty, from my institution (Mayo Clinic), detailed the technique in 1953 (4). Another surgical pathologist from the Mayo Clinic, Dr. D. C. Dahlin (5), updated the philosophy of frozen-section diagnosis in 1980.

---

*Section of Surgical Pathology, Mayo Clinic and Mayo Foundation, Rochester, MN 55905.

J. R. Ryan and L. O. Baker (eds.), Recent Concepts in Sarcoma Treatment, 81–88.

Practice

As with other techniques, experience makes the surgical pathologist more comfortable in providing a diagnosis. Because virtually all specimens are examined by frozen section, members of my department are proficient in this technique. In the two surgical pathology laboratories at the Mayo Clinic in 1986, 58,611 surgical specimens were examined, generating 92,313 frozen-section slides.

Communication between the surgeon and the surgical pathologist is necessary to reduce the chance of a mistake. Our surgical pathology laboratory is on the same floor as the operating rooms and all pathology personnel wear scrub-suits so that they can walk over to the operation theatre and communicate directly with the surgeon. Generally, the orthopedic oncologist carries the biopsy specimen (along with the appropriate roentgenograms) to the surgical pathology laboratory. This helps to avoid mistakes caused by miscommunication.

The technique my colleagues and I use is essentially the same as that described by Dr. Wilson. Fresh samples are frozen on a Spencer freezing microtome using carbon dioxide (Fig. 1). Sections of approximately 10 μm in thickness are stained with polychrome methylene blue and are mounted in a glucose medium (Fig. 2). Freezing, staining, and mounting should require only a minute or less. The laboratory is connected to all operating rooms via an intercommunication system so that the results of pathologic study can be relayed to the surgeon. Generally, there are two technicians cutting

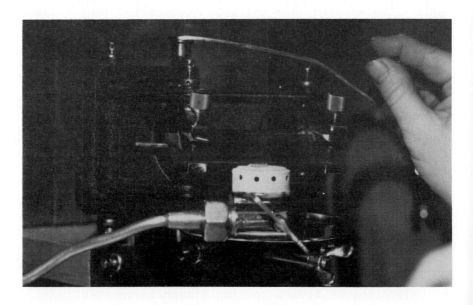

FIGURE 1: Freezing microtome used for preparation of frozen sections.

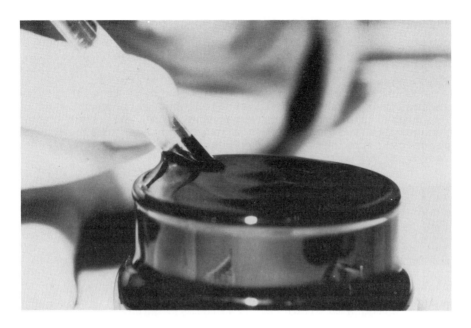

FIGURE 2A: Tissue section is stained by immersing it in polychrome methylene blue for a few seconds.

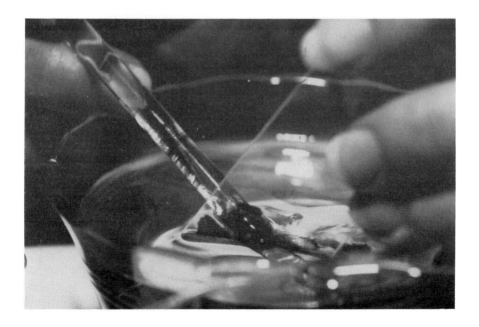

FIGURE 2B: Section is mounted in glucose-water medium.

sections at all times. The surgical report is dictated to a secretary, and a signed report is attached to the patient's chart, usually before the patient leaves the postanesthetic area. Representative sections are embedded in paraffin, and hematoxylin-eosin stained sections are examined the next day. This sequence provides a built-in quality control.

The technique described above pertains to all specimens, including bone and soft-tissue lesions. Pathologists at other institutions may use a cryostat and stain the sections with hematoxylin and eosin. This approach is acceptable but is not practical in our setting because preparing the sections requires too much time.

Many pathologists think of bone tumors as "hard" and, hence, as requiring decalcification. However, most, if not all, bone tumors have soft areas that can be cut without being decalcified. The surgeon who takes the biopsy specimen should be experienced in deducing from the radiologic appearance of the tumor which portion will be unmineralized enough to be cut without being decalcified. (Even if a frozen section is not done, such material should be processed for paraffin sections immediately so that a diagnosis is possible within 24 hours.) If the surgeon provides bone with tumor intermixed, the bony tissue should be separated from the tumor using a scalpel blade (Fig. 3). Rarely is it necessary

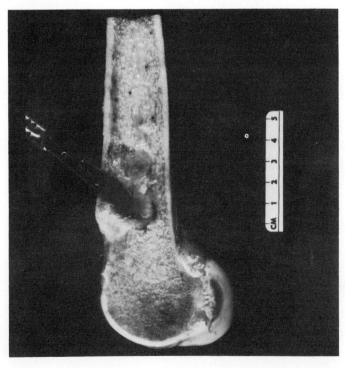

FIGURE 3: Scalpel blade can be inserted into bone, and soft-tumor tissue can be separated from bone.

to decalcify a bone tumor in order to obtain diagnostic material, either on frozen or paraffin section.

Rarely, parosteal osteosarcoma or an extremely sclerotic osteosarcoma will be so hard that an undecalcified section cannot be obtained. If decalcification is necessary, frozen sections can be cut after decalcification, and a diagnosis can be rendered a day earlier than would otherwise be possible (Fig. 4).

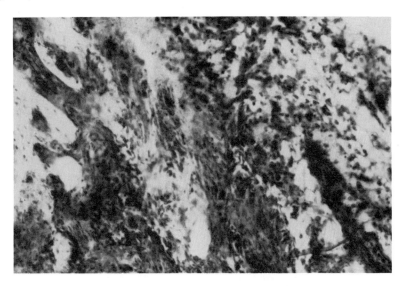

FIGURE 4: Extremely sclerotic osteosarcoma diagnosed on frozen section after decalcification. Photograph seems to be out of focus because of large amount of bone present (unstained). However, malignant spindle cells are clearly evident. (Polychrome methylene blue; x40.)

Advantages of Frozen Sections

The advantages have been detailed by Dahlin (5).

Immediate Diagnosis and Treatment. Although delay of a day or two in treatment probably does not affect prognosis adversely, an immediate definitive diagnosis has other advantages. Most bone sarcomas affect young children, and the family experiences tremendous emotional trauma. A definitive diagnosis, whatever it is, is better tolerated by the patient and the family than is anxiety-producing uncertainty. Also, plans for treatment (such as appropriate staging studies) can be begun immediately. If the specimen is judged to be a focus of metastatic carcinoma, an immediate search for the primary site can be started. Finally, immediate diagnosis can be economically advantageous to the patient by reducing the length of hospital stay.

A Check for Adequacy of Tissue. Even if a definite

diagnosis is not made on frozen section, the pathologist should be able to assure the surgeon that adequate tissue for diagnosis has been obtained. Some sarcomas are necrotic, and the biopsy specimen must include viable tissue; this can be ascertained by frozen section. An attempt to subclassify malignant lymphomas on frozen section need not be made, but the lesion should be recognized as a lymphoma of bone on frozen section so that appropriate material can be obtained for special studies.

The Obtaining of Tissue for Microbiologic Studies. Osteomyelitis can mimic neoplasms of bone. If the process is recognized as infectious while the patient is still in the operating room, material can be obtained for culture and possibly sensitivity studies.

A Check for Surgical Margins. Cortical margins of resection cannot be checked with frozen sections. However, I have found that bone tumors never involve a margin by permeating along the interstices of the cortex. In bone tumors, marrow margin and soft-tissue margins are checked. In large compartmental resections of soft-tissue sarcomas, it is not feasible to check all margins. However, with the cooperation of the surgeon, close margins and margins that are particularly worrisome can be checked.

Problems with Frozen Section

Tiny Biopsy Specimens. The current tendency is to obtain smaller specimens, including needle biopsy specimens. It is reasonable to do a frozen section study on a needle biopsy specimen to ascertain that the lesion in question has been sampled. However, all the diagnostic tissue may be "used up," and adequate tissue may not be available for permanent sections. This problem can be solved to some extent by making a "permanent" slide of the frozen section. However, the quality of such sections is not completely satisfactory.

Inaccurate Sampling of Biopsy Specimen. Frozen sections of a large biopsy specimen may not be representative of the tumor. However, this problem usually can be avoided by careful study of the gross specimen.

Inaccurate Interpretation of the Sections. The biggest problem with the interpretation of frozen sections is that the pathologist may be unfamiliar with the technique. A tentative diagnosis can be made on frozen-section study, and the definitive diagnosis can be deferred until the permanent section is prepared. How often this will be necessary depends on the confidence of the pathologist.

The accuracy of frozen-section diagnosis has been studied (6,7). Although mistakes are unavoidable, they can be minimized if problems are recognized, consultation with colleagues sought, and good communication with the surgeon maintained.

Special Problems with Sarcomas

The stain used by my colleagues and me (polychrome methylene blue) is metachromatic, and, hence, chondroid matrix is stained vividly. This makes it difficult to appreciate the details of the nucleus of the chondrocyte. The problem can be solved by floating the sections in formalin

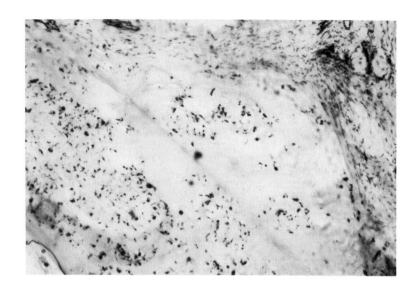

FIGURE 5A: Frozen section of grade 1 chondrosarcoma secondary to osteochondroma in spine of 41-year-old man. (Hematoxylin: x40.)

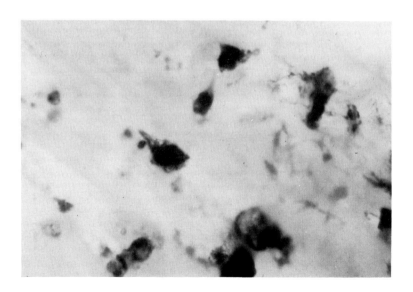

FIGURE 5B: Higher power showing hyperchromatic chondrocyte nuclei. (Hematoxylin; x156.)

for a few seconds and then staining them with hematoxylin (Fig. 5).

Usually, the nuclei can be well visualized with this technique. Most pathologists use hematoxylin and eosin, which obviates this problem. Also, frozen sections are thicker than paraffin sections, and, hence, the tissue may seem to be more cellular than on permanent sections, which may lead to over-diagnosis. The nuclei also tend to appear somewhat larger.

Frozen sections do not "hold together" as well as paraffin-embedded sections, which makes pattern recognition more difficult. For instance, the alveolar pattern of a rhabdomyo-sarcoma or the clustering of a clear-cell sarcoma may not be apparent on frozen sections. However, such subtle subclassifications are probably not urgent.

Summary

Frozen sections are important in the practice of medicine. This importance is highlighted by the recent publication of a textbook on the subject (8). The most important ingredients for success in frozen-section diagnoses are 1) adequate specimen volume (it is impossible for the pathologist to gain confidence if only an occasional frozen section is performed), 2) close proximity of the pathologist to the operating rooms, and 3) open communication between the surgeon and pathologist. A team approach engendering respect among team members helps to avoid mistakes.

REFERENCES

1. Wilson LB: A method for the rapid preparation of fresh tissues for the microscope. JAMA 45:1737, 1905.
2. Mayo WJ: The story of the fresh frozen section. Mayo Clin Proc 4:274-275, 1929.
3. Wilson LB: The microscopic examinations of fresh tissues for the diagnosis of early cancer. St. Paul Med J 15:274-278, 1913.
4. Dockerty MB: Rapid frozen sections: technique of their preparation and staining. Surg Gynecol Obstet 97:113-120, 1953.
5. Dahlin DC: Seventy-five years' experience with frozen sections at the Mayo Clinic (editorial). Mayo Clin Proc 55:721-723, 1980.
6. Holaday WJ, Assor D: Ten thousand consecutive frozen sections. A retrospective study focusing on accuracy and quality control. Am J Clin Pathol 61:769-777, 1974.
7. Lessells AM, Simpson JG: A retrospective analysis of the accuracy of immediate frozen section diagnosis in surgical pathology. Br J Surg 63:327-329, 1976.
8. Silva E, Karemer BB: Intraoperative Pathologic Diagnosis. Frozen Sections and Other Techniques. Baltimore, Williams & Wilkins, 1987.

SURGICAL MANAGEMENT OF SOFT TISSUE SARCOMAS

Dempsey S. Springfield, M.D.*

The appropriate treatment of patients with soft tissue sarcoma remains controversial, but surgery is the principle treatment of the primary tumor in all current protocols. The surgical controversy is how much to remove, with or without irradiation given pre- or postoperatively. There are no definitive answers yet, and oncologists of the future are likely to look back at our work and wonder why we did what we did and marvel at our ignorance. From this perspective, I will discuss the role of surgery in the management of patients with soft tissue sarcomas as of 1987.

Although Morgagni, in the early 1700's, first suggested that soft tissue sarcomas are localized diseases and not systemic illnesses, it was Virchow and Schwann, in the mid 1800's, who classified the sarcomas and distinguished them from carcinomas. They based their classification system on the microscopic characteristics and we still use their classification system today. Limited surgical excision was practiced then but local recurrence was common and some believed surgery was the cause of malignant degeneration of those tumors operated. Seids and McGinnis reviewed the history of the treatment of "fatty tumors" in 1927 and were two of the earliest advocates of wide local resection for the surgical treatment of soft tissue sarcomas. They said that although these tumors seem to be encapsulated and easily enucleated, "simple enucleation is not sufficient - one must go further and extricate thoroughly all the surrounding fat, muscle, and other tissue, in so far as this is possible." They also warned against relying on irradiation to control macroscopic disease left in the patient, stating that attempts to use irradiation to control the primary tumor without surgical resection, or after an inadequate resection, was hopeless. They were most concerned with non-extremity sarcomas, where the surgical margins are limited by surrounding organs, and their recommendations are still appropriate for non-extremity sarcomas, but extremity tumors can be more widely resected.

In 1958, Bowden and Booher published their now oft-cited work regarding the management of extremity soft tissue

----

*Visiting Orthopaedic Surgeon, Massachusetts General Hospital, Boston, MA 02114. Associate Professor in Orthopaedic Surgery, Harvard Medical School, Boston, MA.

J. R. Ryan and L. O. Baker (eds.), Recent Concepts in Sarcoma Treatment, 89–93.
© 1988 by Kluwer Academic Publishers.

sarcomas demonstrating the advantage of resecting the muscles involved by the tumor from their origin to insertion. They were not the first to suggest this principle, but they - probably more than any other surgeons - popularized the concept of longitudinal resection for soft tissue sarcomas. A longitudinal resection of the muscle or muscles involved with the tumor completely surrounded by normal tissue is adequate local treatment for even a high grade soft tissue sarcoma. The major advances in the surgical management of soft tissue sarcomas have been in the field of radiologic examination. The better anatomic localization of the tumor has resulted in fewer amputations without an increase in local recurrences.

Prior to the availability of these sophisticated diagnostic staging tools, oncologic surgeons could not accurately localize the primary tumor and amputations were usually recommended, particularly for the large lesions of the thigh, the most common location of an extremity soft tissue sarcoma. Amputation was favored because of the better local control after an amputation compared to a limb salvage resection. Now the tumor can be accurately localized and the oncologic surgeon is able to determine what has to be resected and what can be saved. When the major neurovascular bundle is involved, an amputation is the only safe means to control the primary tumor with surgery alone. The addition of irradiation with more limited (less than a wide surgical margin, but not an intralesional margin) surgery has been used to permit limb sparing operations without increasing local recurrence. Stener and his group in Sweden, have reaffirmed what Bowden and Booher said thirty years ago. Stener's work shows that if a soft tissue sarcoma is excised with a cuff of uninvolved surrounding tissue, and if the entire muscle or muscles involved are resected from the origin to insertion, local control will be achieved in the vast majority of cases with surgery alone.

Biopsy

An open biopsy is the most common method used to obtain tissue from which to make a diagnosis. "Skinny needle" aspiration and needle biopsy have been, and continue to be, used, but have a minor role in the diagnosis of soft tissue lesions because of the difficulty of making an accurate diagnosis from the limited tissue available from these techniques. This is increasingly true with the routine use of special stains and electron microscopic examinations. Although it is usually possible to decide from a needle biopsy or "skinny needle" aspiration whether a lesion is benign or malignant, it is often difficult to determine the histogenesis or histologic grade. Grading is impossible from a cytologic examination. Therefore, open biopsy is still, and will probably remain, an essential part of the evaluation of a patient with a soft tissue mass.

Biopsy Technique

This audience is aware of the potential problems that can be caused by the poorly planned or poorly performed biopsy. The significance of the surgical approach used for the biopsy has increased during the last few years as we try to salvage more limbs, and often the most difficult part of a limb salvage operation is including the biopsy tract in the resected specimen. The surgeon who does the biopsy must be familiar with limb salvage techniques and assume that every lesion biopsied will require a limb salvage resection. The biopsy should be planned so that it will not compromise a subsequent resection. Skin incisions must be in line with the resection incision, almost always longitudinal (NOT TRANS-VERSE!), major neurovascular bundles should not be exposed, and the dissection should be within muscles - not between muscles. Adequate tissue should be sharply cut from the tumor to include tumor, its pseudocapsule, and a small amount of surrounding normal soft tissue. A frozen section examination should be done to insure that diagnostic tissue has been obtained. The tissue should be sent to the pathologist fresh, not in formalin, so some can be put aside for EM. Hemostasis must be obtained and I drain biopsy wounds to prevent the spread of a hematoma which will contaminate more tissue. The drain tract must be resected with the tumor too, and should be placed in line with and close to the biopsy incision. I routinely use a tourniquet during the biopsy, having elevated the extremity for exsanguination (not a compressive wrap). A bloodless field makes the biopsy easier and more accurate. I deflate the tourniquet before closing the wound. Some surgeons do not use a tourniquet during the biopsy because they suspect that an excess of tumor cells will lodge in the veins just distal to the tourniquet and be released as a tumor emboli when the tourniquet is deflated, increasing the risk of distant metastasis. Although this is a theoretic risk, there is no evidence to suggest that this happens. It should be clear that in order to perform the biopsy correct-ly, it is necessary to have completely evaluated the patient prior to the biopsy. A Thorough knowledge of the anatomic location of the tumor and the structures involved is re-quired. The use of CT scanning and MRI has improved our ability to anatomically localize these usually deep-seated masses and is probably the reason we are doing more limb salvage resections than amputations now compared to the days before these diagnostic tools were available.

Surgical Margin Terminology

Simon and Enneking suggested terminology for describing surgical margins. An `intralesional surgical margin' is a surgical margin which leaves gross tumor in the patient (i.e. incisional biopsy, debulking); a `marginal surgical margin' is an excision through the pseudocapsule which leaves micro-scopic residual tumor in almost all cases (i.e. "shell'em out"); a `wide surgical margin' is a resection of the tumor with a cuff of normal, non-reactive surrounding tissue in all planes (i.e. en bloc resection); and a `radical surgical margin' is obtained when the entire anatomical compartment containing the tumor is resected. Stener and his group have suggested an additional category which is less than `radical' but more than `wide'. They recommend a category for the resection of the tumor and the involved muscles from their origin to insertion with the tumor completely surrounded by normal tissue. This is still a `wide surgical margin' in the Simon-Enneking system, but is more than their minimal wide and probably deserves a separate category.

A `radical surgical margin' provides the best local control with less than 5% local recurrence. A `wide surgical margin' will result in approximately 25% local recurrence, and Stener's longitudinal resection with approximately 10% local recurrence. Although there is a statistical difference between these two margins with respect to local control, there is no difference in survival and, therefore, a longitudinal wide resection is the surgery of choice.

Surgical Technique

The biopsy incision and all tissue exposed during the biopsy must be excised with the tumor. The skin incision should ellipse the biopsy incision and be of sufficient length to permit removal of the muscle(s) from their origin to insertion. The pseudocapsule of the tumor should not be seen during the resection and the entire tumor should be contained within the tissue removed. It is unsafe to "peel" the neurovascular bundle from the tumor's pseudocapsule or "scrape" the tumor off the bone. If it is necessary to do either of these during the resection, an inadequate margin (marginal surgical margin) results. If the preoperative staging studies reveal that the tumor is immediately adjacent to the neurovascular bundle or bone, an amputation should be done or local adjuvant treatment (usually irradiation) can be combined with a 'marginal surgical margin' for limb salvage.

Amputation is still appropriate treatment for some patients and should not be relegated to history. The very elderly with a large tumor is often unable to tolerate the extended preoperative irradiation or the extensive surgery for limb salvage, as limb salvage surgery for a large thigh mass is more demanding on the patient than is an amputation. A patient who had a biopsy which led to contamination of a large portion of the extremity may have an unacceptable risk for local recurrence without an amputation, making limb salvage surgery risky. Soft tissue tumors of the distal lower leg and foot are usually better amputated than treated by limb salvage resection.

The amputation, when done, should be radical and the extremity should be removed one joint proximal to the compartment harboring the tumor. This level of amputation assures local control of the tumor. Patients who have an amputation should be rehabilitated quickly to improve their final level of function, which is usually very good.

Conclusions

Surgery alone should continue to play an important role in the management of patients with soft tissue sarcomas. This is particularly true for the smaller (less than 5 cm) lesions in the extremity. The tumor must be removed with a surrounding cuff of normal, uninvolved tissue and the muscles involved must be resected from their origin to insertion. Whether less surgery should be, or can be, safely done with preoperative irradiation, is still unanswered. Amputation should be done when necessary, but the addition of local irradiation with surgery will save the majority of extremities with a soft tissue sarcoma.

Although there is more work that needs to be done regarding the management of the primary tumor, local control is not the problem with high grade soft tissue tumors of the extremities. The survival from these tumors has not improved over the last three decades due to our inability to control the metastatic disease that most of the patients have at the time of presentation. Further advances must be made in the area of adjuvant treatment.

REFERENCES

1. Abbas JS, Holyoke ED, Morris R, Karabousis CP: The surgical treatment and outcome of soft tissue sarcoma. Arch Surg 116:765-769, 1981.
2. Bowden L, Booher RJ: The principles and techniques of resection of soft parts for sarcoma. Surg 44:963-977, 1958.
3. Cantin J, McNeer GP, Chu FC, Booher RJ: The problem of local recurrence after treatment of soft tissue sarcoma. Ann Surg 168:47-53, 1968.
4. Clark RL Jr, Martin RG, White EC, Wold J: Clinical aspects of soft tissue tumors. Arch Surg 74:859-870, 1957.
5. Collins C, Hajdu SI, Godbold J, Shiu MH, Hilaris BI, Brennan MF: Localized, operable soft tissue sarcoma of the lower extremity. Arch Surg 121:1425-1433, 1986.
6. Markhede G, Angervall L, Stener B: A multivariate analysis of the prognosis after surgical treatment of malignant soft tissue tumors. Cancer 49:1721-1733, 1982.
7. Pack GT: End results in the treatment of sarcomata of the soft somatic tissues. J Bone Joint Surg 36A:241-263, 1954.
8. Potter DA, Kinsella T, Glatstein E, et al.: High grade soft tissue sarcoma of the extremities. Cancer 58:190-205, 1986.
9. Ryholm A: Management of patients with soft tissue tumors. Acta Orthop Scand, Suppl 203, 54: 1983.
10. Sears HF: Soft tissue sarcoma: a historical overview. Semin Oncol 8:129-132, 1981.
11. Seids JV, McGinnis RS: Malignant tumors of fatty tissues. Surg Gynecol Obstet 44:232-243, 1927.
12. Shiu MH, Hajdu SI: Management of soft tissue sarcoma of the extremity. Semin Oncol 8:172-179, 1981.
13. Shiu MH, Hajdu SI, Fortner JG: Surgical treatment of 297 soft tissue sarcomas of the lower extremity. Ann Surg 182:597-602, 1975.
14. Simon MA, Enneking WF: The management of soft tissue sarcomas of the extremities. J Bone Joint Surg 58A:317-327, 1976.

LIMITED SURGERY AND EXTERNAL IRRADIATION IN SOFT TISSUE SARCOMAS

Herman D. Suit[1], Henry J. Mankin[2], Christopher G. Willett[1], Mark C. Gebhardt[2], William C. Wood[3], and Steven Skates[4]

Sarcoma of Soft Tissue

Current management of the primary disease in patients with soft tissue sarcoma is based upon conservative multimodality approaches directed toward limb salvage and reduced resection of grossly uninvolved tissue at torso and head/neck sites. Regrettably, there has not been demonstrated an effective systemic therapy for occult metastatic tumor although, paradoxically, chemotherapy is clearly efficacious in the treatment of an important proportion of patients with gross metastatic disease. Accordingly, there have been clear improvements in the cosmetic and functional results at the primary sites, but no proof of higher long-term survival rates. The superior survival results of recent studies, as compared with historical controls, may merely reflect treatment of progressively more favorable disease with succeeding time periods.

There are several highly effective strategies of management of the primary sarcoma of soft tissue. These are: 1) conservative surgery and radiation given postoperatively (1-5), preoperatively (6-8), or intraoperatively by brachytherapy techniques (9,10); 2) intra-arterial adriamycin, radiation, and resection (11); 3) intra-arterial melphalan $\pm$ actinomycin D, followed by local excision (12); and 4) radical compartmental resection (13,14). The need now is to assess, in a prospective study, the relative quality of the cosmetic and functional results of these diverse treatment strategies, and to do this while investigating further approaches to the treatment of occult metastatic sarcoma.

Such an assessment could be made by a study design in which: 1) participating institutions treated according to the method they judged most effective; 2) an independent group assessed the histological type, grade, size, and site of sarcoma; and 3) an independent group assessed the functional and cosmetic status at, say, 2-5 years after treatment using a standard protocol. The results would then be evalu-

----

[1]Department of Radiation Medicine
[2]Department of Orthopaedic Surgery
[3]General Surgical Service
[4]Department of Medicine
 Massachusetts General Hospital, Harvard Medical School, Boston, MA 02114.

J. R. Ryan and L. O. Baker (eds.), Recent Concepts in Sarcoma Treatment, 94–103.
© 1988 by Kluwer Academic Publishers.

ated according to narrowly defined strata. The MGH would be glad to participate in such a study. Further, there is a clear need for further investigation of the role of size and grade for each histological type of sarcoma on the probability of development of distant metastasis in patients who have control of their primary sarcoma.

In this report, we present: 1) an update of the MGH results in the treatment of patients with Stage M_O sarcoma of soft tissue by radiation given before or following conservative surgery; 2) an assessment of local control and disease-free survival of patients treated for primary or locally recurrent sarcoma; 3) prognostic import of positive resection margins; and 4) prognostic import of tumor size for distant metastases according to grade and histopathologic type of sarcoma.

Clinical Material

From 1971 to June 1986, 258 patients have been treated for their sarcoma of soft tissue by resectional surgery and radiation. Excluded from the analysis, are patients who: 1) received a total radiation dose corresponding to a TDF of ≤ 72.5; 2) had rhabdomyosarcoma and were less than 30 years of age; 3) had Kaposi's sarcoma; 4) had locally malignant, but non-metastatic tumors (aggressive fibromatosis (Desmoid tumors), infiltrating neurofibroma, atypical lipoma, etc.); and 5) had sarcomas of thoracic, abdominal, or pelvic cavities, including retroperitoneal tumors. Results are described in reference to the current and revised AJC staging system (15). In this new system, each tumor is graded on the basis of its histological features, viz., there may be Grade I synovial sarcoma, angiosarcomas, etc. T state is by size only (T_1 refers to a tumor less than 5 cm, T_2 refers to tumors of 5 cm or greater in at least one dimension).

Data are presented as current status, which gives the actual number of patients in each category: NED (no evident disease), LF (local failure), DM (distant metastasis), or ID (intercurrent disease). Further, the data are subjected to an actuarial analysis to yield 5-year local control and disease-free survival rates. For these analyses, patients who are lost to follow-up are censored as of the date of their last examination.

Treatment methods. Radiation therapy has been based upon the shrinking field technique, as described earlier (16). For postoperative treatment, the dose has been an initial ⁻50 Gy given in 25-28 fractions to volumes designed to include subclinical extensions with a boost dose to the site of the primary lesion of ⁻16-18 Gy; the total dose to the central area being 66-68 Gy given over ⁻7 weeks. For patients irradiated preoperatively, the dose was also 50 Gy as for the postoperative series (except that treatment volume was usually smaller); boost dose of ⁻16 Gy was given intra-operatively by brachytherapy technique or postoperatively by small fields directed to the tumor bed as defined by the position of the clips placed at the margin of the residual tumor mass. Several patients have been irradiated on a BID schedule, viz., 1.6-2.0 Gy administered twice per day with

$\geq$4 hours between fractions. For this schedule, the dose has been reduced by 10%. In patients who were to receive adriamycin, the dose was reduced by a further 5-10%.

Results

Tables 1, 2, and 3 present the current status and 5-year actuarial results for the entire series of 258 patients, and separately for 144 patients given postoperative radiation, and the 114 patients who received preoperative radiation. Grade of sarcoma made little impact on local control or disease-free survival (DFS) for patients whose sarcomas were <5 cm in maximum dimension. In marked contrast, DFS decreased sharply with grade for the patients whose sarcomas were $\geq$5 cm in diameter, viz., 88%, 52%, and 39% for Grades 1, 2, and 3, respectively (Table 1). Local control of the $\geq$5 cm

Table 1. Current status and 5-year actuarial results in 258 patients treated by conservative surgery and radiation according to stage

Stages	No. Pts.	NED	LF±DM	DM	ID	5-yr Actuarial Local Control %	DFS %
IA	17	16	–		1	100	100
B	30	24	2	2	2	93	88
IIA	40	28	4	5	3	88	83
B	66	33	8	22	3	85	52
IIIA	33	26	2	2	3	93	87
B	69	25	10	29	5	79	39
IVA	3	3	–	–		100	100
TOTAL	258	155	26	60	17	88	66

NED = No evident disease
LF = Local failure
DM = Distant metastasis
ID = Dead of intercurrent disease
DFS = Disease free survival

Table 2. Current status and 5-year actuarial results in 144 patients treated by surgery and post-operative radiation according to stage

Stages	No. Pts.	NED	LF±DM	DM	ID	5-yr Actuarial Local Control %	DFS %
IA	13	12	–		1	100	100
B	19	16	–	1	2	100	95
IIA	29	19	4	3	3	85	86
B	28	12	7	7	2	71	55
IIIA	26	20	1	2	3	95	87
B	28	9	6	13		·72	31
IVA	1	1	–			100	100
TOTAL	144	89	18	26	11	86	71

NED = No evident disease
LF = Local failure
DM = Distant metastasis
ID = Dead of intercurrent disease
DFS = Disease free survival

Table 3. Current status and 5-year actuarial results in 114 patients treated by pre-operative radiation and conservative surgery according to stage

Stages	No. Pts.	NED	LF±DM	DM	ID	5-yr Actuarial Local Control %	DFS %
IA	4	4			0	100	100
B	11	8	2	1	0	80	73
IIA	11	9	0	2	0	100	67
B	38	21	1	15	1	97	50
IIIA	7	6	1	0	0	86	86
B	41	16	4	16	5	·88	47
IVA	2	2	0	0	0	100	100
TOTAL	114	66	8	34	6	91	60

NED = No evident disease
LF = Local failure
DM = Distant metastasis
ID = Dead of intercurrent disease
DFS = Disease free survival

sarcomas decreased with grade in the postoperative series (100%, 71%, 72% for G1,2, and 3) but not for the pre-operative series (80%, 97%, 91%). There has been substantial improvement in local control results over the past 15 years; namely in the recent period local control rates were 92% and 97% for postoperative and preoperative radiation, respectively, as given in Table 4.

Table 4. Five-year actuarial results among 258 patients treated by radiation and surgery according to time period of treatment

Time Period	Post-op No.Pts.	LC %	DFS %	Pre-op No.Pts.	LC %	DFS %
1971–75	33	81	70	4	100	25
1976–80	48	83.7	69	28	77	54
1980–86	63	92	76	82	97	65
TOTAL	144			114		

LC = Local control
DFS = Disease free survival

The local control results were much less dependent upon size in the preoperative than in the postoperative series, as shown in Table 5. For tumors which were >100 mm, there appeared to be a worthwhile local control advantage to pre-operative radiation therapy. Disease-free survival results, however, deteriorated rapidly with size. In patients with sarcoma of soft tissue tumor, size is an extremely important prognostic factor for development of distant metastasis in patients with Grades 2 or 3 sarcoma. The data in Table 6 show that the frequency of distant metastasis in patients who had achieved local control of their Grade 2 or 3 sarcoma

Table 5. Five-year actuarial local control results according to size

Size (mm)	Post-op No.Pts.	LC %	DFS %	Pre-op No.Pts.	LC %	DFS %
≤ 25	21	86	95	9	100	100
26-49	44	92	85	11	91	65
50-100	57	86	56	48	92	70
101-150	12	91	73	21	100	44
151-200	7	54	43	18	70	37
>200	3	67	67	7	100	21
TOTAL	144	86	71	114	91	60

LC = Local control
DFS = Disease free survival

increased with size from 5% for ≤25 mm sarcoma to 70% and 83% for 151-200 mm and >200 mm sarcomas. This explains the lower survival in the preoperative series: 40% of sarcomas in the preoperative series were >100 mm as compared with 15% in the postoperative series. Similarly, only 17% of the sarcomas in the preoperative series were <50 mm in diameter in contrast with 49% for the postoperative series. Clearly, the preoperative series had much the less favorable group of patients.

Table 6. Five-year actuarial distant metastasis probability as a function of tumo size and grade

Size (mm)	Grade 1 No.Pts.	DM %	Grade 2 & 3 No.Pts.	DM %
≤ 25	5	0	23	5
26-50	11	0	39	14
51-100	17	6	78	42
101-150	5	0	27	52
151-200	4	25	14	70
>200	3	0	6	83
TOTAL	45	6	187	37

DM = Distant metastasis

Status of margins of the resection specimen as a prognostic indicator has been examined. Among patients managed by postoperative radiation, positive margins (tumor spill, tumor removed in pieces, microscopic + margins) had only a slight negative effect on local control or DFS (17). Table 7 is a presentation of local control and DFS rates at 5 years according to margin status of patients given radiation preoperatively. Local control was about the same for M+ and M-status for patients with Stages IIA and IIIA disease. However, for Stages IIB and IIIB, the local control rates were 74% and 95% for M+ and M- resection specimens (the number of patients in the two groups were 14 and 48). The trend for DFS was reversed, viz., apparently higher survival rates for M+ than M- for both Stages IIA, IIIA, and IIB, IIIB.

Table 7.	Status of margins vs local control and disease free survival after pre-operative radiation therapy for primary sarcoma of soft tissue			
	LOCAL CONTROL		DISEASE FREE SURVIVAL	
STAGE	M +	M -	M +	M -
IIA,IIIA	100%(2)*	91%(11)	100%	80%
IIB,IIIB	74%(14)	95%(48)	56%	44%
*Censored a 60/12				

Further, the local control and DFS rates have been determined for patients with primary and recurrent sarcomas. The data in Table 8 show that local control was less frequent following treatment of recurrent rather than primary sarcoma, Stages IIA, IIIA; the reverse obtained for patients with Stages IIB, IIIB disease. With reference to DFS, the results were less satisfactory for patients with recurrent sarcomas for both stages IIA, IIIA, and Stages IIB, IIIB.

Table 8.	Five year actuarial local control and disease free survival for primary and recurrent soft tissue sarcoma			
	LOCAL CONTROL		DISEASE FREE SURVIVAL	
STAGE	PRIMARY	RECURRENT	PRIMARY	RECURRENT
IIA,IIIA	98%(55)	65%(18)	88%	44%
IIB,IIIB	81%(123)	91%(12)	70%	56%

The experience with the 26 patients in this series of 258 patients who have developed local failure was that 7 of the 20 local failures after treatment of primary sarcomas are alive and free of evident tumor (1 died after 5 years of breast cancer); 2 of the 6 patients who failed after treatment of recurrent sarcoma are surviving free of tumor. These indicate a less satisfactory result than obtained for treatment of the primary sarcomas.

In a recent analysis (18) of wound healing delays among 50 patients treated for primary sarcoma of soft tissue by preoperative radiation and resection of the tumor, and who have had a minimum follow-up of >7 months, 10 patients had to have a graft placed (8) or an amputation (2). A multivariate analysis showed significant correlation between wound healing

delay   and: 1) age $\geq$59 years,   2) hypertension;   3) radiation   treatment on a BID   fractionation schedule;   and 4)   a
surgical specimen >205 ml.   Obesity was perhaps a factor, but
below p. 05 level of significance.

Discussion

This update of the experience at MGH in   the   management
of patients (now at 258) with Stage M_O sarcoma of soft tissue
by   moderate   dose radiation   therapy   and less   than radical
compartmental   surgery continues to document   excellent local
control   rates.   This is especially so for the large sarcomas
(>10 cm) treated by preoperative radiation. Our major problem
now is that of eradication of the occult metastatic tumor and
to   refine further the treatment of the local lesion so as to
increase the quality of the functional and cosmetic outcome.

Our   review of the published results of Phase III trials
of   various chemotherapy regimens, featuring   adriamycin, did
not   yield evidence for   a significant increase   in long-term
DFS   rates (17).   The two   trials which reported a   gain also
had unusually low survival rates in their control arm (17,19,
20). Unless there were shown to have been a   good   randomization   as to size and grade, an assumption of comparability of
the control and test arms is not judged   warranted.   Nonetheless,   we are impressed by   the not infrequent important   response of gross disease to the drug/dose schedules similar to
those   employed in the adjuvant   trials. A Phase I   study has
been initiated to assess the feasibility of starting the drug
therapy   earlier   in course   of   management. Namely,   we   are
testing alternating cycles of adriamycin (2-3 cycles of 80-90
mg M^{-2}) and radiation (2 cycles of 21.2 Gy given on a 1.8 Gy
$fraction^{-1}$,   twice   daily with $\geq$4 hours   between fractions)
preoperatively.   The   radiation is   given   at the   mid   point
between the adriamycin cycles. Further work in this direction
is   being planned so   as to develop   a protocol which   yields
acceptable levels of morbidity.

There   have   been   important difficulties   in   achieving
healing of the wound in 10 of 50 patients treated by preoperative radiation. Some delay in healing occurred in 46% of the
patients.   The multivariate analysis by McDonald et al.   (18)
identified   four factors which were   significantly associated
with delay in wound healing: age $\geq$59, hypertension,   BID
treatment   schedule,   and a   surgical   specimen >205   ml. For
example,   9   of 32   patients $\geq$50   years of age   had a wound
healing delay which required a surgical procedure (delay of
4+ to 6+) as compared with 1/18 among patients <50 years old.
They   estimated that   when all   four of   the designated   risk
factors   were present,   some delay   in wound   healing can   be
confidently expected in all patients. Among the   10   patients
with   a 4+ to 6+ delay*,   8 had a surgical specimen >205 ml as
compared with 15 of the 40 who had a lesser or no delay.   Six
of 10 patients with 4+ to 6+ wound healing delay were treated
on a BID basis vs. 12/40 for patients with a 0 to   3+   delay.

----

*Scoring of delay: 4+, grafting required;   6+, amputation.

The observed delays in healing of wounds is not entirely a consequence of the preoperative radiation. In a recent report from the NCI, Skibber et al. (21) reported that 34% of 93 patients had a delay in wound healing and 7 required re-operation to facilitate closure.

Our efforts directed toward reduction of the problem of delayed healing or non-healing include: 1) fill in part of the defect caused by resection of the residual tumor; 2) longer period of drainage; 3) monitor the wounds to ascertain adequacy of drainage; 4) longer immobilization; 5) use myo-cutaneous flaps if feasible where there is any tension on the wound; 6) apply gentle compression on the wound to aid in maintaining contact between superficial and deep tissues. These problems are also discussed by Skibber et al. (21).

Summary

We present an update on the causes of failure, actuarial 5-year local control and disease-free survival among 258 patients treated by radiation and resection of primary or recurrent sarcoma of soft tissue. The analysis was made as of June 1987. For the 145 patients treated during the period 1981-1986, the 5-year actuarial local control rates were 92% and 97% for postoperative and preoperative radiation re-spectively. Among patients with local control after treatment of their Grade 2 or 3 sarcoma, the frequency of distant metastasis increased with size: 5% for $\leq$25 mm sarcoma to 83% for >200 mm sarcomas. Factors associated with delay in wound healing after preoperative radiation are: age $\geq$59 years, specimen volume >205 ml, BID fractionation, and hyper-tension. Efforts to increase ease of healing are described. Also, the Phase I trial of preoperative adriamycin and radia-tion, given in alternating cycles (a minimum of 6 days be-tween adriamycin and radiation) is described.

Acknowledgment: The authors are pleased to acknowledge the important work of Pat McNulty in collating the data.

REFERENCES

1. Suit HD, Russell WO, Martin RG: Sarcoma of soft tissue: clinical and histopathologic parameters and response to treatment. Cancer 35:1478-1483, 1975.

2. Lindberg RD: Conservative surgery and post-operative radiotherapy in 300 adults with soft-tissue sarcomas. Cancer 47:2391-97, 1981.

3. Leibel SA, Tranbaugh RF, Wara WM, Beckstead JH, Bovill EG, Phillips TL: Soft tissue sarcomas of the extremi-ties. Cancer 50:1076-1083, 1982.

4. Coe MA, Maddin FJ, Mould RF: The Role of radiotherapy in the treatment of soft tissue sarcoma: a retrospective study 1958-73. Clin Radiol 32:47-51, 1981.

5. Rosenberg SA, Glatstein EJ: Perspectives on the role of surgery and radiation therapy in the treatment of soft tissue sarcomas of the extremities. Semin Oncol

8:190-200, 1981.

6. Atkinson L, Garvan JM, Newton NC: Behavior and management of soft connective tissue sarcomas. Cancer 16:1552-62, 1963.

7. Suit HD, Mankin HJ, Wood WC, Proppe KH: Radiation and surgery in the treatment of primary sarcoma of soft tissue: pre-operative, intra-operative and post-operative. Cancer 55:2659-2667, 1985.

8. Martin RG, Lindberg RD, Russell WO: Preoperative radiotherapy and surgery in the management of soft tissue sarcoma. In: Management of Primary Bone and Soft Tissue Tumors. Chicago, Year Book Medical Publishers Inc. pp.299-307, 1977.

9. Collins JE, Paine CH, Ellis F: Treatment of connective tissue sarcomas by local excision followed by radioactive implant. Clin Radiol 27:39-41, 1976.

10. Shiu MH, Turnbull AD, Nori D, et al.: Control of locally advanced extremity soft tissue sarcomas by function-saving resection and brachytherapy. Cancer 53:1385-1392, 1984.

11. Eilber FR, Guiliano AE, Huth J, Mirra J, Morton DL: High-grade soft tissue sarcomas of the extremity: UCLA experience with limb salvage. Primary Chemotherapy in Cancer Medicine. Alan R. Liss, Inc. pp.59-74, 1985.

12. Hoekstra HJ, Koops HS, Molenaar WM, Oldhoff J: Results of isolated regional perfusion in the treatment of malignant soft tissue tumors of the extremities. Cancer 60:1703-1707, 1987.

13. Enneking WF, Spanier SS, Malawar MM: The effect of anatomic setting on the results of surgical procedures for soft parts sarcoma of the thigh. Cancer 47:1005, 1981.

14. Markhede G, Angervall L, Stener B: A multivariant analysis of the prognosis after surgical treatment of malignant soft tissue tumors. Cancer 49:1721, 1981.

15. AJC Staging System Manual, in press.

16. Suit HD, Tepper JE, Mankin HJ, Truman JT, Wood WC, Harmon DC, Schiller AL, Rosenberg A: Sarcomas of soft tissue and bone. In: Clinical Radiation Oncology. CC Wang, Ed., Littleton, MA, Wright Pub, in press.

17. Suit HD, Mankin HJ, Wood WC, Gebhardt MC, Harmon DC, Rosenberg A, Tepper JE, Rosenthal D: Treatment of the patient with stage MO sarcoma of soft tissue. Submitted to J Clin Oncol.

18. McDonald J, Suit HD, Skates S, Mankin HJ, Gebhardt MC, Wood WC: Analysis of wound healing in patients treated by pre-operative radiation for primary sarcoma of soft tissue. 1987. Unpublished data.

19. Rosenberg SA, et al.: Prospective randomized evaluation of adjuvant chemotherapy in adults with soft tissue sarcoma of the extremities. Cancer 52:424-34, 1983.

20. Gherlinzone F, et al.: A randomized trial for the treatment of high grade soft tissue sarcomas of the extremities: preliminary observations. J Clin Oncol 4:552-58, 1986.

21. Skibber JM, Lotze MT, Seipp CA, Salcedo R, Rosenberg SA: Limb-sparing surgery for soft tissue sarcomas: wound related morbidity in patients undergoing wide local excision. Surgery 102:447-452, 1987.

BRACHYTHERAPY AND LIMB-SPARING RESECTION IN THE MANAGEMENT OF SOFT TISSUE SARCOMA

Man H. Shiu, M.D.[1], Basil S. Hilaris, M.D.[2],
Murray F. Brennan, M.D.[1]

In the earlier part of the century, surgical efforts focused mainly on the feasibility and safety of the various surgical operations necessary for wide extirpation of soft tissue sarcoma. Major advances were made in the design and safe execution of these complex surgical procedures, such as forequarter amputation and hemipelvectomy. Functional preservation was at that time a secondary goal. In 1953, Bowden and Booher (1) proposed that carefully selected tumors could be treated by en bloc muscle group resection as an alternative to amputation with equally good local tumor control. Local recurrenceswere nevertheless very common with limb-sparing resections in the 1950's and 1960's. Fine et al. (2) reviewed the results of surgical treatment of soft tissue sarcomas up to the late 1960's and noted local recurrence rates of over 50% in various reports, and in some instances up to 90%. Such local failure rates were obviously unacceptable. Surgeons soon recognized the limitations of surgery as an ablative technique in this setting, and sought the additional use of other methods based on entirely different therapeutic principles. Radiation therapy emerged as a feasible means of controlling invisible microscopic residual tumor after resection. Among those who pioneered the combined use of surgery and radiation therapy in the management of soft tissue sarcoma are Lindberg (3), Suit (4,5), Eilber and Morton (6,7) who respectively reported on the successful application of postoperative irradiation, preoperative irradiation and preoperative irradiation combined with intra-arterial infusion of doxorubicin for limb salvage.

At the Memorial Sloan-Kettering Cancer Center, we have favored the use of interstitial radiation (brachytherapy) of the tumor-bed after resection of soft tissue sarcoma, to increase local tumor control and to maximize preservation of function.

The development of this technique resulted from our dissatisfaction with the high local recurrence rates experienced after soft-part resections and the large number of amputations performed (8,9). We considered the use of brachy-

---

[1]Department of Surgery
[2]Department of Radiation Oncology
Memorial Sloan-Kettering Cancer Center, 1275 York Avenue, New York, NY 10021.

J. R. Ryan and L. O. Baker (eds.), Recent Concepts in Sarcoma Treatment, 104–114.
© 1988 by Kluwer Academic Publishers.

therapy because it was a well established technique in the radiation therapy of localized cancers at several anatomic sites, i.e. head and neck, uterine cervix and vagina. Much of the pioneering work on uterine and other cancers had been done by Henschke (10), Hilaris (11) and their colleagues at our institution. Henschke pioneered the afterloading technique in which catheters were inserted at the tumor site during surgery, to be used one or more days later in the early postoperative period for insertion of the radioactive sources, thus preventing exposure of the operating room staff to radiation. A small number of soft tissue sarcomas, mostly in the head and neck, were treated at our center, using radon or radioactive gold implants in the 1950's and 1960's (12). Ellis (13,14) of Oxford University had also used brachytherapy in the management of soft tissue sarcoma with some success in England. Ellis was instrumental in stimulating the surgeons and radiation oncologists to further develop this technique, and a cautious trial was begun at our center in a small number of mostly advanced sarcoma of the limb.

Ellis (13,14) asserted that while postoperative radiation therapy had some merits, it was often doomed to failure, because of inherent lack of radiosensitivity of these tumors, all the more so if therapy was given several weeks after surgery so that the cancer cells would then be trapped by relatively avascular scar tissue. He advocated "implanting radioactive sources in the bed of the operation field at the time of surgery; by this method the cells inadvertently left behind by the surgeon .... may be subjected to a very large dose of radiation. The dose is everywhere greater than 6,000 rads in a layer of tissue." This precise administration of radiation therapy at depth in the tumor-bed also avoided much of the damage to adjacent normal tissues, permitting a higher dose to the tumor site sometimes not possible with standard external-beam radiotherapy.

Brachytherapy and Conservative Resection of Locally Advanced Sarcoma

In 1984, we reported (15) the early experience at the Memorial Sloan-Kettering Cancer Center of treating 33 patients who had locally advanced soft tissue sarcomas of the upper or lower limb using function-saving excision and temporary implants of Iridium-192 sources in the tumor-bed. More than half of these patients had been advised to undergo amputation for control of their tumor, because of large size, deep-seated location, or involvement of adjacent neurovascular bundle, bone or joint. Histopathologically, liposarcoma, tendosynovial sarcoma and fibrosarcoma accounted for more than two-thirds of these tumors. Twenty-three of the 33 tumors were classified as high-grade. Tables 1 and 2 record the extent of invasion and other characteristics of these tumors, most of which possessed several of these adverse features. Surgical resection of these tumors was hampered by the proximity of major neurovascular or skeletal structures. In many instances the surgeon could only remove the grossly visible tumor, leaving behind microscopic or even macroscopic

TABLE 1

Locally advanced sarcoma of limb, Group I: previously untreated tumors

	Size > 5 cm Diameter	High Grade	Tumor abuts or Involves Major Structure	Resection Margin Inadequate(+) or shows tumor(++)	Tumor violated(+) Or Gross Tumor Was left(++)	Status
1.	+			+		NED
2.	+	+		+		NED
3.	+	+			+	NED
4.	+			+		NED
5.	+	+	+ (pubic bone)	++	++	NED
6.		+	+ (radial N)	+		NED
7.		+		+		NED
8.	+	+	+ (popliteal A,V,N)	+		M, DOD
9.	+			+		NED
10.				+	+	NED
11.	+	+		+		NED
12.	+		+ (popliteal A,V,N)	+		NED
13.	+	+	+ (sciatic N)	++		NED
14.		+		++	++	NED
15.	+	+		+		NED
16.		+			+	NED
17.	+	+	+ (femoral A)	++	++	NED

A: artery; N: nerve; V:vein; DOD: dead of disease; M: metastasis; NED: no evidence of disease. Adapted from: Shiu et al. Cancer 53:1385-1392, 1984.

TABLE 2

Locally advanced sarcoma of limb, Group II:previously treated, recurrent tumors

	Size > 5 cm Diameter	High Grade	Tumor abuts or Involves Major Structure	Resection Margin Inadequate(+) or shows tumor(++)	Tumor violated(+) Or Gross Tumor Was left(++)	Status
1.			+ (popliteal N)	+		NED
2.	+	+		+		NED
3.		+	+ (popliteal A)	+		NED
4.	+	+	+ (sciatic N)	+		LR,M,DOD
5.	+	+	+ (sciatic N)	+		LR
6.			+ (brachial A,V)	+		NED
7.	+	+	+ (femur)	+		M,DOD
8.		+	+ (brachial plexus)	+		LR
9.*		+		+		LR,M,NED
10.	+		+ (femoral A,V)	++		NED
11.	+	+	+ (sciatic N)	+	+	M<DOD
12.	+	+	+ (femoral A,V)	+		NED
13.		+	+ (brachial A,V)	++	++	NED
14.			+ (humerus)	+		NED
15.	+		+ (ulna)	+		LR
16.	+	+	+ (femur,saphenous V)			LR,M,DOD

* Patient 9 is free of disease after resection of local recurrence and lung metastasis. A: artery; LR: local recurrence; N: nerve; V:vein; DOD: dead of disease; M: metastasis; NED: no evidence of disease. Adapted from: Shiu et al. Cancer 53:1385-1392, 1984.

fragments of sarcoma, usually on a major nerve, artery or vein, in the interest of preserving limb function.

Technique of Brachytherapy. Immediately after conservative excision of the tumor, the surgeon and the radiation oncologist examine the surgical site and map out the tumor-bed. This encompasses all gross and microscopic tumor, plus a margin of at least 1.5 cm, usually much wider, depending on the size and other characteristics of the lesion. Conceptually, the tumor-bed consists of the tissues over, under and around the tumor, bearing its microscopic ramifications (Fig. 1). After excision of the tumor, the overlying skin and soft tissues including the repaired incision collapse onto the underlying structures, much as the top falls onto the bottom of an empty sac (Fig. 2, left). This composite slab of tissue is the tumor-bed target, for purposes of radiation therapy (Fig. 2, right). Oblong or ovoid in shape, it can be flat or uneven, measuring several centimeters in thickness. The dimensions of this tumor-bed are measured and recorded, and a series of plastic catheters are then inserted percutaneously through 16-gauge hollow needles, to be secured by chromic catgut sutures so that they lie 1 cm apart, covering its entire extent. Postoperative anteroposterior and lateral radiographs, with radiopaque markers in the lumen of the catheters, provide information for computerized dosimetry calculations. In almost all cases, a single-plane array of catheters is sufficient for delivery of the prescribed dose at depth. Based on the radioactivity, number and spatial relationships of the radioactive sources (Iridium-192),

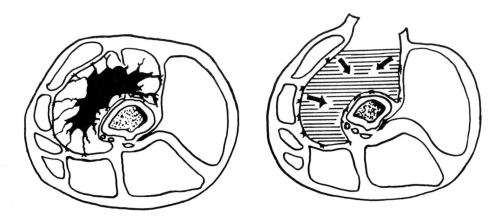

Figure 1: Diagrammatic representation of sarcoma of thigh (left). After excision, the tissues adjacent to the original tumor space collapse onto each other (right). Note microscopic ramifications of tumor left behind. From: Shiu MH and Brennan MF: *Surgical Management of Soft Tissue Sarcoma*. Philadelphia, Lea & Febiger, in press.

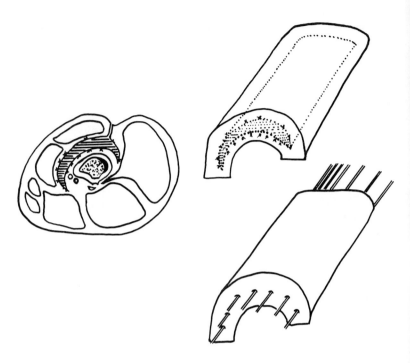

Figure 2: The tumor-bed (left) consists of tissues that surrounded the original tumor, now removed. In three-dimensions (right, upper), it can be considered as an ovoid or oblong slab of tissues. This tumor-bed target can be effectively treated with a single plane array of Iridium-192 sources inserted through afterloading catheters (right, lower). From: Shiu MH and Brennan MF: <u>Surgical Management of Soft Tissue Sarcoma</u>. Philadelphia, Lea & Febiger, in press.

calculations and adjustments can be made of the contour of the radiated target and the number of hours of treatment, increasing the dose in areas of gross tumor, or reducing it where overlying skin is near.

A dose of 4,500 cGy over four to five days has been found to be adequate for microscopic disease in almost all cases. In calculating the implant dose, a reference point near the corner of the implant array at 0.5 cm from the plane of the array is used (16-18). This nominal dose represents the <u>minimal</u> dose within the tumor-bed target, the dose between or nearer the sources being much higher. It is important to consider that radiobiologically, the prescribed interstitial dose of 4,500 cGy over 4-5 days exceeds the equivalent of 6,000 cGy (19) of conventional external irradiation, given in 30 fractions over six weeks.

The sources are loaded through the catheters, usually

six days after surgery, to permit initiation of wound healing
(20). The patient stays confined within a single room while
the Iridium-192 sources, which emit gamma radiation, are in
place. Standard medical and nursing care are provided, but
prolonged exposure of staff was avoided by sharing of nursing
duties and the use of a lead shield. Brachytherapy is avoided
in patients who require close medical or nursing support due
to chronic pulmonary, cardiac, neurologic or other medical
conditions. However, we have found that the use of Iodine-
125 sources as a substitute for Iridium-192 for temporary
implants decreases the need for protection of personnel while
maintaining the same dose distribution as the Iridium-192
(21). Following completion of the prescribed radiation
treatment, the sources and catheters are removed, and the
patient is usually discharged the same or the next day. If
the patient has high-grade soft tissue sarcoma, adjuvant
chemotherapy, using doxorubicin with or without other drugs,
is offered.

    <u>Results</u>. The results of treatment in the series of 33
patients were gratifying (15). These patients had been
followed at the time of the report for a minimum of 19 months
to a maximum of 7 years and 8 months (median follow-up 36
months). Of the 33 patients, 17 had previously untreated
tumors, and none of the 17 developed local tumor recurrence
after combined surgical excision and brachytherapy. The
remaining 16 patients underwent treatment for locally
recurrent tumors, achieving local tumor control in 10, but
six of the 16 patients developed further local recurrence.
Two of the six patients were salvaged by additional resection
and brachytherapy. Thus, 100% local control was achieved for
previously untreated tumors, 62.5% for previously treated,
recurrent tumors, and 89% for the entire group. The extensive
nature of these tumors and the fact that more than half of
the patients had been advised to undergo amputation, leave
little doubt about the efficacy of this method for managing
locally advanced sarcoma of the limb.

    Some concern was raised, however, by the frequency of
wound complications which occurred in 11 of the 33 patients
in this early experience. Wound breakdown with extensive
necrosis of soft tissues or exposed major arteries occurred
in three patients, two of whom had to undergo amputation.
Many of these complications were associated with inadequate
soft tissue closure of the surgical incision, use of excess-
ively high radiation dose (over 5000 cGy, particularly in
patients who had received prior radiation), or loading of the
sources earlier than the 3rd day after surgery (22). With
standardization of radiation dose calculations, planned
loading of the radioactive sources not earlier than the 5th
day, and recognition of the importance of thick, well vascularized skin flaps for closure, these serious, limb-threaten-
ing complications have been avoided.

    The function of the limb after treatment in the 31
patients who did not undergo amputation due to a complication was carefully assessed. Nineteen patients achieved
satisfactory function in terms of power, range of movement,

and capacity for all ordinary activities without discomfort. Four patients stated they had moderate limitation of limb function due to either stiffness, weakness or both. Three patients sustained severe loss of function due to wrist-drop or foot-drop consequent to resection or damage to nerves, and needed tendon grafts or orthotic corrective devices. In all, 26 of the 33 (79%) patients in the study enjoyed good-to-excellent preservation of limb function. With the exception of the two who underwent amputation for complications, all could walk on the treated lower limb, or use the treated upper limb for prehensile purposes.

Brachytherapy proved to be particularly useful in the conservative management of soft tissue sarcomas of the ante-cubital and popliteal space. These anatomical spaces are compact and relatively non-fleshy. Tumors arising in this location often lie close to the main neurovascular bundle of the arm or leg, and may actually invade the major blood vessels, nerves or the adjacent bone or joint. Because of this, wide margin resection is usually anatomically impossible and the standard recommendation for treatment is amputation. In a retrospective study of 24 patients treated with curative intent from 1968 to 1982 at the Memorial Sloan-Kettering Cancer Center (16), 14 underwent surgical treatment only in 1968-1973, while 10 treated in 1974-1982 underwent combined modality therapy including conservative excision, radiation therapy using removable implants of Iridium-192 sources, and adjuvant chemotherapy if the sarcoma was histo-logically high-grade. In the latter group treated by combined modality therapy, local tumor control was achieved in all 10 patients, with no evidence of local recurrence after a follow-up period of 28 months to 9 years. The functional result in the limb was gratifying. This contrasts sharply with the 14 patients treated in 1968-1973 by amputation or excision alone; only two of the 14 survived without re-currence or loss of limb by amputation.

Prospective Randomized Trial of Adjuvant Brachytherapy

While we became convinced of the efficacy of brachy-therapy in controlling locally advanced tumors, including those with microscopic or macroscopic residual tumor after surgery in the limb, we were still concerned by its potential morbidity (22) and hesitated to offer it to many patients after complete resection of soft tissue sarcoma in the limb. To resolve this conflict of potential risk versus potential benefit, we realized a prospective randomized trial of brachytherapy was necessary for patients in this setting. This trial was initiated in 1982 for sarcomas of the limb and superficial trunk. A preliminary analysis of the results has recently been published (23). At this time, overall improve-ment in local control has been demonstrated. This appears due to the effect on patients with high-grade sarcoma (Table 3). The trend in low-grade tumors is not obvious. Many of the patients treated for high-grade sarcoma also received adju-vant chemotherapy, but this was equally distributed between the two groups of patients, i.e. those receiving and those not receiving brachytherapy, suggesting that the improved

TABLE 3

Randomized Trial of Resection versus Resection plus Tumor-Bed Brachytherapy

in Soft Tissue Sarcoma of Limbs and Superficial Trunk

	Number of Patients	Local Recurrence With or Without Metastasis	
High and Low grade tumors:			
Resection plus Iridium-192	52	2	
			p = 0.06
Resection only	65	9	
High grade tumors only:			
Resection plus Iridium-192	41	0	
			p = 0.03
Resection only	47	5	

From: Brennan et al. Local recurrence in adult soft tissue sarcoma: a randomized trial of brachytherapy. Arch Surg (in press, 1987).

local control was not due to the chemotherapy. Survival advantage, however, has not been demonstrated, but follow-up remains short, with a median of 16 months.

Discussion

Brachytherapy offers several theoretical and practical advantages over conventional external radiation therapy in the management of soft tissue sarcoma of the limb (11,15,16):

1. Radiobiologically, applying radiation therapy a few days after surgery may be more effective; this is in contrast to conventional postoperative radiation started several weeks later, when the healing process may have trapped the tumor cells in scar tissue which may be less well oxygenated, rendering them more resistant to radiation.

2. The direct application of radiation sources to the target can give effective dose distribution at depth whatever the shape of the tumor-bed -- a feature not easily emulated by even the most sophisticated external beam treatment facilities. The required high dose can thus be given to the tumor site, with more efficient sparing of adjacent normal tissues.

3. Brachytherapy can be used even in selected patients with recurrent sarcoma who have received previous radiation therapy in the same area; additional external irradiation is often difficult if not impossible in this

setting.

4. Joint attendance of the surgeon and radiation oncologist at the time of surgery assures the most accurate delineation of the tumor-bed, and the most optimal soft tissue closure from both the surgical and radiotherapeutic standpoints, which may not otherwise be possible.

5. The brachytherapy is completed usually within 5 days, and does not substantially prolong the hospital stay. Yet, patients are spared the usual outpatient postoperative radiation treatments that often need transportation and attendance several times a week for 6 weeks.

Brachytherapy does have certain limitations in the management of soft tissue sarcoma. A team of radiation oncologists and physicists experienced in the application of interstitial brachytherapy is necessary. The size of the tumor-bed target must not exceed 30 cm in its greatest diameter. Technical and dosimetric considerations currently limit the size of an implant of Iridium-192 to maximal diameters of approximately 30 cm x 10 cm. Brachytherapy has been found to be useful in the management of sarcoma at almost all sites, but its use is risky in the abdomen in which free moving intestine may directly contact the radioactive sources, resulting in excessive irradiation of the bowel and possible perforation and fistula. Except in these circumstances, we have found brachytherapy to be highly effective in the local control of soft tissue sarcoma when used in combination with conservative resection.

In spite of its theoretical and practical advantages, brachytherapy is by no means the only method that has been successfully used for limb-sparing treatment of soft tissue sarcoma of the limb. As mentioned above, preoperative and postoperative external radiation therapy, and infusion chemotherapy using doxorubicin combined with preoperative radiation, have also been used with considerable success. It is not possible, without a carefully planned randomized clinical trial on a large number of patients, to determine which method offers the best results with the least cost and morbidity in different subsets of patients who have tumors of various characteristics. At the Memorial Sloan-Kettering Cancer Center, we have found brachytherapy to be effective, economical and practical for our patients.

Furthermore, not all patients need adjunctive radiation therapy. For example, a small, superficial tumor overlying a fleshy part of the limb can be excised with a very wide margin of normal tissues. In this setting, the addition of radiation therapy, whether by external beam treatment or by brachytherapy, may not have demonstrable therapeutic benefit, as the predicted local recurrence rates are less than 10% at five years. Our current studies should identify which groups of patients are most likely to benefit from such therapy. The surgeon about to treat a patient with a sarcoma of the limb can determine the risk of local tumor recurrence and offer adjunctive therapy if it is needed. The exact method of adjunctive therapy to use should be determined by what is available in the local geographical region. The only other important consideration is that whichever method is used, it must be administered with the best of equipment and, importantly for radiation therapy, the support of sophisticated dosimetry planning that has enabled the good results reported from the various centers expert in these treatments.

REFERENCES

1. Bowden L, Booher RJ: The principles and techniques of resection of soft parts for sarcomas. Surgery 44:963-977, 1958.
2. Fine G, Ohorodnik JM, Horn RC Jr et al.: Soft tissue sarcomas: their clinical behavior and course and influencing factors. In: Seventh National Cancer Center Conference Proceedings. Philadelphia, Lippincott, p.873-882, 1973.
3. Lindberg R, Martin R, Romsdahl M, et al.: Conservative surgery and postoperative radiotherapy in 300 adults with soft tissue sarcoma. Cancer 47:2391-2397, 1981.
4. Suit HD, Russell WO, Martin RG: Sarcoma of soft tissue: clinical and histologic parameters and response to treatment. Cancer 35:1478-1483, 1975.
5. Suit HD, Proppe KH, Mankin HJ et al.: Preoperative radiation therapy for soft tissue sarcoma. Cancer 47:2269-2274, 1981.
6. Eilber FR, Townsend CM, Weisenberger TH et al.: A clinicopathologic study: preoperative intraarterial adriamycin and radiation therapy for extremity soft tissue sarcoma. In: Management of Primary Soft Tissue Tumors: Proceedings of the Annual Clinical Conference on Cancer, M.D. Anderson Tumor Institute. Chicago, Year Book Medical Publishers, pp. 411-422, 1977.
7. Eilber FR, Mirra JJ, Grant TT, et al: Is amputation necessary for sarcomas? A seven-year experience with limb salvage. Ann Surg 192:431-437, 1980.
8. Shiu MH, Castro EB, Hajdu SI, Fortner JG: Surgical treatment of 297 soft tissue sarcomas of the lower extremity. Ann Surg 182:597-602, 1975.
9. Shiu MH, Hajdu SI: Management of soft tissue sarcomas of the extremity. Seminars in Oncol 8:172-179, 1981.
10. Henschke UK, Hilaris BS, Mahan GD: Afterloading in interstitial and intracavitary radiation therapy. Am J Roentgenol Nucl Med 90:386-395, 1963.
11. Hilaris BS, Nori D: Brachytherapy oncology: concepts and techniques. IN: McKenna RJ, Murphy GP (eds.): Fundamentals of Surgical Oncology. New York, McMillan, pp.335-344, 1986.
12. Hilaris BS: Personal communication.
13. Ellis F: Connective tissue sarcomata. In: Hilaris BS (ed.): Handbook of Interstitial Brachytherapy. Acton, Massachusetts, Publishing Sciences Group, pp.263-273,

1975.
14. Ellis F: Tumor-bed implantation at the time of surgery. In: Hilaris BS (ed.): Afterloading: twenty years of experience, 1955-1975. New York, Memorial Sloan-Kettering Cancer Center, pp.263-273, 1975.
15. Shiu MH, Turnbull AD, Nori D, et al.: Control of locally advanced extremity soft tissue sarcoma by function-saving resection and brachytherapy. Cancer 53:1385-1392, 1984.
16. Shiu MH, Collin C, Hilaris BS et al.: Limb preservation and tumor control in the treatment of popliteal and antecubital soft tissue sarcomas. Cancer 57:1632-1639, 1986.
17. Anderson LL, Hilaris BS, Wagner LK: A nomograph for planar implant planning. Endocurietherapy/Hyperthermia Oncol 1:9-15, 1985.
18. Anderson LL, Wagner LV, Schauer TH: Memorial Hospital methods of dose calculations for Ir-192. In: George FW (ed.): Modern Interstitial and Intracavitary Radiation Cancer Management. New York, Masson Publishing USA Inc, pp.1-7, 1981.
19. Hall EJ, Lam YM: The renaissance in low dose-rate inter-stitial implants: radiobiological considerations. Front Radiat Ther Onc 12:21-34, 1978.
20. Devereux DF, Kent H, Brennan M: Time dependent effects of Adriamycin and x-ray therapy on wound healing in the rat. Cancer 45:2805-2810, 1980.
21. Genest P, Hilaris BS, Nori D et al: Iodine-125 as a substitute for Iridium-192 in temporary interstitial implants. Endocurietherapy/Hyperthermia Oncology 1:223-228, 1985.
22. Arbeit JM, Hilaris BS, Brennan MF: Wound complications in the multimodality modality treatment of extremity and superficial truncal soft tissue sarcomas. J Clin oncol 5:400-408, 1987.
23. Brennan MF, Hilaris BS, Shiu MH, et al.: Local recurrence in adult soft tissue sarcoma. Arch Surg, in press 1987.

NEOADJUVANT CHEMOTHERAPY, RADIATION, AND LIMITED SURGERY FOR HIGH GRADE SOFT TISSUE SARCOMA OF THE EXTREMITY

Frederick Eilber, M.D.[1], Armando Giuliano, M.D.,
James Huth, M.D., Joseph Mirra, M.D., Gerald Rosen, M.D.,
and Donald Morton, M.D.

Malignant soft tissue sarcomas of the extremity continue to present clinical challenges in terms of local tumor control and preservation of a functional extremity. Historically, surgical excision of the primary tumor was the primary mode of therapy and, in order to achieve local tumor control, radical surgical procedures were necessary.(1) This involved amputation in approximately 35% of the cases, or large compartment resections in the remainder.(2) Although these treatment methods were effective in terms of local tumor control, they all resulted in significant functional impairment. Limited surgical excision, which is possible in approximately 75% of cases, followed by high-dose radiation therapy has recently been shown to be equally effective in terms of providing local tumor control and has, in general, provided excellent function.(3-7) The goals of primary therapy in extremity soft tissue sarcomas are to obtain local tumor control, achieve the best functional results with the fewest complications, lower cost both in terms of time, money and function, and finally to design a therapy that is applicable and acceptable to the most patients. In order to improve the historical results of therapy, in 1974 we began a series of consecutive protocols at the UCLA School of Medicine, evaluating the effect of neoadjuvant (preoperative) therapy with intra-arterial chemotherapy, radiation therapy and subsequent surgical excision.

This paper then will summarize the experience in the treatment of high grade soft tissue sarcomas at the University of California at Los Angeles over the past 15 years.

Patients and Methods

From 1972 to 1987, the Division of Surgical Oncology at UCLA School of Medicine evaluated and treated 374 patients with Grade II or III soft tissue sarcomas of the extremity. (8) The patients ranged in age from 13 to 90 years of age and included 189 males and 175 females. The most common anatomic site was the thigh, occurring in 151 patients. The most common histologic types were liposarcoma (87), malignant fibrous histiocytoma (57), synovial cell sarcoma (56), and

---

[1]Division of Surgical Oncology, Department of Surgery,
UCLA School of Medicine, 9th Floor, Factor Building,
10833 LeConte Ave., Los Angeles, CA 90024.

J. R. Ryan and L. O. Baker (eds.), Recent Concepts in Sarcoma Treatment, 115–122.
© 1988 by Kluwer Academic Publishers.

fibrosarcoma (29). All patients had either primary or locally recurrent disease and none had metastatic disease on initial presentation. All patients with low grade (Grade I) soft tissue sarcomas were excluded from the analysis.

Four sequential treatment programs were employed. The first, a historical control group, consisted of 63 patients who were treated from 1972 to 1976. These patients received "standard" surgical therapy which included amputation for 21 patients, wide excision for 11, and in 31 a wide excision followed by 6000cG. Radiation therapy was given at standard 200cG fractions for 5 days over 6 weeks.

A prospective study group (3500cG) was begun in 1974 (Group 1) and received a preoperative treatment regimen consisting of intra-arterial doxorubicin 30mg/day x 3 delivered by an indwelling intra-arterial catheter with 24-hour infusion.(9) The catheter was placed in a high flow vessel such as the common femoral or axillary artery, and immediately following the infusion patients received radiation therapy at 350cG fractions for 10 days (3500cG). The entire region (compartment) of the tumor (e.g., thigh or arm) was treated sparing a strip of skin opposite the primary biopsy site. Approximately 1-2 weeks following radiation therapy the tumor was excised by wide excision.(1) Operations were performed through normal uninvolved tissue planes and pathologic confirmation of tumor-free margins was obtained at the time of operation. In some instances the tumor margin was less than 1 mm., most often when the primary tumor was adjacent to an artery, vein or bone, in which case either adventitia, perineurium, or periosteum was removed. No attempt was made at compartment resection.

A second group (Group 2) of 137 consecutive patients was treated from 1981 to 1984 with an identical chemotherapy regimen of intra-arterial doxorubicin 30mg/day x 3 for the lower extremities and 20mg/day x 3 for the upper extremities, followed by radiation therapy of 350cG fractions for 5 days (1750cG) followed by an identical surgical procedure.(10)

A third group of 97 patients (Group 3) was treated from 1984 to 1987. In this group of patients, the randomization was carried out between intra-arterial chemotherapy (45) versus the same dose of intravenous chemotherapy (51) followed by radiation therapy at 350cG fractions x 8 (2800cG). Again, the preoperative therapy was followed by an identical wide surgical excision.

Postoperative follow-up included physical examination and chest x-ray once a month for the first year, once every two months for the second year, and once every 6 months for the 4th, 5th, and 6th years. Whole lung tomograms or computerized tomographic scans of the chest were done at 6-month intervals. Postoperative adjuvant chemotherapy was given to some patients with high grade sarcomas. Twenty-seven patients received doxorubicin and high-dose methotrexate, and 62 patients received Adriamycin as a single agent.

Statistical evaluation of the overall survival and recurrence rates was done by the Life Table Method of analysis using the Mantell-Cox statistical methods. Pathologic evaluation of resected tumor specimens was performed by one of the authors without prior knowledge of treatment. Ten to 20 sections were taken from different portions of the tumor and at least 10 high power fields for each slide were examined. Necrosis was evaluated on the basis of lack of nuclei.

TABLE 1					(1972-76)	
CONTROL						
(NON-PROTOCOL)						
GRADE #		AMP	PRIMARY RX WIDE EXC	EXC & XRT	RECURRENCE LOCAL	COMPLICATIONS
2	20	2	6	12	4	5
3	43	19	5	19	10	9
	63	21	11	31	14	14
		(33%)			(22%)	(22%)

Results

In the original treatment (control group) of 63 patients treated by standard methods, it was necessary to perform amputative procedures in 21 (33%) of the patients. Fourteen (22%) had complications of treatment including wound slough, edema and neuritis. Fourteen patients (22%) had local disease recurrence (Table 1). Three of the 19 patients (16%) who had amputation had local recurrence, as did 4 of the patients treated by wide excision alone, and 7 treated by wide excision and postoperative radiation therapy.

Group 1. A total of 77 patients were treated with intra-arterial Adriamycin and 3500cG. Twelve patients had Grade II tumors and 65 had Grade III. In 60 patients this was the first treatment of the primary tumor, and in 17 it was the treatment for locally recurrent disease (Table 2). Of these 77 patients, 3 (4%) required amputation and 4 (5%) had local tumor recurrence. Median follow-up of this group of patients is now 8 years. Complications as a result of treatment occurred in 33 (43%) of the patients, and in 18 (23%) of the total group, a second operation was required to treat the complication. The most commonly encountered complication was wound slough in 15 patients. Fracture of adjacent long bones occurred in 8 (10%) and required open intramedullary fixation. In all instances pathologic evaluation showed no evidence of recurrent tumor. Because of this relatively high complication rate, the treatment program was altered in 1981 to reduce the radiation dose by one half from 3500cG to 1750cG.

| TABLE 2 | | | | | | (1974-1984) |

3500 cG

GRADE	#	AMP 1 /2	RECURRENCE LOCAL	COMPLICATIONS # / SURG		NED
2	12	0 1	0	6	2	10
3	65	2 -	4	27	16	38
TOTAL	77	3	4	33	18	48

Group 2. A total of 137 patients were treated with intra-arterial doxorubicin and radiation therapy at 350cG fractions x 5 for a total dose of 1750cG (Table 3). Forty-three patients had Grade II tumors and 94 had Grade III. Of the entire group, 7 (5%) required primary amputation to control their primary tumor, a total of 17 (12%) developed locally recurrent disease. The median follow-up for this group of patients is 48 months. Thirty-five of the 137 (25%) developed a complication following surgery; however, only 8 of the total group (5%) required re-operation for this complication. Only two patients had fractures of adjacent bone. This local recurrence rate of 12% was statistically significantly inferior to the previously noted 5% local recurrence rate of the group treated with 3500cG. In addition, the complication rate requiring re-operation was significantly less. Because of the increased local recurrence rate, the third protocol was begun in 1984.

| TABLE 3 | | | | | | (3|81 - 11|84) |

1750 cG

GRADE	#	AMP 1° /2°	RECURRENCE LOCAL	COMPLICATION # / SURG		NED
2	43	- 1	4	11	2	41
3	94	4 2	13	24	6	64
TOTAL	137	7	17	35	8	105
%		(5)	(12)	(25)	(5)	(77)

GRADE	#	AMP 1°/2°	RECURRENCE LOCAL	COMPLICATION # / SURG		NED
				2800 cG (11/84 - 9/87)		
2	32	- -	1	8	2	32
3	65	1 1	4	17	8	59
TOTAL	97	2	5	23	10	91
%		(2)	(5)	(23)	(10)	(94)

TABLE 4

Group 3. To date, a total of 97 patients have been treated with preoperative doxorubicin and radiation therapy consisting of 350cG fractions x 8 for a total dose of 2800cG. These patients were randomized to receive the same dose of doxorubicin either intravenously (51 patients) or intra-arterially (45 patients). A total of 97 patients have been entered into this study and to date two patients (2%) have required primary amputation, 5 patients (5%) have experienced a local recurrence (Table 4). The median follow-up of this group is now 24 months. Twenty-three (23%) of the patients have had a complication and 10 (10%) of the entire group required surgery to correct this complication.

A preliminary comparison of the intravenous versus intra-arterial route shows no statistical difference in the local recurrence or complication rate in these two groups of patients. Of the 45 patients treated with intra-arterial Adriamycin and 2800cG, 2 have developed a local recurrence, and of the 51 patients treated via the intravenous route, 3 have developed a local recurrence. The complications are similar between the two groups. Sufficient time, however, has not elapsed to make a final statistical comparison of the intra-arterial versus intravenous route of administration.

Local Tumor Control

Of the patients in the three consecutive study groups, a total of 26/311 (8.3%) have developed local recurrence. There are statistical differences between the three groups with 5% local recurrence rate in Groups 1 and 3, and 12% local recurrence rate in Group 2. All three groups, however, have fared better than the historical control groups who had a 25% incidence of local recurrence. Of the patients who developed local recurrence in the three treatment groups, 25% have required amputation in order to control the recurrence, and 75% have had additional local surgical procedures.

TABLE 5				
			SURVIVAL	
DOSE XRT	GRADE	#	LIVING	%
3500	2	12	10	83
1750	2	43	41	95
2800	2	32	32	100
TOTAL		87	83	95%
		#	RANGE	MEDIAN
EXPIRED		4	(27 - 64)	60

Overall Patient Survival

The overall patient survival of the patients in the three protocol treatments is given in Tables 5 and 6. Of the 87 patients with Grade II sarcomas, 83 (95%) remain alive and free of recurrent disease. Four patients have expired at a range of 27 to 64 months, with a median of 60 months. There was a total of 224 patients with high grade (Grade III) extremity soft tissue sarcomas and, of these, a total of 161 (74%) remain alive. Sixty-three patients have expired at a range of 4 to 50 months following initial diagnosis, with a median of 14 months. There was no difference in the overall survival of patients receiving postoperative adjuvant chemotherapy compared to those that did not.(11) A significant increase in death rate was noted for patients with Grade III sarcomas with increasing tumor size, in that of the patients who had 1-5cm tumor 14% have expired, in those with 5-10cm size 20% have expired, 10-15cm in size 34% have expired, and greater than 20cm in size 40% have expired.

The overall results of standard therapy for extremity sarcomas, that is surgery alone or surgery plus postoperative radiation, in our control series are similar to those reported by others.(1-5) The necessity for amputation in 35% of these patients appears to be a relatively constant figure. In addition, the 25% incidence of local disease recurrence also appears common to many reported series.

The protocol of intra-arterial doxorubicin and 3500cG of radiation was very successful in that it allowed nonamputative treatment for 95% of patients. The local recurrence rate of 5% was superior to that of standard methods of therapy. However, the complication rate of 45% and re-operation rate of 23% appeared to be too high. The reduction of the radiation doses to 1750cG did reduce the serious complication rate, requiring re-operation in 5%. However, the local recurrence rate of 12% in Group 2 was statistically inferior to the prior dose of radiation therapy.

TABLE 6	SURVIVAL			
DOSE XRT	GRADE	#	LIVING	%
3500	3	65	38	59%
1750	3	94	64	68%
2800	3	65	59	90%
TOTAL		224	161	74%
		#	RANGE	MEDIAN
	EXPIRED	63	(4-50)	14

Therefore, there does appear to be a dose response to radiation therapy in extremity soft tissue sarcomas. Increasing the total dose of radiation therapy to 2800cG appears to have further reduced the incidence of local recurrence and maintained a relatively low rate of complications requiring re-operation. However, additional follow-up is necessary to make a statistical comparison.

These studies also re-emphasize the importance of tumor grade in terms of overall patient survival.(8) Patients with Grade II soft tissue sarcomas have a low chance of systemic metastases; however, the group of patients with Grade III sarcomas appear to have a significant risk (at least 40%) of distant disease. In addition, the size of the primary tumor also appears to be a major prognostic factor in patients with Grade III sarcomas.

From our studies, it appears that all three preoperative protocols of doxorubicin plus radiation therapy of either 3500cG, 1750cG, or 2800cG allowed us to treat a very high percentage of patients (95%) with nonamputative surgery, compared to patients who received no preoperative therapy. In addition, the local control rate was superior to the control group in both instances. The complication rate was high in all three treatment groups as well as the control group, and has been reduced somewhat by the changing doses of radiation therapy.

The concepts of preoperative therapy have been advocated and described by many investigators. The treatment of a tumor prior to operation allows a clearer definition of the operative margin, and careful preoperative planning with CAT scans allows orderly planning of the surgical approach. In our experience, preoperative treatment with chemotherapy and radiation more clearly defines the tumor limits at the time of operation and also provides the pathologist the opportunity to evaluate the treatment effect on the resected specimen. Finally, all three of these protocols were feasible in that greater than 95% of the patients who were candidates for these protocols complied with them and actually completed treatment.

Finally, we feel that the patient with extremity soft tissue sarcoma is an ideal model system for sequentially testing the various treatment alternatives. With preoperative therapy, evaluation can be made of local tumor control and patient survival, as well as pathologic assessment of the treatment effect on the primary tumor. The use of additional drugs preoperatively, in addition to Adriamycin, would seem a logical extension of these studies.

REFERENCES

1. Enneking WF, Spanier SS, Malawer MM: The effect of the anatomic setting on the results of surgical procedures for soft part sarcomas of the thigh. Cancer 47(5):1005-1022, 1981.
2. Shiu MH, Castro EB, Hajdu S: Surgical treatment of 297 soft tissue sarcomas of the extremity. Ann Surg 182:597-602, 1975.
3. Lindberg RD: The role of radiation therapy in the treatment of soft tissue sarcoma in adults. Proceedings of the 7th National Cancer Congress, Lippincott, 1973.
4. Suit HD, Russell WO, Martin R: Sarcoma of soft tissue. Clinical and histopathologic parameters and response to treatment. Cancer 35:1478-1483, 1975.
5. Suit HD, Proppe KH, Mankin HJ, Woods WC: Preoperative radiation therapy for sarcoma of the soft tissue. Cancer 47:2269-2274, 1981.
6. Lattuada A, Kenda R: Postoperative radiotherapy of soft tissue sarcoma. Tumori 67(2,Suppl A):191, 1981.
7. Rosenberg S, Tepper J, Glatstein E, Costa J, Baker A, Brennan M, DeMoss E, Seipp C, Sindelar W, Sugarbaker P, Wesley R: The treatment of soft tissue sarcomas of the extremities. Prospective randomized evaluations of (1) limb sparing surgery plus radiation compared to amputation, and (2) the role of adjuvant chemotherapy. Ann Surg 96(3):305-315, 1982.
8. Russell WO, Cohen J, Enzinger F, et al.: A clinical and pathologic staging system for soft tissue sarcoma. Cancer 40:1562-1570, 1977.
9. Eilber FR, Mirra JJ, Grant TT, Weisenburger T, Morton DL: Is amputation necessary for sarcoma - a 7-year experiment with limb salvage. Ann Surg 192:431-437, 1980.
10. Eilber FR, Morton DL, Eckardt J, Grant T, Weisenburger T: Limb salvage for skeletal & soft-tissue sarcomas: Multidisciplinary preoperative therapy. Cancer 53:2579-2584, 1984.
11. Eilber FR, Giuliano A, Huth J, Morton DL: Adjuvant Adriamycin in high grade extremity soft tissue sarcoma - a randomized prospective trial. Proc ASCO (C-488):125, 1986.

NATIONAL CANCER INSTITUTE EXPERIENCE IN THE MANAGEMENT OF HIGH-GRADE EXTREMITY SOFT TISSUE SARCOMAS

Alan R. Baker, M.D.[1], Alfred E. Chang, M.D.,
Eli Glatstein, M.D., Steven A. Rosenberg, M.D.

The Surgery Branch of the NCI has had a long-standing interest in the management of patients with soft tissue sarcomas. Table 1 summarizes the succession of clinical trials that we have performed during the past 13 years.

TABLE 1

PROSPECTIVE RANDOMIZED NCI STUDIES OF PATIENTS

WITH SOFT TISSUE SARCOMAS

Study	Patient Entry
1. Randomized and Historical-Control Study of Adjuvant Chemotherapy (extremity)	5/75 - 6/77
2. Role of Adjuvant Chemotherapy (extremity)	6/77 - 7/81
3. Standard Adjuvant Chemotherapy vs "pilot" chemotherapy (extremity)	7/81 - 10/83
4. Limb-sparing surgery vs. amputation (extremity)	5/75 - 7/81
5. Rule of adjuvant radiotherapy (extremity)	10/83 - present

In our initial effort, we sought to explore the impact of adjuvant chemotherapy on patients whose primary high-grade extremity tumor was managed by either amputation or, if clinically indicated, a limb-sparing wide excision of the tumor, coupled with high-dose postoperative local X-ray therapy. All patients received postoperative courses every 28 days of both doxorubicin 50 mg/M^2 i.v. escalating by 10 mg/M^2 increments to 70 mg/M^2) and cyclophosphamide (500 mg/M^2 i.v. escalating by 100 mg/M^2 increments to 700 mg/M^2) until a cumulative dose of between 480 - 530 mg/M^2 of doxorubicin had been reached. Methotrexate (50 mg/kg i.v. escalating at 50 mg/kg increments to 250 mg/kg) with citrovorum factor rescue was then given over 6 successive monthly cycles.

---

[1]National Cancer Institute, Surgery Branch, Bldg. 10 2B06, 9000 Rockville Pike, Bethesda, MD 20205.

J. R. Ryan and L. O. Baker (eds.), Recent Concepts in Sarcoma Treatment, 123–129.
© 1988 by Kluwer Academic Publishers.

124

All patients admitted to this study had high-grade
(Grade II or III) soft tissue sarcomas and were free of
regional lymph node or distant dissemination (AJC Stages
IIa,b and IIIa,b). Patients who had received prior chemotherapy or radiation therapy, as well as those less than 30 years
old with a diagnosis of either embryonal or alveolar rhabdomyosarcoma were excluded from this as well as subsequent
trials. All patients were followed for evidence of local
and/or disseminated recurrent disease at roughly 3 monthly
intervals for the initial 3 years and yearly thereafter: full
lung tomography or chest CAT was done every six months. The
overall results of this trial, details or surgical management, radiation therapy and adjuvant chemotherapy and toxicity have been previously reported (1-3), and are further
updated in this presentation as of December 1, 1986.

Survival curves were computed using the method of Kaplan
and Meier. Comparison of disease-free and overall survival
rates was performed using the test of Mantel and Haenszel.
All P values are two-sided.

Twenty-six patients, accessioned to this initial trial
between May 1975 and June 1977, were all treated with the
above described adjuvant chemotherapy regimen (standard) and
compared to 46 matched historical control patients from our
institution treated prior to 1975 who otherwise met eligibility requirements but did not receive chemotherapy. Recurrence-free and overall survival curves for these patients are
shown in Figures 1 and 2. Substantial, statistically signifi-

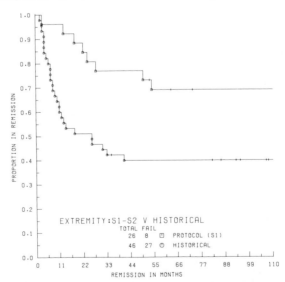

FIGURE 1: Disease-free survival in nonrandomized, historically controlled trial for patients with high-grade extremity
sarcomas. Patients receiving adjuvant chemotherapy had
improved disease-free survival compared to historical
controls (P = 0.008).

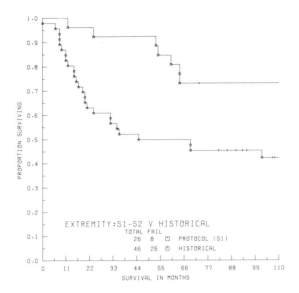

FIGURE   2: True   survival   in   nonrandomized,   historically
  controlled   trial   for   patients with   high-grade extremity
  sarcomas.   Patients   receiving adjuvant   chemotherapy had a
  survival benefit compared to historical controls
  (P = 0.014).

cant   improvement is demonstrated for the adjuvant chemotherapy recipients; recurrence-free survival rates at 5 years are
70%   and 40% for   the chemotherapy recipients   and historical
controls,   respectively (P = 0.008),   while the corresponding
overall survival rates are 73% and 48% (P = 0.014).
     Although   adjuvant drug treatment appeared   quite effec-
tive, we felt a more critically conducted,   prospective   randomized trial was necessary to prove its efficacy.
     In   the   successor   study, patients   were   randomized to
either   receive immediate postoperative adjunctive chemotherapy   or   not. Eligibility   requirements and treatment-related
details   remained   otherwise unchanged.   Sixty-seven patients
were   randomized on   this study   between June   1977 and   July
1981.
     The   results   of   this trial   confirmed the observations
made   in the   pilot study   and are   graphically presented   in
Figures   3 - 5.   The five-year recurrence-free   survival rate
for   the 39 patients   randomized to receive   chemotherapy was
75%   compared to 54% for the 28 patients in the group receiving   no chemotherapy (P = 0.037). The administration of adjuvant chemotherapy led to a statistically significant improvement in local control (P = 0.005) with one   local   recurrence
seen   in chemotherapy   recipients compared   to 4   in the   no-
chemotherapy group. The five-year overall survival rates were
80%   and 60% for the chemotherapy and no-chemotherapy groups,
respectively. This   trend   toward   improved   survival   among

126

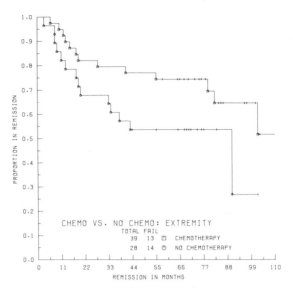

FIGURE 3: Actuarial analysis of disease-free survival in a prospective randomized trial examining adjuvant chemotherapy in high-grade extremity sarcomas. Patients treated with adjuvant chemotherapy had improved disease-free survival compared to those who did not receive chemotherapy (P = 0.037).

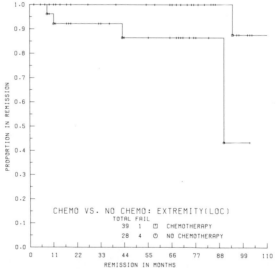

FIGURE 4: Time to local recurrence in high-grade extremity sarcoma patients randomized to receive adjuvant chemotherapy. Patients who developed distant disease as the site of first recurrence are censored on the curves. Patients treated with adjuvant chemotherapy had a reduced incidence of local recurrences compared to patients who did not receive chemotherapy (P = 0.005).

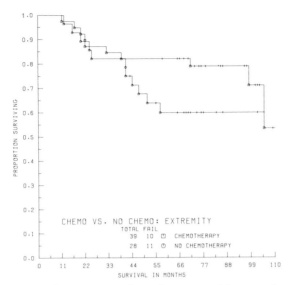

FIGURE 5: Actuarial analysis of overall survival in a prospective randomized trial examining adjuvant chemotherapy in high-grade extremity sarcomas. Patients treated with adjuvant chemotherapy had a trend toward improved overall survival compared to those who did not receive chemotherapy (P = 0.124).

chemotherapy recipients approaches - but does not achieve - statistical significance (P = 0.124).

A substantial amount of doxorubicin-induced cardiomyopathy was noted among adjuvant chemotherapy recipients in this and the prior trial. Almost 15% of our patients developed clinically evident congestive heart failure, while about half of those patients remaining asymptomatic who had received cumulative doses of doxorubicin, between 480 - 530 mg/M^2, were found to have abnormal left ventricular ejection fractions on ECG gaited radionuclide heart scans.

These observations led directly to our third generation trial. In this study, we sought to determine whether an altered adjuvant drug regimen could abrogate the cardiomyopathy while preserving the therapeutic gains noted. Patients were randomized to receive either the standard chemotherapy regimen described previously, or an alternative regimen. Methotrexate was eliminated from the short-course chemotherapy and the dose-intensity of doxorubicin/cyclophosphamide was modified as follows· Doxorubicin (70 mg/M^2 i.v.) and cyclophosphamide (700 mg/M2 i.v.) were administered for 5 monthly cycles such that the maximum cumulative dose of doxorubicin never exceeded 350 mg/m2 for any patient. Between July 1981 and October 1983, 88 patients were randomized on this trial. Recurrence-free and overall survival curves for the 41 patients randomized to receive standard chemotherapy and the 47 patients on the short-course chemotherapy are

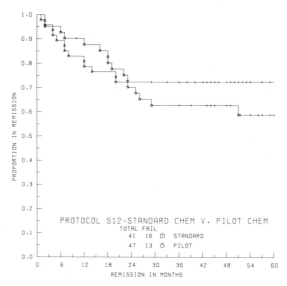

FIGURE 6: Actuarial analysis of disease-free survival in a prospective randomized trail comparing standard chemotherapy versus short-course chemotherapy. There is no significant difference between the curves.

given in Figures 6 and 7. Because no statistically significant difference is apparent between the two groups with regard to either parameter, we concluded that short-course chemotherapy is as good as the standard regimen and have adopted its use in a subsequent trial. Short-course chemotherapy led to actuarial five-year recurrence-free and overall survival rates of 72% and 75%, respectively, in contrast to the 58% and 69% corresponding figures for the standard chemotherapy.

Our experience through this succession of studies has led to the overall conclusion that adjuvant chemotherapy is of benefit to patients with high-grade extremity sarcomas and should be employed accordingly. In an effort to determine the contribution that adjuvant radiotherapy confers on local control, all high-grade sarcoma patients, treated with limb-sparing surgery entering our current trial, are treated with short-course chemotherapy and randomized to either receive or not receive radiotherapy. Given the exceedingly small probability that low-grade (Grade I) extremity sarcomas have for metastasizing, we do not recommend adjunctive chemotherapy in their management. Instead, in an ongoing, randomized trial, the role of surgery alone or surgery and postoperative adjuvant radiotherapy is being evaluated in patients with Grade I lesions.

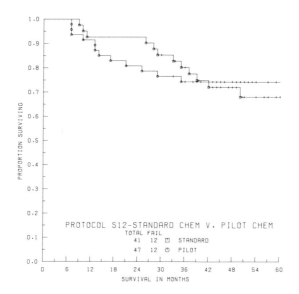

FIGURE 7: Actuarial analysis of overall survival in a prospective randomized trial of standard chemotherapy versus short-course chemotherapy. There is no significant difference between the curves.

REFERENCES

1. Rosenberg SA, Tepper J, Glatstein E, et al.: Treatment of soft tissue sarcomas of the extremities. Prospective randomized evaluations of (1) limb sparing surgery plus radiation therapy compared with amputation and (2) the role of adjuvant chemotherapy. Ann Surg 196:305-315, 1982.
2. Rosenberg SA, Tepper J, Glatstein E, et al.: Prospective randomized evaluation of adjuvant chemotherapy in adults with soft tissue sarcomas of the extremities. Cancer 52:424-434, 1983.
3. Dresdale A, Bonow RO, Wesley R, et al.: Prospective evaluation of doxorubicin induced cardiomyopathy resulting from post-surgical adjuvant treatment of patients with soft tissue sarcomas. Cancer 52:51-60, 1983.

ADJUVANT THERAPY FOR SOFT TISSUE SARCOMAS

Laurence H. Baker, D.O.*

The purpose of this manuscript is to provide an overview of the American experiences with the adjuvant use of chemotherapy for patients with soft tissue sarcomas treated with a curative intent but, nonetheless, at high risk of recurrence and/or dissemination. In addition, an update will be provided of the initial Intergroup Sarcoma Group protocol that addresses this issue. Several clinical trials have addressed this issue and the results are shown in Figures 1 -3). Figure 1 shows the clinical trials with a positive finding or trend

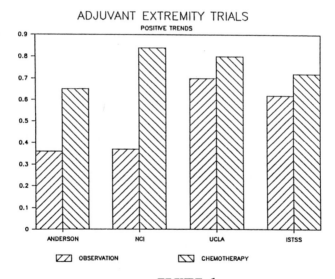

FIGURE 1

(in favor of chemotherapy) in patients with extremity sarcoma. The trials performed at the M.D. Anderson Hospital and the NCI are the most mature of all the studies. Both the Intergroup trial (which will be discussed in greater detail)

----

*Professor of Medicine; Director, Division of Hematology-Oncology, Wayne State University School of Medicine, P.O. Box 02188, Detroit, MI 48201.

J. R. Ryan and L. O. Baker (eds.), Recent Concepts in Sarcoma Treatment, 130–135.
© 1988 by Kluwer Academic Publishers.

and the UCLA trial do not show statistically different results from non-chemotherapy treated controls. "Negative"
trials of extremity sarcoma patients are shown in Figure 2.

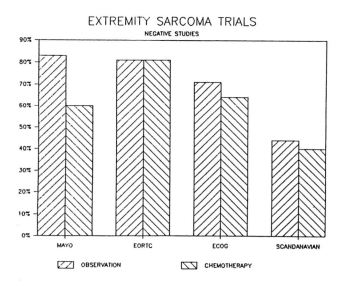

FIGURE 2

In Figure 3, the non-extremity results are shown. Details
for these clinical trials, including the number of patients,
chemotherapies investigated, per cent survival and disease-
free survival are shown in Table 1.

The Intergroup Sarcoma Committee was formed to pool the
resources of the various American cooperative groups to study
this complex clinical issue. In 1983, a clinical protocol was
adopted by the following cooperative groups:
>   Cancer and Acute Leukemia Group B
>   Eastern Cooperative Oncology Group
>   Northern California Oncology Group
>   Piedmont Oncology Group
>   Radiation Therapy Oncology Group
>   Southeastern Oncology Group
>   Southwestern Oncology Group

One hundred fourteen patients were randomly allocated to
either a no-further-treatment group or to receive adriamycin
at doses beginning at 70 mg/m2 Q. 3 weeks and increasing to
90 mg/m2 for a total of 6 doses. This report updates the
initial 81 patients accrued to this study. Eligibility
criteria included: Stage IIB - IVA (American Joint
Commission) soft tissue sarcoma, pathology negative margins,
no prior chemotherapy or radiotherapy, no known contra-
indication of adriamycin, age >16 years. Histological subtypes excluded from this trial included: mesothelioma,

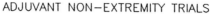

ADJUVANT NON—EXTREMITY TRIALS

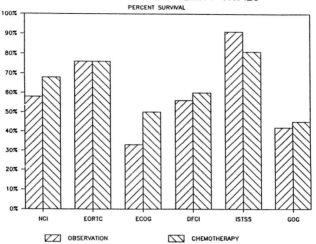

PERCENT SURVIVAL

☐☐ OBSERVATION   ◱◱ CHEMOTHERAPY

FIGURE 3

TABLE 1.

PRIOR EXTREMITY TRIALS

Institution	Drugs	Observation				Chemotherapy		
		N	% LC	% DFS	% S	% LC	% DFS	% S
M.D. Anderson	VACAD	47	100	35	36	93	54	65
Mayo	VACAD	48	67	68	83	67	88	60
NCI	CAM	65	54	64	37	100	73	84
EORTC	A	167	90	65	81	90	65	81
ECOG	A	18	100	71	71	100	72	64
DFCI	A	26	94	81	81	100	90	90
UCLA	A	119	90	52	70	90	56	80
SCAND	A	139	91	55	44	91	52	40
ISTSS	A	41	N/A	50	62	N/A	77	72

Kaposi's sarcoma, embryonal or alveolar rhabdomyosarcoma, and GI and GYN sarcomas. Initial curative therapy was specified in the protocol to be either conservative resection and a specified postoperative radiation therapy, or a radical resection as defined by Enneking.

In this population of patients, the tumor size was less than 5 cm in 30%, 5-10 cm in 43%, and greater than 10 cm in 26%. The primary tumor location was: buttocks/thigh 37%, trunk 28%, arm 15%, knee or below 12%, retroperitoneum 4%, and head and neck region 4%. The most frequent histologic subtypes were: malignant fibrous histiocytoma 31%, lipo-

sarcoma 21%, fibrosarcoma 9%, leiomyosarcoma 8%, and synovial
sarcoma 8%.

Moderate to severe toxicity notations in the initial 41
patients treated with adjuvant doxirubicin included cardiac
toxicity (3 patients), leukopenia (13 patients), thrombocytopenia (2 patients), nausea/vomiting (11 patients), and
stomatitis (4 patients).

Figure 4 shows the disease-free survival and overall
survival by size. Lesions less than 5 cm, despite their high

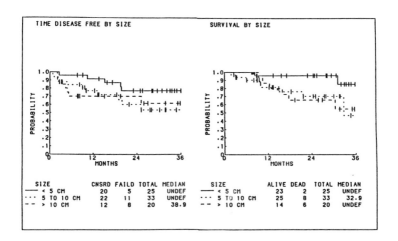

FIGURE 4

grade, did uniformly well. Figure 5 shows the overall survival and disease-free survival in the extremity only patients.
No statistical difference is yet demonstrated between the
adjuvantly-treated patients and the randomized control group.
There is a trend in favor of the chemotherapy-treated group
in disease-free survival (P = .06).

It should be underscored that this is the first preliminary analysis of this trial. Of particular note is that the
two "positive" trials are also the most mature. It is con-
ceivable, with sufficient time, that more trials will yield a
positive outcome in favor of adjuvant chemotherapy. In the
interim, the Intergroup Sarcoma program has launched a second
trial to address this issue. This new trial more precisely
defines the patient population (only patients with Grade 3
tumors will be admitted) and utilizes a more intensive combination chemotherapy regimen consisting of adriamycin, DTIC,
and Ifosphamide (with mesna), all given by continuous intravenous infusion. This trial anticipates randomizing 450
patients and, hopefully, will avoid drawing premature conclusions because of insufficient patient numbers.

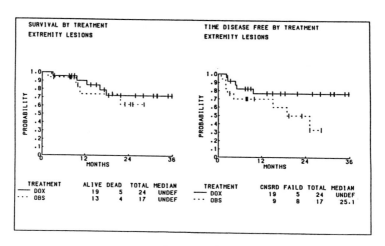

FIGURE 5

REFERENCES

1. Rosenberg SA, Suit HD, Baker LH: Sarcomas of soft tissues. In Cancer: Principles and Practice of Oncology. 2nd edition. DeVita VT, Hellman S, Rosenberg SA (eds.), Philadelphia, JB Lippincott Co., pp.1243-1291, 1985.
2. Antman KH, Blum RH, Wilson RE, Corson JM, Greenberger JS, Amato DA, Ash AS, Canellos GP, Frei E: Survival of patients with localized high grade soft tissue sarcoma with multi-modality therapy: a matched control study. Cancer 51:396-401, 1983.
3. Lindberg RD, Murphy WK, Benjamin RS, et al.: Adjuvant chemotherapy in the treatment of primary soft tissue sarcomas: a preliminary report. In Management of Bone and Soft Tissue Tumors (The University of Texas System Cancer Center, M.D. Anderson Hospital and Tumor Institute, 21st Annual Clinical Conference on Cancer). Chicago, IL, Year Book Medical Publishers, Inc., pp.343-352, 1977.
4. Muss HB, Bundy B, Disaia PJ, Homesley HD, Fowler WC, Creasman W, Yordan E: Treatment of recurrent or advanced uterine sarcoma. A randomized trial of doxorubicin versus doxorubicin and cyclophosphamide (A phase III trial of the Gynecologic Oncology Group), Cancer 55:1648-1653, 1985.
5. Borden EC, Amato D, Enterline HT, Lerner H, Carbone PP: Randomized comparison of adriamycin regimens for treatment of metastatic soft tissue sarcomas. Proc ASCO, 1983:231 (C902).
6. Omura GA, Major FJ, Blessing JA, et al.: A randomized study of adriamycin with and without dimethyl triazenoimidazole carboxamide in advanced uterine sarcomas. Cancer 52:626-632, 1983.

7. Benjamin RS, Terjanian TO, Barkley, et al.: The importance of combination chemotherapy for adjuvant treatment of high-risk patients with soft-tissue sarcomas of the extremities. In Adjuvant Therapy of Cancer. VS Salman (Ed.), Grune & Stratton Inc., 1987.

8. Edmonson JH: Systemic chemotherapy following complete excision of nonosseous sarcomas: Mayo Clinic experience. Cancer Treat Symp 3:89-97, 1985.

9. Rosenberg SA, Chang AE, Glatstein E: Adjuvant chemotherapy for treatment of extremity soft tissue sarcomas: review of National Cancer Institute experience. Cancer Treat Symp 3:83-88, 1985.

10. Glenn J, Kinsella T, Glatstein E, et al.: A randomized prospective trial of adjuvant chemotherapy in adults with soft tissue sarcomas of the head and neck, breast and trunk. Cancer 55:1206-1214, 1985.

11. Glenn J, Sindelar WF, Kinsella T, Glatstein E, Tepper J, Costa J, Baker A, Sugarbaker P, Brennan MF, Seipp C, et al.: Results of multimodality therapy of resectable soft-tissue sarcomas of the retroperitoneum.

12. Bramwell VHC, Rouessé J, Santoro A, et al.: European experience of adjuvant chemotherapy for soft tissue sarcoma: preliminary report of randomized trial of cyclophosphamide, vincristine, doxorubicin, and dacarbazine. Cancer Treat Symp 3:99-107, 1985.

13. Gherlinzoni F, Bacci G, Picci P, et al.: A randomized trial for the treatment of high-grade soft-tissue sarcomas of the extremities: preliminary observations. J Clin Oncol 4:552-558, 1986.

14. Eilber FR, Guiliano AE, Huth JF, Morton DL: Adjuvant adriamycin in high-grade extremity soft-tissue sarcoma - a randomized prospective trial. Proc ASCO 5:C-488, 1986.

15. Alvegard TA (for the Scandinavian Sarcoma Group): Adjuvant chemotherapy with adriamycin in high grade malignant soft tissue sarcoma - A Scandinavian randomized study. Proc ASCO 5:C-485, 1986.

16. Omura GA, Blessing JA, Major F, et al.: A randomized clinical trial of adjuvant adriamycin in uterine sarcomas: a Gynecological Oncology Group study. J Clin Oncol 3:1240-1245, 1985.

17. Antman K, Amato D, Pilepich M: A preliminary analysis of a randomized intergroup (SWOG, ECOG, CALGB, NCOG) trial of adjuvant doxorubicin for soft tissue sarcomas adjuvant chemotherapy, Tucson, AZ, 1986.

PEDIATRIC EXPERIENCE IN RHABDOMYOSARCOMA

Harold M. Maurer, M.D.*

Rhabdomyosarcoma (RMS) is the most common soft tissue sarcoma in the pediatric age group. Less than 500 new cases are seen each year in the United States, however. Because of this relatively low incidence, Phase III treatment strategies and various clinical-pathological characteristics of this malignancy are studied most effectively through a collaborative intergroup mechanism. In 1972, the multidisciplinary Intergroup Rhabdomyosarcoma Study (IRS) was initiated by Cancer and Leukemia Group B (CALGB), Children's Cancer Study Group (CCSG) and the Southwest Oncology Group (SWOG). The IRS has completed two studies (1972-78; 1978-84) and is in midst of the third (1984-present). The current participating cooperative groups are CCSG, the Pediatric Oncology Group (formerly the pediatric divisions of CALGB and SWOG) and, since 1980, the United Kingdom Children's Cancer Study Group.

IRS-I (1972-1978)

A total of 799 patients were registered on this study (Figure 1).(1) Of these, 686 were eligible, previously untreated patients under 21 years of age with RMS or undifferentiated sarcoma. These patients had a minimum potential follow-up time of 7 years at the last report.

Fifteen per cent of the patients were in clinical group (stage) I (localized disease, completely resected). They were randomized to receive either VAC (vincristine, actinomycin D, cyclophosphamide) or VAC + radiation. Approximately 80% of patients on either treatment were still disease-free (DFS) at 5 years and the survival rates of 93% and 81%, respectively (p = 0.67), also were not significantly different between treatments.

Clinical group II (regional disease, grossly resected) comprised 25% of the patients; they were randomized to receive either VA + radiation or VAC + radiation. At 5 years, the DFS and overall survival rates were not significantly different between treatments, 72% vs. 65% (p = 0.46) and 72% vs. 72%, respectively.

---

*Professor and Chairman, Department of Pediatrics, Children's Medical Center, Medical College of Virginia, Virginia Commonwealth University, P.O. Box 646, Richmond, Virginia 23298.

J. R. Ryan and L. O. Baker (eds.), Recent Concepts in Sarcoma Treatment, 136–143.
© 1988 by Kluwer Academic Publishers.

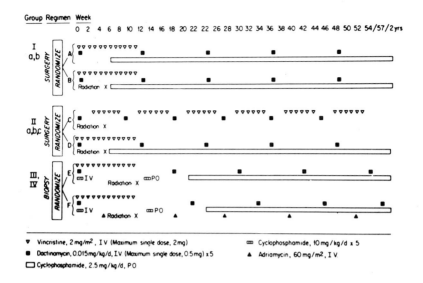

FIGURE 1: Intergroup Rhabdomyosarcoma Study-I therapy regimens (1972-78).

Patients in clinical groups III (gross residual disease after surgery; 41% of the total) and IV (metastatic disease at diagnosis; 19% of total) were randomized to receive either "pulse" VAC + radiation or "pulse" VAC + Adriamycin + radiation. The complete remission (CR) rate was 69% in group III and 50% in Group IV, with no statistically significant difference between treatments in either group. Those in CR in group III had a 60% chance of staying in remission for 5 years compared to 30% in group IV. The percentage alive at 5 years was 52% in group III compared to 20% in group IV (p < .0001). The 5-year survival rate for the entire cohort of 686 patients was 55%. With relapse, survival was poor, being 32% at 1 year and 17% at 2 years. Distant relapse occurred more often than local recurrence within each clinical group. Orbit and GU tumors carried the best prognosis and retroperitoneal tumors the worst prognosis.

In summary, for the treatments evaluated in IRS-I, there was no therapeutic advantage to including local radiation in the treatment of group I disease, or cyclophosphamide given as a daily low dose oral regimen in the treatment of group II disease, or Adriamycin in the treatment of groups III and IV diseases.

IRS-II (1978-84)

The study design of IRS-II was based upon the findings of IRS-I (Figure 2).(2,3) A total of 1115 patients were entered on study, of which 1002 patients were eligible. There were certain subcategories of patients that were handled

138

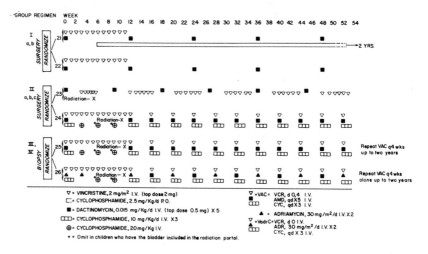

FIGURE 2: Intergroup Rhabdomyosarcoma Study-II
therapy regimens (1978-84).

differently in IRS-II than in IRS-I where they were treated
only according to disease grouping. Patients with extremity
alveolar disease in clinical groups I and II were treated
more intensively than other group I and some group II patients because of their relatively unfavorable outcome in
IRS-I. Patients with cranial parameningeal tumors (primaries
of the nasopharynx, nasal cavity, nasal sinuses, middle ear-
mastoid region, pterygopalatine-infratemporal fossa) with or
without bone erosion at the base of the skull, cranial nerve
palsy or intracranial extension were given CNS prophylaxis in
addition to systemic therapy, because of the approximately
35% incidence of CNS extension and nearly 100% mortality rate
from this complication in IRS-I. Patients with primary tumors
of the bladder, prostate, vagina and uterus were treated with
primary chemotherapy followed as needed by radiation therapy
and surgery in an attempt to improve bladder salvage while
maintaining the approximately 70% survival rate achieved with
all three modalities used in combination in IRS-I.

Patients in clinical group I (excluding alveolar extremity cases) were randomized to receive either VAC or VA (same
regimen minus cyclophosphamide), without radiation. Patients
in clinical group II (excluding alveolar extremity cases)
were randomized to receive either intensive VA + radiation or
repetitive courses of "pulse" VAC + radiation. Patients in
clinical groups I and II with extremity alveolar tumors
received repetitive "pulse" VAC ± radiation (according to
group). Clinical groups III and IV patients were treated with
repetitive "pulse" VAC ± Adriamycin + radiation. Addition-

ally, patients with cranial parameningeal tumors at risk of CNS extension received cranial radiation plus courses of methotrexate, hydrocortisone and cytosine arabinoside in combination intrathecally.

Patients with special pelvic tumors (bladder, prostate, vagina and uterus) were treated with primary repetitive "pulse" VAC followed as needed with radiation and/or surgery to obtain CR status, in hope of preserving the bladder, while not jeopardizing survival.

The results of IRS-II for the treatments evaluated may be summarized as follows:

1. Deletion of cyclophosphamide from the standard VAC regimen for group I patients was detrimental to local tumor control. Thus, one should not delete cyclophosphamide + radiation from this regimen. However, a more intensive VA schedule should be tried.

2. When intensive VA + radiation were given for Group II disease, they did as well as repetitive "pulse" VAC + radiation.

3. Both repetitive "pulse" VAC and VadrC-VAC regimens for two years, plus radiation, improved survival in group III patients as did CNS prophylaxis for cranial parameningeal tumors. The beneficial effect of these treatments for group IV was less obvious and the outcome for group IV remains poor.

4. Patients with alveolar extremity tumors in groups I and II did better when they were treated with therapy designed for more advanced disease groups.

5. Repetitive "pulse" VAC primary chemotherapy for special pelvic tumors lacked sufficient tumoricidal activity to significantly improve bladder salvage.

Comparing IRS-II vs. I by clinical group from I-IV, survival rates at 3 years were: 87% vs. 87%, 79% vs. 74%, 67% vs. 57% (p $<$.001) and 32% vs. 23% (p = .12), respectively. Comparing IRS-II vs. I at 3 years, the overall survival experience was significantly (p < .001) superior for IRS-II, being 66% for IRS-II vs. 60% for IRS-I.

IRS-III (1984-Present)

The results of IRS-II led to the design of IRS-III, which is still in progress (Figure 3). Patients are assigned or randomized by tumor histology (favorable vs. unfavorable), primary site (orbit, special pelvic, paratesticular, cranial parameningeal, head non-parameningeal, other) and clinical group. The results are too early to report.

Other Studies

The first SIOP study of RMS (1975-83) included only stages II and III (TNM staging) patients in the trial.(4,5) One hundred sixty-two patients were randomized to primary VAC-Vadr chemotherapy given until maximum tumor regression was obtained versus one course of VAC, either arm followed by surgery or radiation to the residual tumor. Maintenance chemotherapy was VAC-Vadr given for up to 18 months from the

140

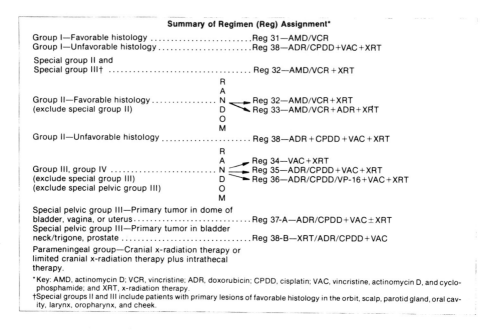

Summary of Regimen (Reg) Assignment*

Group I—Favorable histology ....Reg 31—AMD/VCR
Group I—Unfavorable histology ....Reg 38—ADR/CPDD+VAC+XRT

Special group II and
Special group III† ....Reg 32—AMD/VCR+XRT

Group II—Favorable histology ....R A N D O M → Reg 32—AMD/VCR+XRT / Reg 33—AMD/VCR+ADR+XRT
(exclude special group II)

Group II—Unfavorable histology ....Reg 38—ADR+CPDD+VAC+XRT

Group III, group IV ....R A N D O M → Reg 34—VAC+XRT / Reg 35—ADR/CPDD+VAC+XRT / Reg 36—ADR/CPDD/VP-16+VAC+XRT
(exclude special group III)
(exclude special pelvic group III)

Special pelvic group III—Primary tumor in dome of
bladder, vagina, or uterus............................Reg 37-A—ADR/CPDD+VAC±XRT
Special pelvic group III—Primary tumor in bladder
neck/trigone, prostate ....Reg 38-B—XRT/ADR/CPDD+VAC

Parameningeal group—Cranial x-radiation therapy or
limited cranial x-radiation therapy plus intrathecal
therapy.

*Key: AMD, actinomycin D; VCR, vincristine; ADR, doxorubicin; CPDD, cisplatin; VAC, vincristine, actinomycin D, and cyclo-
phosphamide; and XRT, x-radiation therapy.
†Special groups II and III include patients with primary lesions of favorable histology in the orbit, scalp, parotid gland, oral cavity, larynx, oropharynx, and cheek.

**FIGURE 3: Randomization schema for Intergroup
Rhabdomyosarcoma Study-III (1984-   )**

start of chemotherapy. There was no significant difference in
outcome between treatments. The overall survival rate at 3
years was 42%. Stages I and IV were treated with VAC-Vadr +
surgery + radiation without randomization. Survival at 3
years was 76% and 33%, respectively.

In the second SIOP study which began in 1984, IVA
(ifosfamide, vincristine and actinomycin D) is the mainstay
of chemotherapy for all stages. Cisplatin + Adriamycin are
added for patients who achieve less than a CR. Surgery and
radiation are added for residual disease in stage I and as
part of the treatment plan for stages II-IV. A preliminary
report on the IVA induction regimen (pilot study) in 33
patients with stages II-IV disease indicated a CR rate of
79%, with an overall response rate of 94%, clearly superior
to any induction combination previously reported.

The Italian Cooperative Group entered 117 evaluable
patients on study between 1979-85.(7) All patients were under
15 years of age. The study compared VAC vs. VAC-M (modified)
in which somewhat higher doses of each drug were given.
Surgery and radiation therapy were added to eradicate residual tumor. Maintenance therapy consisted of alternate courses
of C-Adr-V and VAC-M for a total treatment period of 12-18
months. At 3 years, the overall survival rates were 86% in
IRS group I, 65% in group II, 60% in group III and 31% in
group IV, with no significant difference between treatments

in each group. The CR rate to primary chemotherapy was 74%.

The results of the German Oncology Group studies of RMS are reported elsewhere in this publication by Dr. Jorn Treuner.

The St. Jude Children's Research Hospital reported their experience using the combination of dacarbazine + Adriamycin in 26 children with untreated RMS, 14 with local or regional disease and 12 with disseminated disease.(8) Responders continued to receive this drug combination during maintenance therapy in alternating sequence with VAC. After three course of therapy, 17 patients (65%) achieved PR status and 9 failed to respond. The lack of CR's to this combination indicated that it was less effective than VAC as frontline therapy.

The National Cancer Institute treated 68 newly-diagnosed, high-risk sarcoma patients in their first complete remission with an intensive consolidation including vincristine, Adriamycin and cyclophosphamide and total body irradiation (4.0 Gy/d x 2d) followed by reinfusion of unpurged autologous bone marrow. Eighteen of the 68 patients had RMS, groups III and IV diseases. The overall actuarial survival at 24 months for the entire study group was 60% and DFS was 40%. This intensive regimen, although it included total body irradiation with autologous marrow rescue, appeared to offer no advantage over conventional treatment for these two groups of patients.

Because human RMS xenograft studies proved melphalan (LPAM) superior to conventional drugs inducing CR, Horowitz, et al., gave previously untreated RMS patients with poor prognoses LPAM, 45 mg/m^2 I.V. bolus for 2 doses each separated by 3 weeks.(10) LPAM produced 6 PR in 7 patients, a promising result. This agent deserves further study as frontline chemotherapy with other active agents.

Chemotherapy for Recurrent RMS

Survival after relapse is poor being 32% at 1 year and 17% at 2 years in the IRS-I. Table 1 lists the results of treatment of small series of relapsed patients with different agents. Promising agents for incorporation into frontline protocols include cisplatin + VP16 (11,12), ifosfamide (13, 14), ifosfamide + VP-16 (15), and high-dose methotrexate given as a 42-hour infusion.(16) Some of these already are in frontline studies or such studies are being planned. While not effective for recurrent disease, LPAM is active in newly diagnosed patients.

TABLE 1
Chemotherapy for Recurrent Rhabdomyosarcoma

Drugs	No.	CR	PR	Ref.
CPDD + VP-16	13	3	4	11
CPDD + VP-16	9	2	1	12
IFOSF	5	0	2	13
IFOSF + VCR	6	2	4	14
IFOSF + VP-16	13	3	6	15
MELPHAN	13	0	1	10
HD MTX	4	1	2	16

Conclusion

VAC chemotherapy remains the most active combination against RMS in childhood. Although Adriamycin is an active agent, it has not been shown to add benefit when combined with VAC. Adriamycin's place in therapy has yet to be determined. Promising agents for further study are cisplatin, VP-16, ifosfamide, melphalan and high-dose continuous infusion methotrexate. Bone marrow transplantation has not changed the outcome of advanced RMS thus far, but the experience is still limited with this approach.

REFERENCES

1. Maurer HM, Beltangady M, Gehan EA, et al.: The Intergroup Rhabdomyosarcoma Study-I: A final report. Cancer (in press).
2. Maurer HM, Foulkes M, Gehan E (for the IRS Committee of CCSG and POG): Intergroup Rhabdomyosarcoma Study-II (IRS-II): A preliminary report. Proc Am Soc Clin Oncol 2:70, 1983.
3. Maurer HM, Raney RB, Rogab A, et al.: Improved survival of children with group III rhabdomyosarcoma (non-special pelvic sites): A report of IRS-II. Proc Am Soc Clin Oncol 5:202, 1986.
4. Rodary C, Rey A, Rezvani A, et al.: Prognostic factors in children with rhabdomyosarcoma. Proc XVII Intl Soc Pediatr Oncol, Venice, Italy, p.98, 1985.
5. Flamant F, Hill C: The improvement in survival associated with combined chemotherapy in childhood rhabdomyosarcoma. Cancer 53:2417, 1984.
6. Otten J, Flamant F, Rodary C, et al.: Effectiveness of combination of ifosfamide, vincristine and actinomycin D in inducing remission in rhabdomyosarcoma in children. Proc Am Soc Clin Oncol 4:236, 1985.
7. Carli M, Perilongo G, Guglielmi M, et al.: Rhabdomyosarcoma in childhood: A report from the Italian Cooperative Group. Proc XVII Intl Soc Pediatr Oncol, Venice, Italy, p.89, 1985.
8. Etcubanas E, Horowitz M, Vogel R: Combination of dacarbazine and doxorubicin in the treatment of childhood rhabdomyosarcoma. Cancer Treat Rep 69:999, 1985.
9. Miser J, Kinsella T, Triche T, et al.: Treatment of high-risk sarcomas with an intensive consolidation followed by autologous bone marrow transplantation. Proc Am Soc Clin Oncol 6:218, 1987.
10. Horowitz M, Etcubanas E, Christensen M, et al.: Melphalan (LPAM), a clinically effective agent for rhabdomyosarcoma as predicted by the xenograft model. Proc Am Soc Clin Oncol 5:206, 1986.
11. Carli M, Perilongo G, Montezemolo L, et al.: Phase II trials of cis-platin and VP-16 in children with advanced soft tissue sarcoma: A report from the Italian Cooperative Rhabdomyosarcoma Group. Cancer Treat Rep 71:525, 1987.

12. Maurer HM, Russell EC: Personal communication.
13. Pratt CB, Horowitz M, Meyer WH, et al.: Phase II trial of ifosfamide in children with malignant solid tumors. Cancer Treat Rep 71:131, 1987.
14. de Kraker J, Voute PA: Ifosfamide, Mesna and vincristine in paediatric oncology. Cancer Treat Rev 10:165, 1983.
15. Miser J, Kinsella T, Tsokos, M, et al.: High response rate of recurrent childhood tumors to etoposide (VP-16), Ifosfamide (ifos) and mesna (mes) uroprotection. Proc Am Soc Clin Oncol 5:209, 1986.
16. Bode U: Methotrexate, a relapse therapy for rhabdomyosarcoma. Am J Pediatr Oncol 8:70, 1986.

RESULTS OF A RANDOMIZED TRIAL FOR THE TREATMENT OF LOCALIZED SOFT TISSUE TUMORS (STS) OF THE EXTREMITIES IN ADULT PATIENTS*

P. Picci[1], G. Bacci, F. Gherlinzoni, R. Capanna, M. Mercuri
P. Ruggieri, N. Baldini, M. Avella, G. Pignatti, M. Manfrini

The purpose of the protocol was to obtain a homogeneous group of adult patients with localized and high grade STS in an extremity (including pelvic and shoulder girdle) treated with three different local surgical procedures chosen depending on the presentation of the tumor. Once local control was obtained, the patients were randomized to receive or not to receive adjuvant chemotherapy with Adriamycin (total dose 450 mg/m2).

Protocol

1. _Ablative surgery_. Patients judged unsuitable for limb salvage surgery were amputated without any previous treatment and then randomized to receive or not six cycles of ADM (90 mg/m2 in 3 consecutive days).

2. _Conservative surgery_. When a tumor appeared amenable to conservative surgery, this was preceded by radiotherapy (4500 rads, 3 weeks) plus two cycles of ADM at the doses previously reported. After surgery, patients were randomized to receive or not four more cycles of ADM.

3. _Re-excision of the scar of the previous surgical bed_. This group includes patients treated elsewhere within three months from inadequate surgery (usually excisional biopsy). After the re-excision of the scar, these patients were randomized to receive or not the six cycles of ADM. If foci of tumoral cells were found in the scar, postoperative radiotherapy was also administered (4500 rads in 3 weeks). Randomization for each group was pair matched with stratification for age (older or younger than 45), site (girdle or extremity), size of the tumor (less or greater than 5 cm), and stage intra- or extracompartmental).

Patients

From 8/81 to 9/86, 187 soft tissue sarcomas were observed. One hundred and ten cases were excluded due to: age, younger than 16 or older than 70 (27 cases), metastases at diagnosis (21 cases), low grade of malignancy (18 cases), refused the protocol (17 cases), inoperable (9 cases), previous radiation or chemotherapy treatment (8 cases),

---

[1]Istituto Ortopedico Rizzoli, Via Codivilla 9, Bologna 40136 Italy.

---

*Supported by grant n.86.02679.44 from the Italian National Research Council, Special Project "Oncology".

J. R. Ryan and L. O. Baker (eds.), Recent Concepts in Sarcoma Treatment, 144–148.
© 1988 by Kluwer Academic Publishers.

contraindications to ADM (4 cases). Six patients were also excluded because, having been sent to our institution only for surgery, they were randomized and sent back to the original institution for further treatment. For these patients, we cannot confirm the exact treatment and follow-up. The remaining 77 patients are the subject of this report. Thirty-three received chemotherapy, and 44 no further treatment. Twenty-eight were treated with ablative surgery, 29 with conservative surgery, and 20 with re-excision of the scar. The histology of the 77 comprises: 24 malignant fibrous histiocytomas, 22 synovial sarcomas, 9 fibrosarcomas, 5 pleomorphic or undifferentiated liposarcomas, 3 rhabdomyosarcomas, and 3 epithelioid sarcomas, 2 high grade hemangiopericytomas and 2 soft tissue osteosarcomas, 1 alveolar sarcoma, mesenchymal chondrosarcoma and undifferentiated sarcoma.

Results

Table 1 reports the overall results. The difference of continuously disease-free patients with and without chemotherapy (73% vs. 45%) is statistically significant (p<0.02).

TABLE 1

OVERALL RESULTS

	CHEMO 33 cases	NO CHEMO 44 cases	TOTAL 77 cases
CONT. NED	24 (73%)	20 (45%)	44 (57%)
LOC. REC.	4 (12%)	7 (16%)	11 (14%)
METAST.	7 (21%)	22 (50%)	29 (38%)
DEATH	3 (9%)	13 (30%)	16 (21%)

Figures 1 and 2 report the actuarial curves (Kaplan and Meyer method) for continuously disease-free survival, respectively. Both differences are statistically significant.

Figures 3, 4 and 5 report the actuarial curves for the three different local treatments. No statistical analysis was performed due to the small number in each subgroup.

Complications

No severe complications were caused by chemotherapy. All patients completed the scheduled cycles. In a few cases, it was necessary to delay some cycles, but for no longer than one week.

146

FIGURE 1

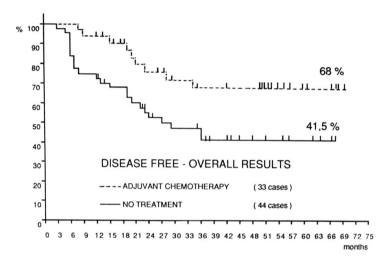

DISEASE FREE - OVERALL RESULTS

---- ADJUVANT CHEMOTHERAPY   (33 cases)
—— NO TREATMENT   (44 cases)

FIGURE 2

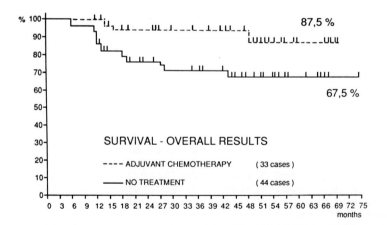

SURVIVAL - OVERALL RESULTS

---- ADJUVANT CHEMOTHERAPY   (33 cases)
—— NO TREATMENT   (44 cases)

FIGURE 3

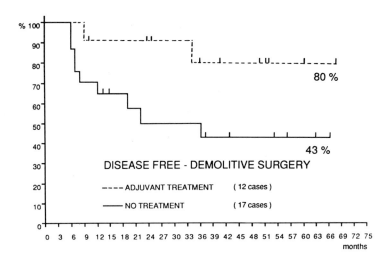

80 %

43 %

DISEASE FREE - DEMOLITIVE SURGERY

- - - - ADJUVANT TREATMENT (12 cases)

——— NO TREATMENT (17 cases)

FIGURE 4

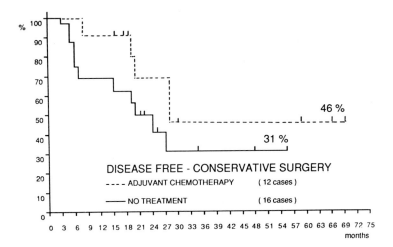

46 %

31 %

DISEASE FREE - CONSERVATIVE SURGERY

- - - - ADJUVANT CHEMOTHERAPY (12 cases)

——— NO TREATMENT (16 cases)

148

FIGURE 5

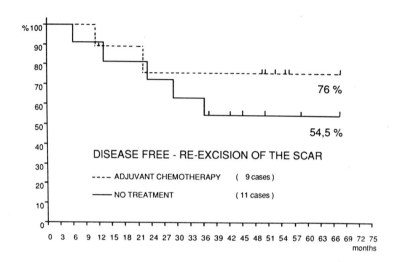

Other complications included four wound infections, all healed (in two cases with surgical debridement), and two fractures on irradiated bones that healed with plaster.

Conclusions

Adjuvant chemotherapy with ADM seems to increase both disease-free and survival in localized high grades STS of the extremity in adult patients.

This protocol does not seem to cause important side effects. Patients treated with conservative surgery seem to have a worse prognosis. This fact has to be confirmed by further studies.

SOFT TISSUE SARCOMAS - JAPANESE EXPERIENCE

Kiyoo Furuse, M.D.*

Between 1971 and 1980, Kyushu University, Jikei University and the NCCH collected 1556 cases of STS, which were classified (in decreasing order) as: malignant fibrous histiocytoma (MFH) (305 cases, 19.6%); liposarcoma (LS) (220 cases, 14.1%); rhabdomyosarcoma (RMS) (210 cases, 13.5%); and leiomyosarcoma (LMS) (125 cases, 8.0%), unclassified STS (111 cases, 7.1%).(1) These tumors appeared as predominant in various age groups. MFH and LMS predominated in late adult life (mean age, 59 and 57.5 years, respectively); LS in middle adult life (mean age 48.5 years); and RMS, especially of the embryonal type, in childhood. Although many tumor types had a slight predilection for males, LMS, malignant schwannoma and alveolar soft part sarcoma were more frequent in females. The most common primary site for each tumor type in Japan does not differ with that in other countries. An organization of five orthopedic institutions (2) reported a study on 414 patients with STS treated between 1972 and 1983. (3) The 5-year cumulative survival rates were, in the order of whole STS's, LS, MFH, LMS and RMS, 55.8%, 73.7%, 63.0%, 32.4% and 26.8%, respectively.

This paper deals with the results of treatment in two large series in Japan for STS's. Current status and future problems in the treatment of STS's, classified by the type of tumor, is also described.

Experience at the National Cancer Center Hospital (NCCH) (4)

Between 1962 and 1984, Fukuma and his co-workers (4) treated 145 patients, aged 1 to 92 years (mean 34 years) with nonmetastatic STS's of the limbs. Adjuvant chemotherapy was carried out in 78 (54%) of the 145: to classify by the subtype of STS's, 17 (81.0%) of 21 patients with RMS, 12 (75.0%) of 16 with neurogenic sarcoma, 7 (46.7%) of 15 with angiosarcoma, 10 (41.7%) of 24 with MFH, 12 (32.4%) of 37 with LS, and 12 with other subtypes.

The route of administration was intra-arterial (IA) in 38 patients, intravenous (IV) in 24 patients, IA + IV in 14 patients, and regional perfusion (RP) in two.

Continuous IA chemotherapy was carried out in 51 patients (1 with one-shot IA infusion). Seventy-eight per cent of the 51 were given either vincristine and carbazilquinone

---

*Department of Orthopedic Surgery, Tottori University School of Medicine, Yonago 683, Japan.

J. R. Ryan and L. O. Baker (eds.), Recent Concepts in Sarcoma Treatment, 149–155.
© 1988 by Kluwer Academic Publishers.

(VCQ) or VCQ plus adriamycin (VCQA). The period of infusion ranged from three to 74 days (mean 36 days). In patients with measurable lesions, the overall response rate (complete and partial) was only 14% (6/42); however, IA chemotherapy was very effective in most patients of RMS. The primary toxicities of continuous IA chemotherapy were numbness and pain in 27 patients (52.9%), nausea and vomiting in five patients (9.8%), and various other toxicities in 11 patients, including an especially severe case of interstitial pneumonia. Only eight patients (15.7%) were free from side effects. However, many patients were tolerable for IA chemotherapy.

Table 1 shows the relationship between local recurrence and distant metastasis to adjuvant chemotherapy: 44 patients underwent various surgical procedures from marginal resection to radical amputation after IA chemotherapy. IA chemotherapy seemed to contribute to a decrease in the local recurrence rate, with 27.3% in the IA group, 50.0% in the IA+IV group, and 41.7% in the IV group. The incidence of distant metastasis was similar among the 3 groups.

TABLE 1.

Incidences of Local Recurrence and Distant Metastasis
in Soft Tissue Sarcomas at National Cancer Center
(1962-Mar.1984)

Continuous IA Inf.

Total Cases	Cases with Local Recurrence	Cases with Distant Metastases
44	12(27.3%)	21(47.7%)

Continuous IA Inf. + Sys.Chemo.

Total Cases	Cases with Local Recurrence	Cases with Distant Metastasis
14	7(50.0%)	7(50.0%)

Sys.Chemo.

Total Cases	Cases with Local Recurrence	Cases with Distant Metastasis
24	10(41.7%)	14(58.3%)

(Fukuma,H.,1984)

In comparing the 5-year cumulative survival rates between patients receiving and not receiving chemotherapy, chemotherapy-treated patients showed slightly greater survival for LS, RMS and LMS.

Figure 1 shows the comparison of the survival rates between groups treated before 1975 and after 1976 (unpublished data by the NCCH in 1986). The 10-year survival rate differed significantly between the groups: of 160 patients with nonmetastatic STS, the survival rate for 77 patients treated before 1975 was 39%, and the rate of 83 patients treated after 1976 was 65%. It has been suggested that this significant difference may be due to the markedly improved prognosis of LS after 1976, and because of changes in

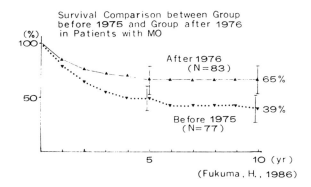

Survival Comparison between Group
before 1975 and Group after 1976
in Patients with MO

(Fukuma, H., 1986)

FIGURE 1.

characteristics of patients with STS at the NCCH during the 25 years between 1962 and 1986. At the NCCH, the proportion of patients without prior treatment showed a gradual increase from the 1960's to the 1970's. During the late 1970's, the level reached twice that in the 1960's. On the other hand, the number of pretreated patients decreased from 82% to 62% with the number of local recurrence, patients decreasing from 64% to 38%.

Experience at the Cancer Institute Hospital (CIH) (5-8)

A series of studies by Kawaguchi and his colleagues (5-8) have mainly dealt with the surgical treatment of STS's. They suggested a curative surgical margin for primary tumors. This margin lies between the radical and wide margins, as proposed by Enneking et al.(9) A curative wide margin is generally judged to be about 2 or 3 cm. outside the biological barrier that covers the tip of the tumor, or, in the case of no barrier, about 5 cm. outside the tip of the tumor. Biological barriers include the fascia, tendon, periosteum and joint capsule, and have potential resistance against the growth of the tumor.

Figure 2 shows the myriad kinds of curative wide resections for variously located STS's. During the 11 years between 1976 and 1986, 141 patients with or without prior treatment were treated at the CIH with curative resection of tumor. The rates of 5-year cumulative survival, local recurrence and distant metastasis were 62%, 12%, and 43%, respectively.

Table 2 shows comparison results between the CIH study and either Group Study I (1962-1976) (10) or II (1972-1983). (2,3,8) The CIH described better results than in the two-group studies, particularly in local recurrence rate. However, the level of distant metastasis did not differ between the CIH and Group Study II. The 5-year survival rate in the CIH study did not differ much with that in the study by the

Curative Resection for Soft Tissue Sarcoma

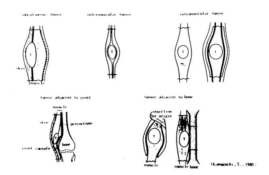

FIGURE 2.

TABLE 2.

Treatment Results of Soft Part Tissue Sarcomas

	Local Recurrence	Distant Metastasis	5-yr Survival Rate
Group Study[1] (318 Cases) 1962-1976	52%	63%	42%
Group Study[1] (414 Cases) 1972-1983	23%	45%	56%
CIH[2] (141 Cases) 1976-1986	12%	43%	62%

1) by the Grant-in-Aid for Cancer Research from the Ministry of Health and Welfare
2) Cancer Institute Hospital

(Amino,K.and Kawaguchi,T.,1986)

NCCH in 1986.

Amino and co-workers (8) studied 85 previously untreated patients with neither metastasis in the regional lymph nodes nor distant distant metastasis who were treated with curative resection between 1976 and 1986. The rates of local recurrence, distant metastasis and 5-year cumulative survival for 55 of these patients were favorable (5.5%, 21.8% and 79.3%, respectively (Figure 3)). Thirty patients were re-resected due to apparent relapse or suspected remaining local tumor, with local recurrence, distant metastasis and 5-year cumulative survival rates of 20.0%, 36.7%, and 61.8%, respectively. Thus, patients with prior treatment elsewhere belonged to a high-risk group, but at the CIH, 102 (81.8%) of 126 patients

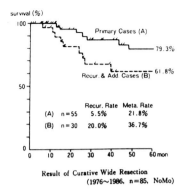

FIGURE 3.

with STS of the limbs could be controlled with limb-salvage surgery.

As these CIH studies reported, most of the patients could be controlled by the curative wide resection, but a small number of them were often treated with either ablative surgery alone or in combination with preoperative radiotherapy or chemotherapy. Preoperative treatment is indicated for patients having: 1) tumors prohibiting surgery alone because they are situated near major nerves, vessels and/or bone; 2) high-risk distant metastasis; 3) metastasis in the regional lymph nodes; 4) age as a factor limiting surgery; and 5) refused amputation.

At the CIH, for patients requiring preoperative treatment, preoperative irradiation was done at 70 time-dose-fractionation for two to four weeks, and a modified CYVADIC regimen was given as adjuvant chemotherapy (Gottlieb and co-workers (11)). From their experiences at the NCCH, Fukuma and colleagues (4) summarized the types of tumors indicating a need for adjuvant chemotherapy as Das Gupta (12) suggested a similar idea: an absolute indication -RMS, extraskeletal osteosarcoma, Ewing's sarcoma, and peripheral neuroblastoma; a subordinate indication - all tumors of 5 cm. or more in size in LMS, synovial sarcoma, MFH, LS of the round-cell and pleomorphic types, neurogenic sarcoma, angiosarcoma and fibrosarcoma except infantile one.

Current Status and Future Problems in Japan

In treating STS's, pathological diagnosis should be established before treatment because clinical diagnosis alone is limited. Diagnostic techniques, including aspiration needle biopsy and/or incisional biopsy are the first priority in managing STS's. Imaging techniques including xeroradiography, angiography, computed tomography, isotope scanning, thermography and ultrasound become necessary to determine surgical staging.

154

We believe that the strategy in treating STS's lies in the prevention of local recurrence and limb preservation. Therefore, radical removal by adequate surgery is the most important treatment/step.

Recent treatments have produced better results in Japan as well. The reasons behind this are multifaceted: increased knowledge about STS; orthopedists have become more skillful in tumor surgery aided by improved imaging diagnostic techniques; and the number of new cases we see has increased.

On the other hand, because STS's are collections of various histological subtypes that differ in biological behavior, it is invalid to discuss the results of treatment as a whole.

The role of adjuvant chemotherapy has not been fully identified, though its efficacy on STS's was clearly proven in RMS in childhood, and is gradually becoming more clear in other subtypes. Long-term follow-up is needed for identifying the effects of adjuvant chemotherapy.

Detailed data about regional lymph node metastasis has not yet been reported in Japan. We should treat certain types of tumors such as alveolar RMS, clear cell sarcoma, epithelioid sarcoma and angiosarcoma more carefully because regional lymph node metastases are not infrequent in these lesions. (13)

REFERENCES

1. Committee on Bone and Soft Tissue Tumors, Japanese Orthopedic Association. General rules for clinical and pathological studies on malignant soft tissue tumors. Kanahara, Tokyo, 1985 (in Japanese).
2. Furuse K, et al.: In Ogawa M, Muggia FM, Rosencweig M (eds.): Adriamycin, its expanding role in cancer treatment. Proceedings of the International Symposium on Adriamycin, Japan, 1983. Excerpta Medica, Amsterdam, pp. 307-318, 1984.
3. Furuya K: In Seikeigeka Mook No. 38. pp. 141-142, 1985 (in Japanese).
4. Fukuma K, Beppu Y, Nishikawa K: Nippon Gan Chiryo Gakkaishi 11:1729-1735, 1984 (in Japanese).
5. Kawaguchi N, Wada S, et al.: Rinsho Seikeigeka 17:1192-1206, 1982 (in Japanese).
6. Kawaguchi N, Amino K, et al.: Nippon Gan Chiryo Gakkaishi 11 (pt. 1):1736-1745, 1984 (in Japanese).
7. Kawaguchi N, Amino K, et al.: Seikeigeka Mook 38:98-119, 1985 (in Japanese).
8. Amino K, Kawaguchi N, et al.: Nippon Gan Chiryo Gakkaishi 14 (pt. 2):1589-1596, 1987 (in Japanese).
9. Enneking WF, Spanier SS, Goodman MA: Clin Orthop 153: 106-120, 1980.
10. Furuya K, Fukuma H, et al.: In Abstracts of Interim Report on Study by Grant-in-Aid for Cancer Research. p 119, National Cancer Center, Tokyo, 1983.

11. Gottlieb JA, Baker LH et al.: Cancer Chemother Rep 3:271-282, 1975.
12. Das Gupta TK: Tumors of the Soft Tissues, Norwalk, Connecticut, Appleton-Century-Crofts, 1983.
13. Enzinger FM, Weiss SW: Soft Tissue Tumors. St. Louis, CV Mosby Co, 1983.

EUROPEAN EXPERIENCE OF ADJUVANT CHEMOTHERAPY FOR SOFT TISSUE
SARCOMA: INTERIM REPORT OF A RANDOMIZED TRIAL OF CYVADIC
VERSUS CONTROL*

Vivien Bramwell[1]., J. Rouessé, W. Steward, A. Santoro,
J. Buesa, H. Strafford-Koops, T. Wagener, R. Somers, W. Ruka,
D. Markham, M. Burgers, J. van Unnik, G. Contesso, D. Thomas,
R. Sylvester, H. Pinedo

Introduction
    A Multidisciplinary approach to the management of soft
tissue sarcomas has led to improvements in the rates of local
control, despite increasing use of limb salvage procedures.
However, metastasis, which seems to correlate with higher
histological grade, remains a distressingly frequent problem,
occurring in approximately 30% of individuals, often in the
absence of local failure.
    In advanced disease, combination chemotherapy has pro-
duced response rates ranging from 20-60% (1). Various sched-
ulings of CYVADIC (Cyclophosphamide, Vincristine, Adriamycin,
DTIC) have been evaluated in more than 750 patients, and the
average response rate is 48%, range 15-68% (1). The first
positive results for CYVADIC (overall response rate 59%) were
published by the Southwest Oncology Group in 1975 (2), and
prompted the EORTC to plan a randomized adjuvant trial,
CYVADIC chemotherapy versus control, which commenced accrual
in 1978.

Materials and Methods
    Criteria for eligibility. Patients, aged 15-70 years,
with histologically proven soft tissue sarcoma were eligible
for this study. They were required to have adequate hemato-
logical function (WBC $\geq$ 4.0×10^9/L, platelets $\geq$ 120×10^9/L)
and no evidence of metastases, either hematogenous or in
regional nodes. Patients who had received previous
chemotherapy or radiotherapy were excluded, as were those in
poor physical or psychological condition. Other criteria for
exclusion were severe hepatic dysfunction, bleeding
disorders, significant symptomatic cardiac disease, serious
infections and a history of other malignant disease,
excluding basal cell skin cancer. All histological types were
included, with the exception of borderline/very low grade
tumors such as fibromatoses and well-differentiated liposarcomas.

----

[1]London Regional Cancer Centre, 391 South St., London,
Ontario, N6A 4G5, Canada.
----

*A study conducted by the Soft Tissue & Bone Sarcoma Group of
the European Organization for Research and Treatment of
Cancer.

156

J. R. Ryan and L. O. Baker (eds.), Recent Concepts in Sarcoma Treatment, 156–163.
© *1988 by Kluwer Academic Publishers.*

Guidelines for surgery and radiotherapy have been described previously (3).

Trial design. After adequate surgery $\pm$ radiotherapy, patients were stratified by: (a) institution, (b) site of primary, (c) local recurrence before entry, (d) postoperative radiotherapy; and then randomized to a control group (no further treatment) or a chemotherapy group receiving CYVADIC (Cyclophosphamide 500 mg/m^2, Vincristine 1.5 mg/m^2, Adriamycin 50 mg/m^2, all IV day 1, and Dacarbazine 400 mg/m^2 IV days 1-3; repeated every 4 weeks x 8).

The statistical design has been described previously (3).

Results

This study opened to accrual in 1978 and 446 patients had been entered as of July 31, 1987. Two Hundred and twenty-five patients were randomized to receive CYVADIC and 221 to the control arm. Eighty-eight patients were ineligible for the following reasons: inadequate radiotherapy 23/14 (CYVADIC/CONTROL), pathology not sarcoma 9/8, advanced disease 6/5, inadequate surgery 6/2, no data 2/5, poor general condition 3/1, late randomization 2/1, previous chemotherapy 1/0. Thus, 358 patients (80%) were eligible, 173 on CYVADIC and 185 control. Stratification prior to randomization ensured that the treatment groups were well balanced according to site, local recurrence before entry and administration of postoperative radiotherapy (Table 1).

Patient characteristics for the 332 eligible patients, documented by an on-study form, are also shown in Table 1. The median time from definitive surgery to entry on study was 42 days. To date, central pathology review has been performed on 255 eligible cases and the cell types, by treatment group, are shown in Table 2. Tumor size (largest diameter on histopathology) has been documented for 292 patients, and the numbers of patients in each size category are well balanced between the two arms (Table 2). North & South pathology panels have each carried out a detailed analysis of grade (reported elsewhere in these Proceedings), but as the number of mitoses proved to be the most important prognostic factor, Table 2 shows the distribution of patients in the three groups (mitotic count < 3/10 HPF; 3-20); > 20). Again, the treatment arms are well balanced.

Table 3 details the outcome for all 358 eligible patients, and also for the 233 patients with limb sarcomas only. Three year progression free survivals (Fig. 1) are 67% for CYVADIC versus 52% for control (p=0.01). However, survival at 3 years is not significantly different between the two arms; 79% versus 74%, p=0.12 (Fig. 2). It appears that CYVADIC reduced local recurrence (p=0.005), but did not prevent metastasis (p=0.28). The influence of CYVADIC on local recurrence was most apparent in head, neck and trunk tumors (p=0.038), rather than limb sarcomas (p=0.32). The incidence of distant metastases was similar in both arms of the study for head, neck and trunk tumors (p=0.97) and limb sarcomas (p=0.20), and this was paralleled by survival. Although the group receiving radiotherapy theoretically were

TABLE 1

STRATIFICATION GROUPS Eligible patients 358

	CYVADIC	CONTROL	TOTAL (%)
Site			
Head, neck, trunk	59	66	125 (35)
Limbs	114	119	233 (65)
Local Recurrence (prior to entry)			
No	141	148	289 (81)
Yes	32	37	69 (19)
Radiotherapy			
No	93	98	191 (53)
Yes	80	87	167 (47)
PATIENT CHARACTERISTICS	Eligible, documented 332		
Sex M:F	1.26	1.17	
Age Median	44	42	
Range	15-70	15-70	
Surgical procedure			
Local recurrence	121	140	261 (79)
Amputation	35	36	71 (21)
Resectability			
Microscopic residual	17	20	37 (11)
Total resection	139	156	295 (89)

at higher risk of recurrence because many had narrow or contaminated margins, there were no significant differences in local recurrence, metastases, overall progression or survival between irradiated versus nonirradiated patients.

Eighty-three patients (23%) have died, of whom 73 succumbed to malignant disease. One eligible patient in the CYVADIC arm died of toxicity (infection, hemorrhage), and one ineligible patient died of infection. There have been two intercurrent deaths on CYVADIC (both cardiovascular) and six in the control arm (2 cardiovascular, 2 postoperative complications, one each lung cancer and pancreatitis).

Eighty-two (47%) of the 173 eligible patients in the CYVADIC arm have completed eight courses of chemotherapy, and 50 (29%) are still receiving treatment. Chemotherapy was discontinued early in 41 patients (24%) because of progression (14 pts.), refusal (8 pts.), toxicity (7 pts.), loss to follow-up (3 pts.), intercurrent death (2 pts.), missing data (5 pts.), and miscellaneous (2 pts.).

Discussion

Accrual to this study is in its tenth year, and is nearing completion. This interim analysis does not

TABLE 2

HISTOPATHOLOGY	Central Review		
CELL TYPE	CYVADIC No. (%)	CONTROL No. (%)	TOTAL No. (%)
Malignant fibrous			
histiocytoma	22 (19)	32 (23)	54 (21)
Synovial sarcoma	25 (22)	15 (11)	40 (15)
Liposarcoma	9 (8)	26 (18)	35 (14)
Leiomyosarcoma	19 (17)	14 (10)	33 (13)
Neurogenic sarcoma	10 (9)	12 (8.5)	22 (8.5)
Fibrosarcoma	7 (6)	8 (6)	15 (6)
Angiosarcoma	5 (4)	3 (2)	8 (3)
Rhabdomyosarcoma	0 (0)	6 (4)	6 (2.5)
Undifferentiated	0 (0)	5 (3.5)	5 (2)
Unclassified	11 (10)	13 (9)	24 (10)
Miscellaneous	6 (5)	7 (5)	13 (5)
TOTAL	114 (100)	141 (100)	255 (100)
Not yet reviewed	55	40	95
Material unavailable/			
inadequate	4	4	8
Tumor size (292 pts)			
1-5 cms.	55 (40)	71 (46)	126 (43)
6-10 cms.	52 (38)	53 (33)	105 (36)
11-15 cms.	12 (9)	15 (10)	27 (9)
> 15 cms.	18 (13)	16 (11)	34 (12)
Grade-mitoses (187 pts)			
< 3	17 (20)	17 (17)	34 (18)
3-20	46 (54)	58 (57)	104 (56)
> 20	22 (26)	27 (26)	49 (26)

demonstrate any significant survival benefit for patients receiving CYVADIC, regardless of site. Reduced local recurrence, rather than a reduction in metastases, as might be expected, accounts for the prolonged progression free interval in the CYVADIC arm. Although it appears that the reduction in local recurrence is only significant for head, neck and trunk tumors, this result of subgroup analysis should be viewed with caution. Nevertheless, one could speculate that, as surgery is more often suboptimal in this group, with a consequent higher incidence of local recurrence, the contribution of chemotherapy is more likely to be evident.

Only one small study (4) in the literature has demonstrated a survival benefit for patients with limb sarcomas receiving adjuvant combination chemotherapy. The results of the first randomized adjuvant study, from the M.D. Anderson (5) have recently been updated and are remarkably similar to our own. Disease-free survival was significantly prolonged in the chemotherapy arm (p=0.04), but this was entirely accounted for by a reduction in local recurrence. Metastases

```
┌──────────────────────────────────────────────────────────────────────┐
│                              TABLE 3                                   │
│                                                                        │
│                                                                        │
│  OUTCOME          Average follow up:   3 years (0-9.5)                 │
│                                                                        │
│                                                                        │
│                        CYVADIC          CONTROL          TOTAL         │
│                        No. (%)          No. (%)          No. (%)       │
│                                                                        │
│                                                                        │
│  All eligible patients  173              185             358  (100)    │
│                                                                        │
│  Local recurrence only    6  (3.5)        24 (13)         30  (8.5)    │
│  Metastases only         30 (17)          36 (19.5)       66 (18.5)    │
│  Both                    12  (7)          14  (7.5)       26  (7)      │
│  Total relapse           48 (28)          74 (40)        122 (34)      │
│  Died                    33 (19)          50 (27)         83 (23)      │
│                                                                        │
│                                                                        │
│  Limb only              114              119             233           │
│                                                                        │
│  Local recurrence only    2  (2)           8  (7)         10  (4)      │
│  Metastases only         17 (15)          28 (23.5)       45 (19)      │
│  Both                     7  (6)           5  (4)         12  (5)      │
│  Total relapse           26 (23)          41 (34)         67 (29)      │
│  Died                    22 (19)          31 (26)         53 (23)      │
│                                                                        │
└──────────────────────────────────────────────────────────────────────┘
```

occurred with similar frequency in both arms, and survival was not significantly different (p=0.25). In contrast, Edmonson et al. (6) showed no effect of adjuvant chemotherapy on the rate of local recurrence (which was high at 30%), possibly because radiotherapy was not used), although chemotherapy did delay the appearance of metastases. Survival was similar for control and chemotherapy groups, 82% at 5 years. Randomized studies evaluating adjuvant Adriamycin (7-10) have not shown significant benefit in terms of overall survival. Gherlinzoni et al. (7) reported a significant improvement in disease-free survival, associated with fewer metastases in patients receiving Adriamycin. Median follow-up (27.6 months) for this small study was short and overall survival was not reported. The results and methodology have been criticized (11).

As there are many theoretical reasons to support commencing adjuvant chemotherapy as soon as possible after diagnosis, a criticism that could be levelled at the present study is the considerable delay, median six weeks, in commencing chemotherapy. This issue is addressed in a new EORTC study currently in the planning stages.

Based on this interim analysis, we see no reason to alter our conclusion from an earlier analysis (3), that we cannot recommend adjuvant chemotherapy with CYVADIC outside the context of a randomized clinical trial. Reviewing the tenuous data currently available in the literature, this

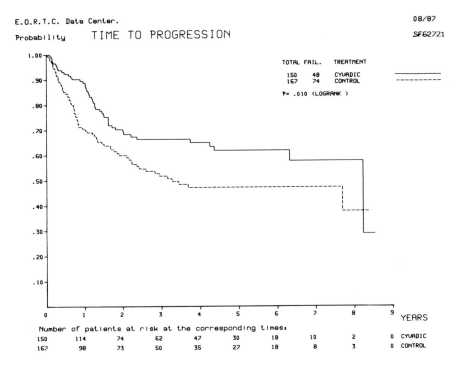

E.O.R.T.C. Data Center.

Probability   TIME TO PROGRESSION

08/87

SF62721

FIGURE 1:   Time to progression - all eligible patients -
CYVADIC vs. control.

162

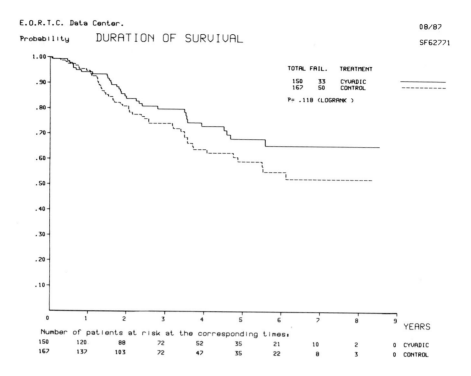

E.O.R.T.C. Data Center.   08/87

FIGURE 2.   Survival - all eligible patients - CYVADIC vs. control.

conclusion could well be extended to all types of adjuvant chemotherapy for soft tissue sarcoma.

REFERENCES

1. Bramwell VHC: The role of chemotherapy in multi-disci-plinary treatment. Can J Surg (in press) 1987.
2. Gottlieb JA, Baker LH, O'Bryan RM, et al.: Adriamycin (NSC-123127) used alone and in combination for soft tissue and bone sarcomas. Cancer Chemother Rep 6:271-282, 1975.
3. Bramwell VHC, Rouessé J, Santoro A, et al.: European experience of adjuvant chemotherapy for soft tissue sarcoma: a randomized trial comparing CYVADIC with control (preliminary report). Cancer Treat Symposia 3:99-107, 1985.
4. Rosenberg SA, Chang AE, Glatstein E: Adjuvant chemother-apy for treatment of extremity soft tissue sarcomas: review of the National Cancer Institute Experience. Cancer Treat Symposia 3:83-88, 1985.

5. Benjamin RS, Terjanian TO, Fenoglio CJ, et al.: The importance of combination chemotherapy for adjuvant treatment of high risk patients with soft tissue sarcomas of the extremities. Adjuvant Therapy of Cancer V, Grune & Stratton, pp. 735-744, 1987.

6. Edmonson JH, Fleming TR, Ivins JC, et al.: Randomized study of systemic chemotherapy following complete excision of non-osseous sarcomas. J Clin Oncol 2:1390-1396, 1984.

7. Gherlinzoni F, Bacci G, Picci P, et al.: A randomized trial for the treatment of high grade soft tissue sarcomas of the extremities: preliminary observations. J Clin Oncol 4:552-558, 1986.

8. Alvegard TA: Adjuvant chemotherapy with Adriamycin in high grade malignant soft tissue sarcoma - A Scandinavian randomized study. Proc Am Soc Clin Oncol 5:125, 1986.

9. Antman, K, Amato D, Lerner H, et al.: Adjuvant Doxorubicin for sarcoma: Data from the Eastern Cooperative Oncology Group and Dana-Farber Cancer Institute/ Massachusetts General Hospital studies. Cancer Treat Symposia 3:109-116, 1985.

10. Eilber FR, Giuliano AE, Huth JF, Morton DL: Adjuvant Adriamycin in high grade extremity soft tissue sarcoma - a randomized prospective trial. Proc Am Soc Clin Oncol 5:125, 1986.

11. Sylvester R: Soft tissue sarcomas of the extremities. J Clin Oncol 5:321-322, 1987.

RESULTS OF THE GERMAN SOFT-TISSUE SARCOMA STUDY[*]

J. Treuner[1], M. Keim[1], E. Koscielniak[1], D. Bürger[2],
M. Herbst[3], K. Winkler[4], H. Jürgens[5], J. Ritter[6],
D. Niethammer[1]

Between 1981 and the end of 1985, 352 children and teen-
agers with all types of soft-tissue sarcomas were registered
in a national multi-center study. Of these, 293 patients were
classified under chemosensitive sarcomas and were treated
according to a uniform therapeutic concept. The other 59
patients had generally non-chemosensitive sarcomas and were
not given treatment under the guidelines.

The treatment regimen was assigned to the primary postsurgical stage following the IRS staging system. In all four
stages, the initial chemotherapy combination, which included
vincristine, actinomycin, cyclophosphamide and adriamycin
(VACA), was administered over seven weeks. For non-responders, defined as less than 1/3 tumor reduction or tumor progression, the chemotherapy was altered. For patients who
manifested a degree of response, a chemotherapy combination
was continued up to week 16, followed by second-look surgery.
Patients without any evidence of tumor residue after 16 weeks
of chemotherapy did not receive radiotherapy. Patients with
microscopic or macroscopic residue were irradiated with 40 Gy
or 50 Gy, respectively, after resection of the residual
tumor. In the case of chemosensitive sarcoma patients, 222
out of 293 received treatment which strictly adhered to the
protocol guidelines. The following data were compiled using
this group, called protocol patients (PP), as the base.

Figure 1 delineates the event-free survival rate (EFS)
and the survival rate of all the chemosensitive sarcoma
patients. The latter included rhabdomyosarcoma (RMS), synovial sarcoma (Sy-Sa), extraskeletal Ewing's sarcoma (EES),
and undifferentiated sarcoma (US). As is evident, both curves
become similar after 50 months, and only the early drop in
the case of patients in a state of continuous remission
differs from the survival curves. In the case of patients
with a relapse, it is immediately apparent that they have a
highly unfavorable prognosis.

The event-free survival rate for the chemosensitive

---

[1]Department of Pediatric Hematology and Oncology, University
Hospital, Tübingen.
[2]Hannover, [3]Erlangen, [4]Hamburg, [5]Düsseldorf, [6]Münster (FRG)

---

[*]Supported by the Bundesministerium für Forschung und
Technologie, Bonn (FRG). Grant No. 01 ZP 0831.

J. R. Ryan and L. O. Baker (eds.), Recent Concepts in Sarcoma Treatment, 164–167.
© 1988 by Kluwer Academic Publishers.

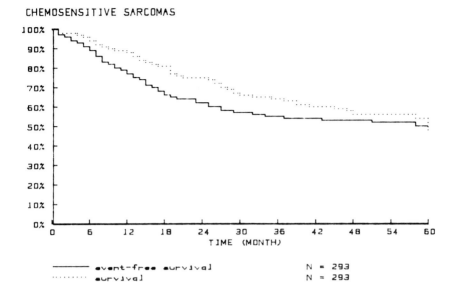

CHEMOSENSITIVE SARCOMAS

FIGURE 1: Survival curve and event-free survival curve of chemosensitive mesenchymal sarcoma in the CWS-81 study. Life table analysis according to Kaplan and Meier.

sarcoma patients, according to their histological subtype, is illustrated in Figure 2. For three groups, the EFS rate may be regarded as being roughly identical: 55% for RMS, 49% EES, and 55% US. What is exceptionally noteworthy is that EES and US patients experience a relapse earlier than RMS patients. Sy-Sa is the best so far, with a 72% EFS rate, but the difference between Sy-Sa and RMS is not statistically significant.

In the case of chemosensitive sarcoma patients, we found a difference of 13% in the EFS rate in Stages II and III in the final outcome. RMS Stage II (EFS rate 63%), however, had nearly the same outcome as III (EFS rate 59%) (Figure 3).

The primary tumor reduction, down to microscopic residues, does not improve the final outcome when compared with the patients who had primary unresectable RMS. As mentioned above, the study concept for primary unresectable tumors (Stage III) prescribed cytostatic pre-treatment for 16 weeks. After this period, the patients were re-staged, following the second-look operation and an evaluation of the effect of chemotherapy. Radiation therapy was additionally administered: patients without histologically-proven microscopic residues (Ipc) received no radiotherapy and had an 84% EFS rate; patients with microscopic residue (IIpc) received 40 Gy and had an EFS rate of 47%; patients with macroscopic residue (IIIpc) received 50 Gy after tumor resection and their EFS rate was 38%. Concerning the pattern of failure in

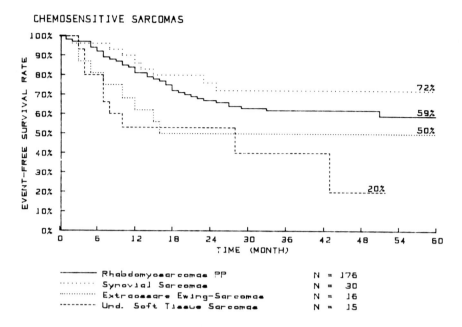

FIGURE 2: Event-free survival by histological subtype. Life
table analysis according to Kaplan and Meier.

these three groups, it is worth mentioning that patients with
macroscopic residue have a higher rate of metastasis formation and tumor progression.

In a prospective way, all patients with Stage III RMS
were monitored by CT scan after seven weeks of chemotherapy
(first VACA cycle) concerning the degree of tumor reduction.
Out of 93 patients, 13 were non-responders, 80 (86%) responded to chemotherapy, 23 (25%) clinically complete, 25 (27%)
achieved a partial remission of more than 2/3 of tumor volume, but not complete reduction, and in 26 patients (28%) a
tumor reduction of between 1/3 and 2/3 was registered.

Table 1 illustrates the correlation between the EFS rate
and the degree of clinical response in RMS Stage III patients
after seven weeks of VACA chemotherapy.

Another point, which led to the tumor reduction prognosis correlation, is the observation that the patients with
partial response by week seven, who achieved complete remission by week 16, showed a reduction in the final outcome in
comparison to the patients who had a complete remission by
week seven (70% versus 95% EFS rate).

We concluded from this data that the time factor involved in the tumor reduction under chemotherapy is of considerable importance. There is a qualitative difference
between achieving a complete remission by an early point in
time and achieving the same by a later point in time.

By means of single multivariate analysis (Cox regression

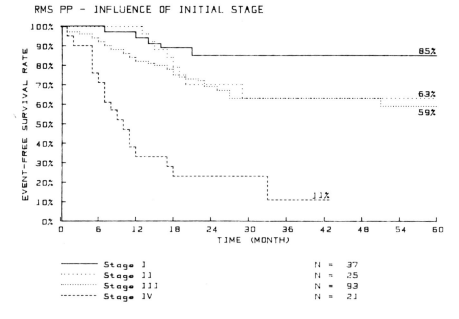

RMS PP - INFLUENCE OF INITIAL STAGE

———————	Stage I	N = 37
··········	Stage II	N = 25
··············	Stage III	N = 93
---------	Stage IV	N = 21

FIGURE 3: Event-free survival by primary post-surgery stage of RMS patients. Life table according to Kaplan and Meier.

TABLE 1: RMS Stage III, response at week 7, under initial chemotherapy, pattern of failure and EFS rate.

response group at week 7	n	local relapse	loc.relapse +metastasis	metastasis	tumor progression	death	EFS rate
complete	23	1	-	-	-	-	95%
> 2/3	25	6	1	1	-	1	61%
< 2/3	26	8	1	3	-	1	31%
no resp.	13	2	1	2	2	-	46%
total	87	17	3	6	2	2	59%

model) it was possible to show that the cytostatic time response factor takes precedence over well-known prognostic factors as histological subtype, tumor size or location. The tumor size, however, indicated the greatest influence on the response behavior of the tumor in comparison to other risk factors.

The kinetic relationship between the degree of initial cytostatic response under chemotherapy in RMS is a new aspect and the concept of the study which followed, CWS-86, is based on these findings.

A PILOT STUDY OF ADRIAMYCIN, DACARBAZINE AND IFOSFAMIDE IN ADVANCED ADULT SOFT TISSUE SARCOMAS[*]

Vivien Bramwell, M.D.[1] and Elizabeth Eisenhauer, M.D.[2]

Introduction

An extensive literature documents the efficacy of combination chemotherapy in locally advanced and metastatic sarcomas (1-3). Response rates in larger studies range from 20-60%, but complete remission rates are rarely above 15%. The most effective combinations generally contain Doxorubicin and Dacarbazine (DTIC), which were, until recently, the most active single agents. Average response rates, in collected series (3) for Adriamycin were 24% (range 16-41) and DTIC 17.5% (range 15-25). An analogue of Cyclophosphamide, Ifosfamide has shown promising results producing remission rates ranging from 18-38%, with an average of 28% (3,4).

The optimum use of these three agents in combination is of considerable interest, particularly as Ifosfamide and DTIC are relatively marrow sparing. Elias et al. (5) have explored a four-day infusion schedule (necessitating placement of a central venous catheter in all patients) but, as chemotherapy for metastatic soft tissue sarcoma is essentially palliative, the Canadian Sarcoma Group elected to investigate a shorter schedule of the same drugs administered by peripheral vein over 36 hours (Figure 1).

Materials and Methods

Criteria for eligibility. Patients, aged 15-75 years, with histologically proven advanced and/or metastatic soft tissue sarcomas were eligible for this study. They were required to have measurable progressive disease and an ECOG performance status of 0-2. Recurrent tumor in irradiated areas was not permitted as the sole evaluable lesion, and pleural effusions or bony metastases were not considered to be measurable. Other criteria for exclusion were previous chemotherapy, a previous or concomitant different malignant tumor, significant organic heart disease or other serious

---
[1]London Regional Cancer Centre, 391 South St., London, Ontario, N6A 4G5, Canada.

[2]National Cancer Institute of Canada, Clinical Trials Group, Queen's University, 82-84 Barrie Street, Kingston, Ontario K7L 3N6, Canada.
---

[*]A Preliminary Report from the Canadian Sarcoma Group/ National Cancer Institute of Canada Clinical Trials Group.

J. R. Ryan and L. O. Baker (eds.), Recent Concepts in Sarcoma Treatment, 168–173.
© 1988 by Kluwer Academic Publishers.

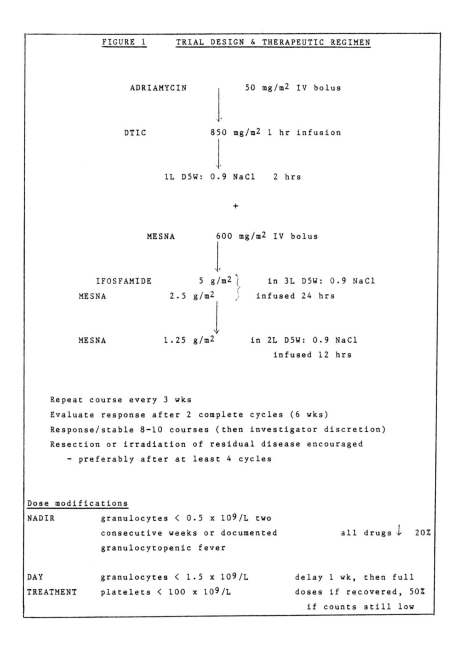

FIGURE 1   TRIAL DESIGN & THERAPEUTIC REGIMEN

ADRIAMYCIN   50 mg/m^2 IV bolus

DTIC   850 mg/m^2 1 hr infusion

1L D5W: 0.9 NaCl   2 hrs

+

MESNA   600 mg/m^2 IV bolus

IFOSFAMIDE   5 g/m^2 in 3L D5W: 0.9 NaCl
MESNA   2.5 g/m^2 infused 24 hrs

MESNA   1.25 g/m^2 in 2L D5W: 0.9 NaCl
                                      infused 12 hrs

Repeat course every 3 wks
Evaluate response after 2 complete cycles (6 wks)
Response/stable 8-10 courses (then investigator discretion)
Resection or irradiation of residual disease encouraged
   - preferably after at least 4 cycles

Dose modifications

NADIR   granulocytes < 0.5 x 10^9/L two
         consecutive weeks or documented   all drugs ↓ 20%
         granulocytopenic fever

DAY   granulocytes < 1.5 x 10^9/L   delay 1 wk, then full
TREATMENT   platelets < 100 x 10^9/L   doses if recovered, 50%
                                        if counts still low

concomitant illness, and central nervous system metastases. At entry, patients were required to have adequate renal function (serum creatinine ≤130 umol/L), hepatic function (serum bilirubin ≤20 umol/L) and bone marrow reserve (granulocytes ≥2.0 x 10^9/L, platelets ≥125 x 10^9/L).

Pretreatment and follow-up investigations. Baseline studies included history and physical examination, performance status, tumor measurements, CBC, biochemical profile, urinalysis, microscopy, chest radiograph and ECG. Radionucleide ejection fraction studies were optional. Other investigations to aid in tumor measurement were performed as indicated. Blood counts were performed at weekly intervals between treatments, and all baseline investigations were repeated after two courses of chemotherapy, and when the patient completed chemotherapy or went off study. Central pathology review will be performed.

Statistical design. Inclusion of 36 evaluable patients would be sufficient to adequately assess the toxicity of this pilot combination. A new regimen showing a response rate of >40% would be worth further study. Eleven responses in 36 patients would be sufficient to exclude a true response rate of 20% or less with a 10% probability of error, and has a 90% probability of occurring if the true response rate is 40% or greater.

Results

By the end of August 1987 (18 mos.), 39 patients had been accrued, and an on-study form had been received for 33. At present, two patients are regarded as ineligible; in one, the pathology is uncertain, and the other received radiotherapy to the sole index lesion. It is too early to evaluate four patients for response or toxicity. One patient went off study after one course because of a cardiac event, and the disease was not measured, leaving 26 patients evaluable for response. One patient died as a result of tumor progression six days after the start of chemotherapy, leaving 26 patients evaluable for toxicity.

The characteristics of eligible patients are described in Tables 1 and 2. The median age was 52 years (range 18-71). Sixty-three courses were administered at full dose (level A), with patients receiving 1-6 courses. Twenty-seven courses were administered at 80% doses (level B), the number of courses ranging from 1-5. Fifty-two courses were evaluable for hematologic toxicity at level A, and 23 at level B. Median nadir neutrophil counts for levels A and B were 0.26 (0.01-1.8) and 0.30 (0.02-1.5) x 10^9/L, respectively. The corresponding figures for platelet nadirs were 158 (3-520) and 174 (29-287) x 10^9/L, respectively. The nadir for hematological toxicity was around d 15. In all, 39/52 (75%) courses at level A and 14/23 (61%) courses at level B were associated with a neutrophil nadir of < 0.5 x 10^9/L. Infections occurred in 15/90 (17%) cycles. Eight episodes of neutropenic fever were clearly related to chemotherapy and three respiratory infections were probably related. Two wound infections and one pustular rash were less obviously attributable to chemotherapy. One infection was not described. Nine infections required parenteral antibiotics.

The majority of patients had some degree of alopecia, and nausea/vomiting. Grade 2 stomatitis occurred in three patients, and grade 3 in two patients. One severe episode of Ifosfamide encephalopathy causing coma occurred, but resolved

TABLE 1   PATIENT CHARACTERISTICS   N=31

		Number Patients (%)
Sex M/F		23/8
Performance status	0	15
	1	9
	2	7
Previous XRT		13
Primary site:	limb	10
	bowel	7
	trunk	5
	retroperitoneum	3
	urogenital	3
	head	1
	thorax	1
	uncertain	1
Site of disease:	locoregional only	3 (10)
	metastases only	23 ⎫
	both	5 ⎭ (90)
Sites of metastases[*]:	lung $\pm$ pleura	19 (61)
	liver	8 (26)
	intra-abdominal	4 (13)
	nodes/soft tissue	3 (10)
	bone	3 (10)
	extradural	2 (6)

[*] range number sites/patient 1-4

without sequelae. This patient responded to treatment, but relapsed when ADR/DTIC only was given for the second course and was not counted as a response. Mild CNS effects, such as drowsiness, confusion or personality change occurred in six other patients. Hematuria, and mild reversible elevation of serum creatinine occurred in one patient each. One patient had an episode of severe chest pain and flushing 24 hours after the start of the first course. ECG and enzymes did not show any evidence of myocardial infarction. There was a dramatic drop in left ventricular ejection fraction, which slowly recovered. The patient was taken off study.

Seven of 26 patients (27%) have shown partial response. Thirteen showed disease stabilization and six progressed. Ninety-five percent confidence intervals for this response rate are 11-47%. Lung metastases responded in six patients (one of whom had regression of a soft tissue metastasis) and mediastinal nodes were the site of response in one patient. There were no responses of primary tumor, nor of bone or liver metastases. Three responders had lesions measuring more than 5 cms, which regressed by more than 50%. Responses were

TABLE 2   PATHOLOGY   n=31

*Cell Type	Number Patients
Leiomyosarcoma	10
Liposarcoma	5
Malignant fibrous histiocytoma	4
Neurofibrosarcoma	3
Rhabdomyosarcoma	2
Synovial sarcoma	2
Undifferentiated	2
Fibrosarcoma	1
Haemangiopericytoma	1
Alveolar soft parts sarcoma	1

Bulk of Disease

⊗Diameter lesions (cm)

< 2 cms	2
2-4 cms	5
5-10 cms	10 ⎱ 73%
> 10 cms	9 ⎰

* according to local pathologist

⊗ largest size one of multiple lesions

seen in the following histological types: liposarcoma (two) and one each of malignant fibrous histiocytoma, neurofibrosarcoma, synovial sarcoma, rhabdomyosarcoma, undifferentiated sarcoma. There were no responses in the ten leiomyosarcomas.

Discussion

A preliminary response rate of 27% is somewhat disappointing, but the 95% confidence intervals for this value are wide: 11-47%. We require responses in 11 of 36 patients to determine that this combination of ADR/IFOS/DTIC is worth pursuing (see statistical section), and a further four responses could occur in the remaining ten evaluable patients; a 36-hour schedule would have obvious advantages over more prolonged 4-day infusional therapy, if response rates and durations were similar. A later analysis will be more informative.

Myelosuppression was severe, with granulocyte nadirs $<0.5 \times 10^9/L$ in approximately 70% of courses. The incidence of infection was comparable to another study of ADR/IFOS/DTIC (6), and none of these episodes were life threatening.

It is interesting to note that although leiomyosarcoma was the most common histological type in the study, 0/10 responded to chemotherapy. Bramwell et al. (4), in a randomized phase II study comparing Ifosfamide with Cyclophosphamide, noted 1/31 responses in patients with leiomyosarcomas despite overall response rates of 18% (IFOS) and 8% (CYCLO). Elias et al. (6) noted a much higher rate of response in patients with locoregional disease only (82% versus 48% for those with metastases), but very few of our patients fell into this category. In general, our patients had bulky metastases - 73% had one or more metastases measuring 5 cms. or greater, and Antman et al. (unpublished data) found this to be an adverse factor p=0.05 in their study of AID.

REFERENCES

1. Bramwell VHC, Pinedo HM: Bone and soft tissue sarcomas. In: Cancer Chemotherapy. The EORTC Cancer Chemotherapy Annual 1. HM Pinedo (ed.). Exerpta Medicas pp. 424-450, 1979.
2. Bonadonna G, Santoro A: Bone and soft tissue sarcomas. In: Cancer Chemotherapy Annual 6. HM Pinedo, BA Chabner (eds.). Elsevier, pp. 436-449, 1984.
3. Bramwell VHC: The role of chemotherapy in multi-disciplinary treatment of soft tissue sarcomas. Canadian J Surg (in press).
4. Bramwell VHC, Mouridsen HT, Santoro A et al.: Cyclophosphamide versus Ifosfamide: final report of a randomized phase II trial in adult soft tissue sarcomas. Eur J Cancer Clin Oncol 23:311-322, 1986.
5. Elias AD, Antman KH: Doxorubicin, Ifosfamide and Dacarbazine (AID) with Mesna uroprotection for advanced untreated sarcoma: a phase I study. Cancer Treat Rep 70: 827-833, 1986.
6. Elias AD, Ryan L, Aisner J, Antman KH: Doxorubicin, Ifosfamide and DTIC (AID) for advanced untreated sarcomas. Proc Am Soc Clin Oncol 6:134, 1987.

CHEMOTHERAPY OF ADVANCED SOFT TISSUE SARCOMAS

Karen H. Antman, M.D.[*]

Abstract: Doxorubicin (Adriamycin) and ifosfamide are the most active single agents in soft tissue sarcoma, with response rates of 15-35% in various trials. Dacarbazine (DTIC), frequently used in combinations, has a response rate as a single agent of 16%.

Both published randomized studies of doxorubicin with or without DTIC observed an increased response rate for the combination. All three randomized trials of doxorubicin based regimens with and without cyclophosphamide have failed to detect an advantage for the addition of cyclophosphamide. Thus, the most active standard combination for soft tissue sarcomas is doxorubicin and DTIC. A randomized trial of 5 gm/m^2 of ifosfamide versus 1.5 gm/m^2 of cyclophosphamide noted a higher response rate for ifosfamide with less myelosuppression. A randomized study of doxorubicin and DTIC with and without ifosfamide is currently underway.

Commercially Available Single Agent Chemotherapy for Soft Tissue Sarcoma

Table 1 summarizes the activity of commercially available single agents in soft tissue sarcoma. Doxorubicin (Adriamycin) alone has a response rate of 15-35% in various studies.(14-21) Both randomized (17,45,46) and nonrandomized (20) studies document higher response rates at doses greater than 50 mg/sqM every 3 weeks, suggesting a steep dose response relationship. Continuous infusion of doxorubicin over 4 days appears equally effective as bolus dosing and may be less cardiotoxic.(21)

Dacarbazine (DTIC) has a single agent response rate of 16%.(23) Administration as a continuous infusion substantially decreases the major toxicity, nausea and vomiting. Other commercially available drugs in adult soft tissue sarcomas (other than rhabdomyosarcoma) have response rates of less than 20%.

The most active investigational agent is ifosfamide, with response rates in Phase II trials in previously treated patients consistently between 15 and 40%.(1-13) The European Organization for Research in the Treatment of Cancer (EORTC) compared cyclophosphamide at 1.5 gm/sqM with 5 gm/sqM

---

*Division of Medicine, Dana Farber Cancer Institute, 44 Binney Street, Boston, MA 02115.

J. R. Ryan and L. O. Baker (eds.), Recent Concepts in Sarcoma Treatment, 174–182.
© 1988 by Kluwer Academic Publishers.

```
┌─────────────────────────────────────────────┐
│ Table 1: Single Agents in Soft Tissue Sarcoma│
│ (in order of response rate)                  │
│                                              │
│                    Reference  Cases    %RR   │
│ Ifosfamide         1-13       188       35   │
│ Doxorubicin        14-21      356       26   │
│ Actinomycin-D      22          30       17   │
│ Dacarbazine(DTIC)  23         109       16   │
│ Methotrexate,                                │
│   standard dose    24-25       49       18   │
│   high dose        26-32       44       10   │
│ Cisplatin          33-36       85       13   │
│ Cyclophosphamide   37,38       15       13   │
│ 5-Fluorouracil     44           8       12   │
│ CCNU               23          19       10   │
│ Etoposide(VP-16)   39,40       41        7   │
│ Bleomycin          41          32        6   │
│ Vincristine        42,43       19        5   │
└─────────────────────────────────────────────┘
```

of ifosfamide in a total of 123 patients with sarcoma (59% with no prior chemotherapy) and observed less hematologic toxicity (p=0.04) and double the response rate for ifosfamide in sarcomas.(13)

Combination Chemotherapy in Soft Tissue Sarcoma

Randomized studies. Table 2 summarizes published data evaluating combination chemotherapy in measurable soft tissue sarcomas. Doxorubicin appears to be the most active standard single agent with a response rate of 20-40%. The combination of doxorubicin and DTIC has been advocated by investigators of M.D. Anderson Hospital in Houston (51,53) and the Southwest Oncology Group, initially as part of the CYVADIC (cyclophosphamide/vincristine/Adriamycin/DTIC) regimen.

Two randomized studies have compared single agent doxorubicin with a combination of doxorubicin and DTIC.(18,47,48) Doxorubicin 60 mg/sqM with or without 250 mg/m^2/day x 5 of DTIC resulted in response rates in measurable gynecologic sarcomas of 24% versus 16%, lasting a median of 5.3 and 4.2 months, respectively.(47) The authors concluded that the increased gastrointestinal toxicity of DTIC was not justified by any significant increase in survival. In the ECOG randomized study (18,48) of doxorubicin versus doxorubicin and DTIC for soft tissue sarcomas, the response rate of the combination was significantly better than that of the single agent given every 21 days or in divided doses weekly.

In contrast, when doxorubicin (50 mg/m^2), cyclophosphamide and vincristine were compared to single agent doxorubicin (70 mg/m^2) in an ECOG study (17), the cyclophosphamide arm was inferior, presumably because of compromise of the dose of doxorubicin. The addition of cyclophosphamide to doxorubicin alone (GOG,50) or to doxorubicin & DTIC (SWOG,49) was not significantly better in either study (Table 2).

Table 2: Randomized Chemotherapy Trials in Soft-Tissue Sarcoma
(Modified from Cancer Treatment Symposia 3:110, 1985)

	Group	Regimen	No	CR	PR	RR%	Comments
Omura	GOG 47	A	80	5	8	16	Uterine sarcomas only
		AD	66	7	9	24	
Lerner	ECOG 48	A	34	1	5	18	
		AD	32	1	13	44	Leiomyosarcomas only
Borden	ECOG 18	A q 3 wk	93	6	12	19	A 15 mg/m^2/wk
		A q wk	92	4	11	16	A 70 mg/^{2} q 3 wks
		AD	95	4	25	30	
Schoenfeld	ECOG 17	A	66	4	14	27	Also included bone sarcomas
		ACV	70	3	10	19	
		CVAd	64	1	6	11	
Baker	SWOG 49	AD	79	11	14	32	
		ADC	95	12	11	35	
		ADAd	98	9	15	24	
Muss	GOG 50	A	50	1	4	19	
		AC	54	2	3	20	
Benjamin	SWOG 51	ADCV	221	31	84	52	
		AAdCV	224	27	63	40	
Bodey	SWOG 45	ADCV	27	4	14	67	A 50 mg/sqM C 500 mg/sqM
		ADCV	24	8	9	71	A 80 mg/sqM C 800 mg/sqM
Pinedo	EORTC 46	ADCV	71	14	18	38	full dose
		AD-CV	74	4	7	14	half dose
Bramwell	EORTC 13	I	68	2	10	18	5gm/sqM
		C	67	1	4	8	1.5 gm/sqM
Baker	SWOG 52	AD	135	9	16	19	Bolus
		AD	143	14	11	18	Continuous Infusion

A: Doxorubicin   D: DTIC
Ad: Actinomycin D I: Ifosfamide
C: Cyclophosphamide V: Vincristine

Nonrandomized Combination Chemotherapy Regimens (Table 3)

A series of nonrandomized studies from M.D. Anderson Hospital in Houston have suggested an improved response rate for soft tissue sarcomas with combination therapy, although the addition of vincristine has never been shown to improve the response rate.(51,53) The Dana Farber Cancer Institute in Boston (DFCI) confirmed a response rate of 55% for a combination of cyclophosphamide, doxorubicin and DTIC.(54) Follow-up of this study reveals a small percentage of long-term disease-free survivors in patients with metastases. A few long-term disease-free survivors, after intensive chemotherapy (approximately one third of the complete responders), have also been observed in a series from The Royal Marsden Hospital in England (55) and the M.D. Anderson Hospital series in Houston.(56)

The role of the addition of ifosfamide to standard sarcoma regimens is not yet defined. Of 33 previously untreated patients with Stages III and IV rhabdomyosarcoma given vincristine, actinomycin D and ifosfamide, 3 g/m^2/dx2,

Table 3: Nonrandomized Combination Chemotherapy in Untreated Sarcomas

Combinations	References	CR(%)	PR	Evaluable	%RR
AD	18,23,47,61	48(10)	120	476	35
ADV	62,63	11(7)	40	161	32
ADVC	51,64,65	62(15)	136	414	48
ADC	21,23,54	20(14)	38	139	42
ADCVM	66	0	7	29	24
ACV	17	3	10	70	19
ACM	67	4	38	140	30
AAdVC	51	25(11)	55	224	36
AAdD	23	9	15	98	24
AAdVMD	66	0	13	41	32
AAdVM	66	0	14	32	44
A + methyl-CCNU	68	3	17	41	49
AV + methyl-CCNU	66	0	10	22	45
A + streptozotocin	69	0	2	14	14
AV-HDM	70	1	2	14	21
ADV-HDM	70	0	2	5	46
AdVC	17,70,63	3(2)	17	142	11
AdL	19	0	1	26	0
AdL + cycloleucine	22	0	0	25	0
Ad + chlorambucil	22	0	5	40	13
AdM + chlorambucil	22	0	8	40	20
IVAd	57	27	4	33	94**
IA	58	NA	NA	125	36
IAD	59,60	6	26	62	52

*	Continuous infusion
**	Rhabdomyosarcoma only
A	Doxorubicin
Ad	Actinomycin C
C	Cyclophosphamide
D	Dacarbazine (DTIC)
(HD)M	(High dose) Methotrexate
I	Ifosfamide
L	(L PAM) Melphalan

27 responded completely and 4 partially. The response rate of 94% with 79% complete responses was "superior" to their prior standard regimens.(57) A Scandinavian study documented a response rate of 36% for a combination of doxorubicin and ifosfamide against previously untreated sarcomas.(58) A Dana Farber Cancer Institute study (59,60) of doxorubicin, ifosfamide and DTIC (AID) in 62 previously untreated sarcoma patients resulted in 6 complete (10%) and 26 partial responses (42%) (overall response rate 52%). Seventy-seven per cent of the inoperable primaries responded versus 42% of metastatic lesions (p=.026). WBC nadirs <500/ul occurred in 26% of courses. Thrombocytopenia <50,000/ul, seen in 19% of patients, was significantly associated with the DTIC dose (p=.03).

REFERENCES

1. Klein HO, Wickramanayake PD, Dias P, Coerper CL, et al.: High-dose ifosfamide and mesna as continuous infusion over five days - a phase I/II trial. Cancer Treat Rev 10(Suppl.A):167-173, 1983.

2. Czownicki Z, Utracka-Hatka B: Clinical studies with uromitexan - an antidote against urotoxicity of holoxan. Preliminary results. Nowotwory 30:377-383, 1980.

3. Czownicki A, Utracka-Hutka B: Contribution to the treatment of malignant tumors with ifosfamide. In Burkert H, Voight HC, eds. Proc Intl Holoxan Symposium. Dusseldorf, W. Germany, Asta-Werke AG. pp.109-111, 1987.

4. Scheulen M, Niederle N, Seeber S: Results of a clinical phase II study on the use of ifosfamide in refractory malignant diseases. Comparison of the uroprotective effect of uromitexan and forced diuresis with alkalization of the urine. New Experience with the Oxazaphosphorines with Special Reference to the Uroprotector Uromitexan, H. Burkert, Bielefeld, and GA Nagel, Gottingen, eds., pp.40, 1980.

5. Magrath IT, Sandlund JT, Rayner A, et al.: Treatment of recurrent sarcomas with ifosfamide (IF). ASCO. 4:136, 1985.

6. Bierbaum W, BHremer K, Firusian N, High M, et al.: Chemotherapeutische Behandlungsmoglichkeiten Bei Forgeschrittenen Sarkomen. Dtsch Med Wochenschr 106: 1181-1185, 1981.

7. Antman K, Montella D, et al.: Phase II trial of ifosfamide with mesna in previously treated metastatic sarcoma. Cancer Treat Rep (in press).

8. Stuart-Harris R, Harper PG, Kaye SB, Wiltshaw E: High-dose ifosfamide by infusion with mesna in advanced soft tissue sarcoma. Cancer Treat Rev 10(Suppl.A):163-164, 1983.

9. Pratt C, Horowitz M, Meyer W, et al.: Phase II trial of ifosfamide (IFOS) with Mesna in patients with pediatric malignant solid tumors. ASCO 4:234, 1985.

10. Wellens W, Mussgnug G, Havets L, et al.: The combination ifosfamide/VP 16-213 in therapy of small cell bronchogenic carcinoma and other malignant tumors. In Burkert H, Nagel G, eds. Beitrage zur Onkologie, Vol 5, Basel and Munchen. Karger, pp. 81-87, 1980.

11. Wellens W, Donhuijsen-Ant R, Habets L, et al.: Therapie progredienter Sarkome mit Etososid und Ifosfamide. Etoposide Symposium, Aktuelle Onkologie, Zuckschwerdt Munchen. 4:159-164, 1981.

12. de Kraker J, Voute PA: Ifosfamide and vincristine in pediatric tumors. A phase II study. Eur Pediatr Haematol Oncol 1:47-50, 1984.

13. Bramwell V, Mouridsen H, Santoro G, et al.: Cyclophosphamide (DP) versus ifosfamide (IF): A randomized phase II trial in adult soft tissue sarcoma (STS). Preliminary report of EORTC Soft Tissue and Bone Sarcomas Group. ASCO 4:143, 1985.

14. Blum RH: An overview of studies in adriamycin (NSC-123127) in the United States. Cancer Chemother Rep 6:247-251, 1975.

15. O'Bryan RM, Luce JK, Talley RW, et al.: Phase II evaluation of adriamycin in human neoplasia. Cancer 32:1-8, 1973.

16. Creagan ET, Hahn RG, Ahmann DL, et al.: A clinical trial, adriamycin (NSC-123127) in advanced sarcomas. Oncology 34:90-91, 1977.

17. Schoenfeld D, Rosenbaum C, Horton J, et al.: A comparison of adriamycin versus vincristine and adriamycin, and cyclophosphamide for advanced sarcoma. Cancer 50:2757-2762, 1982.

18. Borden EC, Amato D, Enterline HT, Lerner H, Carbone PP: Randomized comparison of adriamycin regimens for treatment of metastatic soft tissue sarcomas. Proc ASCO 1983:231(C902).

19. Cruz AB Jr, Thames EA Jr, Aust JB, et al.: Combination chemotherapy for soft tissue sarcomas: A phase III study. J Surg Oncol 11:313-323, 1979.

20. O'Bryan RM, Baker LH, Gottlieb JE, et al.: Dose response evaluation of adriamycin in human neoplasia. Cancer 39:1940-1948, 1977.

21. Legha S, Benjamin RS, Mackay B, et al.: Reduction of doxorubicin cardiotoxicity by prolonged continuous intravenous infusion. Ann Int Med 96:133-139, 1982.

22. Golbey R, Li MC, Kaufman RF: Actinomycin in the treatment of soft part sarcomas. James Ewing Society Scientific Program (abstr.), 1968.

23. Rosenberg SA, Suit HD, Baker LH: Sarcomas of Soft Tissue. In Cancer, Principals & Practice of Oncology, 2nd ed., Philadelphia, JB Lippincott, p.1243.

24. Andrews N, Wilson W: Phase II study of methotrexate (NSC 740) in solid tumors. Cancer Chemother Rep 51:471-474, 1967.

25. Subramanian S, Wiltshaw E: Chemotherapy of sarcoma - A comparison of three regimens. Lancet pp.683-686, 1978.

26. Rosen G, Caparros B, Nirenberg A, et al.: High dose methotrexate (HDMTX) with citrovorum factor rescue (CFR) in the treatment of radiation-induced sarcomas. Proc AACR 1983:194, 1981.

27. Frei E, Blum R, Pitman S, et al.: High dose methotrexate with leucovorin rescue: Rationale and spectrum of antitumor activity, Am J Med 68:370-375, 1979.

28. Vaughn C, McKelvey E, Balcerzak S, et al.: High dose methotrexate with leucovorin rescue plus vincristine in advanced sarcoma: A Southwest Oncology Group Study. Cancer Treat Rep 68:409-410, 1984.

29. Ambinder EP, Perloff M, Ohnuma T, et al.: High-dose methotrexate followed by citrovorum factor reversal in patients with advanced cancer. Cancer 43:1177-1182, 1979.

30. Karakousis CP, Rao U, Carlson M: High-dose methotrexate as secondary chemotherapy in metastatic soft-tissue sarcomas. Cancer 46:1345-2=1348, 1980.

31. Von Hoff DD, Rozencwieg M, Louie AC, et al: "Single"-agent activity of high-dose methotrexate therapy with citrovorum factor rescue. Cancer Treat Rep 62:233-235, 1978.

32. Isacoff WH, Eilber F, Tabbarah H, et al.: Phase II clinical trial with high-dose methotrexate therapy and

citrovorum factor rescue. Cancer Treat Rep 62:1295-1304, 1978.

33. Bramwell VHC, Brugarols A, Mouridsen HT, et al.: EORTC. Phase II study of cisplatinum CYVADIC-resistant soft tissue sarcoma. Eur J Cancer 15:1511-1513, 1979.

34. Karakousis CP, Holterman OA, Holyoke ED: Cisdichloro-diammineplatinum (II) in metastatic soft tissue sarcomas. Cancer Treat Rep 63:2071-2075, 1979.

35. Samson MK, Baker LH, Benhamin RS, et al.: Cis-dichloro-diammineplatinum (II) in advanced soft tissue and bony sarcomas. A Southwest Oncology Group Study. Cancer Treat Rep 63:2027-2028, 1979.

36. Gershenson DM, Kavanagh JJ, Copeland LJ, et al.: Cis-platin therapy for disseminated mixed mesodermal sarcoma of the uterus. J Clin Oncol (in press).

37. Bergsagel DE, Levin WC: A prelusive clinical trial of cyclophosphamide. Cancer Chemother Rep 8:120-134, 1960.

38. Korst DR, Johnson D, Frenkel EP, et al.: Preliminary evaluation of the effect of cyclophosphamide on the course of human neoplasms. Cancer Chemother Rep 7:1-12, 1960.

39. Radice PA, Bunn PA Jr, Ihde DC: Therapeutic trials with VP-16 and VM26. Cancer Treat Rep 63:1231-1239, 1979.

40. Bleyer WA, Chard R, Krivit W, et al.: Epipodophyllotoxin therapy of childhood neoplasia. A comparative phase II analysis of VM-26 and VP 16-213. Proc Am Assoc Cancer Res 19:373, 1978.

41. Amato DA, Borden EC, Shiraki M, et al.: Evaluation of bleomycin, chlorozotocin, MGBG, and bruceantin in patients with advanced soft tissue sarcoma, bone sarcoma, or mesothelioma. Investigational New Drugs 3:397-401, 1985.

42. Selawry OS, Holland JF, Wolman IJ: Effect of vincristine (NSC-67574) on malignant solid tumors in children. Cancer Chemother Rep 52:497-499, 1968.

43. Korbitz BC, Davis HL Jr, Ramirez G, et al.: Low doses of vincristine (NSC-67574) for malignant disease. Cancer Chemother Rep 53:249-254, 1969.

44. Gold G, Hall T, Shnider B, et al.: A clinical study of 5-fluorouracil. Cancer Research 19:935-939, 1959.

45. Bodey GP, et al.: Protected environment - prophylactic antibiotic program for malignant sarcoma: randomized trial during remission induction chemotherapy. Cancer 47:2422-2429, 1981.

46. Pinedo HM, Bramwell VHC, et al.: CYVADIC in advanced soft tissue sarcoma: a randomized study comparing two schedules. A study of the EORTC Soft Tissue and Bone Sarcoma Group. Cancer 53:1825-1832, 1984.

47. Omura GA, et al.: A randomized study of adriamycin with and without dimethyl trazenoimidazole carboxamide in advanced uterine sarcomas. Cancer 52:626-632, 1983.

48. Lerner H, Amato D, Stevens C, et al.: Leiomyosarcoma: the Eastern Cooperative Oncology Group experience with 222 patients. Proc Am Assoc Cancer Res 24:142(C-561), 1983.

49. Baker, LH: Personal communication.
50. Muss HB, Bundy B, DeSaia P, et al.: Treatment of recurrent or advanced uterine sarcoma - a randomized trial of doxorubicin versus doxorubicin and cyclophosphamide (a phase III trial of the Gynecologic Oncology Group). Cancer 55:1648-1653, 1985.
51. Benjamin RS, Gottlieb JA, Baker LH, et al.: CYVADIC vs CYVADACT- a randomized trial of cyclophosphamide (CY), vincristine (V), and adriamycin (A) plus either dacarbazine 'DIC) or actinomycin-D (DACT) in metastatic sarcomas. Proc Am Assoc Cancer Res, Am Soc Clin Oncol 17:256, 1976.
52. Baker L, Green S, Ryan J, et al.: SWOG 8024: Combined modality therapy for disseminated soft tissue sarcoma, Phase III. Proceeding of ASCO 6:138 (abstr. no.542), 1987.
53. Gottlieb JA, Baker LH, et al.: Adriamycin (NSC-123127) used alone and in combination for soft tissue and bony sarcomas. Cancer Chemother Rep. 6:271-282, 1975.
54. Blum R, Corson J, et al.: Successful treatment of metastatic sarcomas with cyclophosphamide, adriamycin, and DTIC (CAD). Cancer 46:1722-1726, 1980.
55. Subramanian S, Wiltshaw E: Chemotherapy of sarcoma. A Comparison of three regimens. The Lancet pp.683, 1978.
56. Yap BS, Sinkovics JG, Benjamim RS, et al.: Survival and relapse patterns of complete responders in adults with advanced soft tissue sarcomas (ASTS). Proc Am Assoc Cancer Res and ASCO 20:352, 1979.
57. Otten J, Flamant F, Rodary C, et al: Effectiveness of combination of ifosfamide, vincristine and actinomycine D in inducing remission in rhabdomyosarcoma in children. For the RMS group of the International Society of Pediatric Oncology (SIOP). ASCO 4:236, 1985.
58. Schutte J, Dombernowsky P, Santoro A, et al.: Adriamycin (A) and ifosfamide (I), a new effective combination in advanced soft tissue sarcoma; preliminary report of a phase II study of the EORTC Soft Tissue and Bone Sarcoma Group. Proc of ASCO 5:145, 1986.
59. Elias AD, Antman K, Ryan L: Doxorubicin (DOX), ifosfamide (IFF), and DTIC with mesna uroprotection for advanced untreated sarcoma. Proc of ASCO, 1987.
60. Elias A, Antman K: Doxorubicin, ifosfamide, and dacarbazine (AID) with mesna uroprotection for advanced untreated sarcoma: a Phase I study. Cancer Treat Rep, 70:827-833, 1986.
61. Gottlieb JA, Maker LH, Quagliana JM, et al.: Chemotherapy of sarcomas with a combination of adriamycin and diemthyltrazenoimidazolecarboxamide. Cancer 30:1632-1638, 1972.
62. Gottlieb JA, Baker LH, Burgess MA, et al.: Sarcoma Chemotherapy. In Cancer Chemotherapy Fundamental Concepts and Recent Advances. 19th Annual Clinical Conference in Cancer, 1974, M.D. Anderson Hospital, Year Book Medical Publishers, 1975.
63. Creagan ET, Hahn JRG, Ahmann DL, et al.: A comparative

clinical trial evaluating the combination of actinomycin D, cyclophosphamide, and vincristine, and a single agent, methyl-CCNU, in advanced sarcomas. Cancer Treat Rep 60:1385-1386, 1976.

64. Yap B, Baker LH, Sinkovics JG, et al.: Cyclophosphamide, vincristine, adriamycin, and DTIC (CYVADIC) combination chemotherapy for the treatment of advanced sarcomas. Cancer Treat Rep 64:93-98, 1980.

65. Pinedo HM, Vendrik CPJ, Bramwell VHC, et al.: Re-evaluation of the CYVADIC regimen for metastatic soft tissue sarcoma. Proc AACR and ASCO (abstr.) C-228, 1979.

66. Shiv MH, Magill GB, Hopfan S: Recent Trends in Treatment of Soft Tissue Sarcomas-Appendix A. In Hajdu SI (ed.): Pathology of Soft Tumors, Philadelphia, Lea & Febiger, pp.537-542. 1979.

67. Lowenbraun S, Moffitt JS, Smalley R, et al.: Combination chemotherapy with adriamycin, cyclophosphamide and methotrexate in metastatic sarcomas. ASCO (abstr.) 18:289, 1977.

68. Rivkin SE, Gottlieb JA, Thigpen T, et al: Methyl CCNU and adriamycin for patients with metastatic sarcomas. A Southwest Oncology Group Study. Cancer 46:446-451, 1980.

69. Chang P, Wiernik PH: Combination chemotherapy with adriamycin and streptozotocin. Clin Pharmacol Ther 20:605-610, 1976.

70. Kaufman JH, Catane R, Douglass HO: Combined adriamycin, vincristine, and methotrexate. NY State J Med 742-743, 1977.

71. Jacobs EM: Combination chemotherapy of metastatic testicular germinal cell tumors and soft part sarcomas. Cancer 25:324-332, 1970.

CHEMOTHERAPY IN ADVANCED SOFT TISSUE SARCOMA - THE EORTC EXPERIENCE

A.T. Van Oosterom[1], A. Santoro[2], J. Rouessé[3],
H.T. Mouridsen[4], W.P. Steward[5], R. Somers[6], J. Buesa[7],
G. Blackledge[8], J. Schütte[9], T. Wagener[10], J.H. Mulder[11],
V.H.C. Bramwell[12], H.M. Pinedo[13], D. Thomas[14], R. Sylvester[14]

The Soft Tissue and Bone Sarcoma Group (STBSG) is one of the 17 clinical cooperative groups of the European Organization for Research and Treatment of Cancer (EORTC). It was constituted in 1975 and increased from nine full members in 1976 to 21 full and 11 probational members from nine European countries by 1987.

Over 2000 patients have been entered into the first and second line studies. The Group meets three times a year and has surgical and radiotherapy subcommittees and two regional pathology review committees who meet at least twice a year. Slides of every patient entered in any study are reviewed.

Eligibility criteria are now standardized for both studies of advanced disease and adjuvant therapy.

Entry criteria include age ≥ 15 years, histologically proven advanced or metastatic sarcoma with measurable pro-

----

[1]Department of Oncology, University Hospital Antwerp, 10 Wilrijkstraat, 2520 Edegem, BELGIUM.

[2]1st. Nazionale per lo Studio e la Cura dei Tumori, Milano, ITALY.

[3]Centre René Huguenin, St. Cloud, FRANCE.

[4]Dept. of Medicine, Finsen Institutet, Copenhagen, DENMARK.

[5]Christie Hospital, Medical Oncology Department, Manchester, UNITED KINGDOM.

[6]Antoni van Leeuwenhoek Ziekenhuis, Amsterdam, THE NETHERLANDS.

[7]Hospital General de Asturias, Servicio de Quimioterapia, Oviedo, SPAIN.

[8]West Midlands CRC Clinical Trial Unit, Queen Elizabeth Hospital, Birmingham, UNITED KINGDOM.

[9]Dept. Oncology, West German Cancer Center, Essen, FED. REP. GERMANY.

[10]Radboudziekenhuis, University Hospital Nijmegen, Nijmegen, THE NETHERLANDS.

[11]Daniel den Hoedkliniek, R.R.T.I., Rotterdam, THE NETHERLANDS.

[12]Ontario Cancer Foundation London Clinic, London, Ontario, CANADA.

[13]Dept. of Oncology, Free University Hospital, Amsterdam, THE NETHERLANDS.

[14]EORTC Datacenter, Brussels, BELGIUM.

J. R. Ryan and L. O. Baker (eds.), Recent Concepts in Sarcoma Treatment, 183–190.
© 1988 by Kluwer Academic Publishers.

gressive disease, WHO performance status 0,1 or 2, and adequate renal function (serum creatinine < 150 µmol/1), hepatic excretory function (serum bilirubin < 20 µmol/1) and bone marrow reserve (leucocytes > $3,5.10^9/1$ and platelets > $100.10^9/1$). Recurrent tumor in an irradiated area is not permitted as the sole evaluable lesion, and pleural effusions and bone metastases are not considered measurable.

Other criteria for exclusion are a previous or concomitant different malignant tumor, any serious concurrent disease and central nervous system metastases.

Informed consent is obtained according to local institutional/national requirements.

The upper age limit and specifications regarding previous chemotherapy vary between protocols.

Response and toxicity are graded according to the WHO criteria (1).

The sarcoma types included in the soft tissue sarcoma studies are of the following cell types: malignant fibrous histiocytoma, liposarcoma, rhabdomyosarcoma, synovial sarcoma, fibrosarcoma, leiomyosarcoma, angiosarcoma including hemangiopericytoma, neurogenic sarcoma, unclassified sarcoma and miscellaneous sarcomas including mixed mesodermal tumors of the uterus.

The following cell types have always been excluded: malignant mesothelioma, paraganglioma, chondrosarcoma, neuroblastoma, osteosarcoma, Ewing's sarcoma/embryonal rhabdomyosarcoma.

Patients are registered by telephone, telex or via the Eurocode system at the EORTC data center in Brussels (Belgium), where all data are collected and analyzed.

First Line Studies

In the five finalized and one ongoing first-line studies about 1000 patients fulfilling all eligibility criteria and fully evaluable at pathological and clinical review have been entered.

In the first study (2) the CyVADic regimen, which had produced impressive results in the SWOG (3) report, has been compared with the alternating regimen consisting of Adriamycin/DTIC and Cyclophosphamide/Vincristine.

The response rate of 38% for the classical regimen was disappointing in comparison with the first SWOG publication which, however, later could not be confirmed.(4) It was more interesting that, in spite of the difference in response rate (only 14%) with the alternating regimen, no difference in time to progression or survival between the two arms could be observed.

The most important finding was the striking influence of the patients' Karnofsky Performance status (KP) at the start of treatment on the response. The response rate was respectively: 46% for KP 100%, 38% for KP 90%, and less than 20% for all other performance scores.

The Group had long discussions about these results, the inconvenience and toxicity of the regimen, and finally decided to start investigating less inconvenient and, hopefully, less toxic regimens which might have similar response rates.

In the next two studies, Adriamycin was selected as the control arm since it was, at that time, the only available drug with a repeatedly confirmed 25-30% response rate if given at adequate dosage (≥ 70 mg/m^2) (5,6). The first drug it was compared with was Carminomycin, a drug with a suggested similar response rate and less toxicity. (7) The toxicity was lower (8), but so also was the activity. See Table 1.

Table 1						
First line chemotherapy studies, EORTC ST + BS group.						
Drugs	n(ev)	CR	PR	CR + PR	RR%	Ref.
CyVADic	84	14	11	32	38	2
vs CyV-Adic	78	4	7	11	14	
Adriamycin	38	1	10	11	29	8
vs Carminomycin	33	0	1	1	3	
Adriamycin	83	6	15	21	25	9
vs Epirubicin	84	4	11	15	18	
Cyclophosphamid	38	1	4	5	13	11
vs Ifosfamid	40	2	8	10	25	
Adria+Ifos.	178	16	48	64	36	12
Adriamycin Adria+Ifos CyVADic	started nov'85	june 1	'87: entered 326.			13

The second randomized tested single agent was Epirubicin which also was less toxic and less active, but not significantly. The conclusion from this study (9) must be that Epirubicin should be re-tested at a higher dose to produce the same myelotoxicity and, hence, better activity might result. The activity of Adriamycin in these studies was 26% but with considerable toxicity and only 8% complete responses. (9)

During the last study, a second line randomized phase II study revealed the already published (10) activity of Ifosfamide with some good and several minor responses. (11) This led the Group into a study where Cyclophosphamide, a drug extensively used in combinations in sarcomas, but with scarce single agent data, was investigated versus Ifosfamide.

The response rate observed was 25% in non-pretreated patients, which was very similar to the Group's previous experience with Adriamycin. Cyclophosphamide was less active, with a response rate of 13%, but the difference was not significant. The higher response rate for Ifosfamide with less myelo-suppression suggested that this drug might have advantages over Cyclophosphamide in combination with

Adriamycin.

The Group then decided to go back to a combination and selected Adriamycin 50 mg/m^2, the same dose as in the CyVADic combination, and Ifosfamide 5 g/m^2 over 24 hours. This pilot study raised great enthusiasm and accrued very rapidly.

In 16 months, over 200 patients were entered, of whom, 178 proved eligible and evaluable. The response rate was 36% with 9% complete responders. (12) The preliminary results of this study were encouraging and so a study (which is still open) was started in 1985 to compare the Adriamycin/Ifosfamide combination with the different options from the past CyVADic and Adriamycin single agent.

This study will be closed in November 1987 if the two-year accrual is over 400 patients. This should certainly be achieved since the monthly accrual has been 18-19 patients in the last six months and, as of June 1, 326 patients had been entered.

Second Line Studies

After finding that the results of treatment with CyVADic (in the study initiated in 1976) were disappointing as compared with previous reports in the literature, we were left with a group of patients with good performance status for whom no further treatment was available. Up to that time, only a small number of drugs had been tested in adequate phase II studies. Therefore, in 1977, the Group decided to start a phase II program, which has resulted in the data presented in Table 2. In nine years, 13 drugs have been adequately tested in about 400 patients of whom, 337 proved fully evaluable. Several important data have evolved. Firstly, the activity of Ifosfamide (already demonstrated by others) could be confirmed because patients entered into the studies had a progression arrest in over 50%. (26)

The phase II studies require measurable disease which is progressive (at least 25% increase) in the two months prior to entry. So, if patients have a response or remain stable (less than 50% decrease and less than 25% increase), This means that the drug has at least some activity. The demonstration of a progression-arrest in >50% of patients suggests that the drug should be tested as a first-line agent in further patients. We found this progression arrest for three drugs: respectively, 72% for Adriamycin (21), 64% for Ifosfamide (11), and very recently 52% for DTIC (given in a bolus injection of 1200 mg/m^2 on day 1 every 3 weeks). (22) Secondly, the activity observed for DTIC justifies its inclusion in future combinations where it can be given on one day only (as it is in the CyVADic arm of our ongoing phase III study). It also justifies its use in combination with Ifosfamide and Adriamycin (as a two-day treatment) - a regimen we will shortly be testing as a first line treatment. (27)

Thirdly, many have suggested that this type of phase II testing in pretreated or advanced patients will not result in the discovery of new active drugs. We believe this to be incorrect because all three known active drugs could be identified with the progression-arrest >50% rule, and DTIC

Table 2

Second-line phase II studies, EORTC ST + BS Group.

Drug	Dose	N	CR	PR	No Ch.	Ref
Cisplatin	100 mg/m^2 q 3 wks	17	-	-	4	14
Chlorozotocin	120 mg/m^2 q 4 wks	17	-	-	3	15
Methotrexate	40 mg/m^2 weekly	26	-	-	4	16
PALA	2,5g/m^{2}d1,2 q 2 wks	27	-	1	4	17
Elliptinium	100mg/m^2 weekly	19	-	-	8	18
Mitomycin C	12mg/m^2 q 3 wks	34	-	-	12	19
Cyclophosphamide	1.5g/m^2 q 3 wks	29	-	-	11	11
Ifosfamide	5g/m^2 q 3 wks	28	1	1	16	11
Vepesid (oral)	130mg/m^{2}d1-5 q 3 wks	26	-	1	7	20
Adriamycin	75mg/m^2 q 3 wks	18	-	3	10	21
DTIC	1.2 g/m^2 q 3 wks	42	1	7	14	22
TGU	600mg/m^2 q 4 wks	21	-	-	3	23
MDMS	125mg/m^2 q 5 wks	33	-	-	8	24
Mitozolomide	90mg/m^2 q 6 wks	25	too early			25

and Adriamycin even had, respectively, a 19% and 17% WHO response rate.

We have, therefore, decided to continue phase II testing in this way including patients with a WHO performance score of 0 or 1, measurable disease, which has progressed over the two months prior to study entry, and who have not received more than four cytotoxic agents previously. No more than 25 patients are entered unless responses are reported to the study coordinator.

It is our belief that with the cooperation which has been established within the Group in the past ten years, with the increasing numbers of patients included in studies, and the rising number of new drugs available, the discovery of more active agents for use in this disease will grow.

Inclusion of one or more of these into new combinations could, hopefully, result in similar advances being made as have already occurred in the treatment of Hodgkin's disease and testicular cancer.

REFERENCES

1. WHO. Handbook for Reporting Results of Cancer Treatment. WHO Offset Publication, Number 48, Geneva, 1979.
2. Pinedo HM, Bramwell VHC, Mouridsen HT, Somers R, Vendrik CPJ, Santoro A, Buesa J, Wagener Th, van Oosterom AT, van Unnik JAM, Sylvester R, De Pauw M, Thomas D,

Bonadonna G: Cyvadic in advanced soft tissue sarcoma: a randomized study comparing two schedules. A study of the EORTC Soft Tissue and Bone Sarcoma Group. Cancer 53:1825-1832, 1984.

3. Gottlieb JA, Baker LH, O'Bryan RM, et al.: Adriamycin (NSC-123127) used alone and in combination for soft tissue and bone sarcomas. Cancer Chemother Rep 6:271-282, 1975.

4. Yap BS, Baker LH, Sinkovics JG, et al.: Cyclophosphamide, vincristine, adriamycin and DTIC (CYVADIC) combination chemotherapy for the treatment of advanced sarcomas. Cancer Treat Rep 64:93-98, 1980.

5. Bramwell VHC, Pinedo HM: Bone and soft tissue sarcomas. In HM Pinedo, (ed.): Cancer Chemotherapy. The EORTC Cancer Chemotherapy Annual 1. Excerpta Medica 1979:424-450.

6. Bramwell VHC, Pinedo HM: Bone and soft tissue sarcomas. In HM Pinedo (ed.): Cancer Chemotherapy. The EORTC Cancer Chemotherapy Annual 2. Excerpta Medica 1980:393-414.

7. Perevudchikova NI, Lichinityer MR, Gorbunova VA: Phase I clinical study of carminomycin: its activity against soft tissue sarcoma. Cancer Treat Rep 61:1705, 1977.

8. Bramwell VHC, Mouridsen HT, Mulder JH, Somers R, Van Oosterom AT, Santoro A, Thomas D, Sylvester R, Markham D: Carminomycin versus Adriamycin in advanced soft tissue sarcomas: an EORTC randomised phase II study. Eur J of Cancer and Clin Oncol 19:1097-1104, 1983.

9. Mouridsen HT, Somers R, Santoro A, Mulder JH, Bramwell V, Van Oosterom AT, Sylvester R, Thomas D, Pinedo HM: Doxorubicin versus epirubicin in advanced soft tissue sarcomas. An EORTC randomized phase II study. In Advances in anthracycline chemotherapy: epirubicin. G. Bonadonna (Ed.), pp. 95-103, 1984. ISBN 88.214.1715.8.

10. Stuart-Harris RC, Harper PG, Parsons CA et al.: High dose alkylation therapy using Ifosfamide infusion with Mesna in the treatment of adult advanced soft tissue sarcoma. Cancer Chemother Pharm 11:69-72, 1983.

11. Bramwell VHC, Mouridsen HT, Santoro A, Blackledge G, Somers R, Verwey J, Dombernowsky P, Onsrud M, Thomas D, Sylvester R, Van Oosterom AT (for the European Organization for Research and Treatment of Cancer, Soft Tissue and Bone Sarcoma Group: Cyclophosphamide versus Ifosfamide: final report of a randomized phase II trial in adult soft tissue sarcomas. Eur J Cancer and Clin Oncol 23:311-323, 1987.

12. Schütte J, Dombernowsky P, Santoro A, Stewart W, Mouridsen HT, Somers R, Van Oosterom AT, Blackledge G, Thomas D, Sylvester R (1986): Adriamycin (A) and ifosfamide (I), a new effective combination in advanced soft tissue sarcoma. Preliminary report of a phase II study of the EORTC Soft Tissue and Bone Sarcoma Group. Proc Eur Conf Clin Oncol, 4:232, 1987.

13. Santoro A: Personal communication, 1987.

14. Bramwell VHC, Brugarolas A, Mouridsen HT, Cheix F,

de Jager R, Van Oosterom AT, Vendrik CPJ, Pinedo HM, Sylvester R, De Pauw M: EORTC phase II study of Cisplatin in CyVADIC resistant soft tissue sarcomas. Eur J Cancer 15:1511-1513, 1979.

15. Mouridsen HT, Bramwell VHC, Lacave J, Metz R, Vendrik CPJ, Hild J, Mc Creanney J, Sylvester R: Treatment of advanced soft tissue sarcomas with chlorozotocin. a phase II trial of the EORTC Soft Tissue and Bone Sarcoma Group. Cancer Treat Rep 65:509-511, 1981.

16. Buesa JM, Mouridsen HT, Santoro A, Somers R, Bramwell V, Van Oosterom AT, Wagener Th, Vendrik C, Thomas D: Treatment of advanced soft tissue sarcomas with low-dose Methotrexate: a phase II trial by the European Organization for Research and Treatment of Cancer (EORTC) Soft Tissue and Bone Sarcoma Group, Cancer Treat Rep, 68:683, 1984.

17. Bramwell V, Van Oosterom AT, Mouridsen HT, Cheix F, Somers R, Thomas D, Rozencweig MN: -(Phosphonacetyl)-L-Aspartate (PALA) in advanced soft tissue sarcoma: a phase II trial of the EORTC Soft Tissue and Bone Sarcoma Group. Eur J Cancer and Clin Oncol 18:81-84, 1982.

18. Somers R, Rouessé J, Van Oosterom AT, Thomas D: Phase II study of elliptinium in metastatic soft tissue sarcoma. Eur J Cancer Clin Oncol 21:591-593, 1985.

19. Van Oosterom AT, Santoro A, Bramwell V, Davy M, Mouridsen HT, Thomas D, Sylvester R: Mitomycin C (MMc) in advanced soft tissue sarcoma: a phase II study of the EORTC Soft Tissue and Bone Sarcoma Group. Eur J Cancer Clin Oncol 21:459-461, 1985.

20. Dombernowsky P, Buesa J, Pinedo HM, Santoro A, Mouridsen H, Somers R, Bramwell V, Onsrud M, Rouessé J, Thomas D, Sylvester R: VP 16 (Etoposide) in advanced soft tissue sarcoma: a phase II study of the EORTC Soft Tissue and Bone Sarcoma Group. Eur J Cancer Clin Oncol 23:579, 1987.

21. Blackledge G, Van Oosterom AT, Mouridsen HT, et al.: Treatment of advanced soft tissue sarcomas with adriamycin in second line. A phase II study of the EORTC Soft Tissue and Bone Sarcoma Group. Submitted for publication.

22. Buesa JM, Mouridsen H, Van Oosterom AT, Steward WT, Verwey J, Thomas D: High-dose DTIC in advanced soft-tissue sarcomas (STS) of the adult. A phase II study of the EORTC Soft-Tissue and Bone Sarcoma Group. Program and Abstracts, fifth NCI EORTC Symposium on new drugs in cancer therapy. Amsterdam nr. 2.20, 1986.

23. Rouessé J, Van Oosterom AT, Kerbrat P, Cappelaere P, Pinedo H, Thomas D, Benshahar D: Phase II study of 1,2,4 triglycidyl urasol (TGU) in advanced soft tissue sarcoma. A trial of EORTC's Soft Tissue and Bone Sarcoma Cooperative Group. Eur J Cancer Clin Oncol 21:1413-1414, 1987.

24 Steward WP, Somers R, Kerbrat P, Verwey J, Buesa J, et al: Phase II study of Methyleen dimethane sulphonate (MDMS) in advanced soft tissue sarcomas of the adults.

(in preparation).

25. Somers R: Personal communication.
26. Van Oosterom AT, Bramwell VHC, Mouridsen HT, Somers R, Santoro A, Buesa J, Vendrik CP, Rouessé J, Dombernowsky P, Pinedo HM, Thomas D, Sylvester R: Review of the EORTC Soft Tissue and Bone Sarcoma Group's Phase II studies in advanced soft tissue sarcomas. In Management of Soft Tissue and Bone Sarcomas. Van Oosterom AT, van Unnik JAM (eds.), EORTC monograph, vol. 16, Raven Press, New York, pp. 161-167, 1986.
27. Verwey J: Personal communication.

PROGNOSTIC INDICATORS FOR SOFT TISSUE SARCOMA PATIENTS WITH
PULMONARY METASTASES

Jack A. Roth, M.D.*

Twenty to 30% of patients with soft tissue sarcomas
metastatic to the lungs will achieve disease-free survival of
three years or more following resection.(1-3) However, in
all series, a significant number of patients have
unresectable pulmonary metastases at the time of exploration
or develop recurrence of their metastases rapidly following
resection. Therefore, it would be useful to be able to
predict a patient's prognosis and resectability prior to
surgical exploration of the chest.

Criteria such as patient age, sex, primary tumor location, and radiographic involvement of one or both lungs are
generally not predictive. Several criteria, including the
number of pulmonary metastases, tumor doubling time, and
disease-free interval, are predictive of prognosis in one or
more previous studies.

Of nine studies encompassing a variety of tumors that
investigated disease-free interval, seven found a positive
correlation with survival.(2-10) Nine studies analyzed the
correlation between the number of metastases and survival.
(3,5,8,9,11-15) Five of the studies found that more metastases correlated with poorer survival for several types of
cancers. The four studies that did not show a correlation
compared only single with multiple metastases, rather than
determining a value that discriminated between good and poor
prognosis patients. The tumor doubling time also correlated
with prognosis in three of four studies.(3,5,9,16) One study
that examined tumor doubling time for osteogenic sarcoma
patients did not find a correlation.(5)

I will review the application of the above prognostic
indicators for patients with adult soft tissue sarcomas. This
review includes patients evaluated by the staff of the
Surgery Branch of the National Cancer Institute between 1974
and 1985. A group of 67 patients with histologically confirmed, isolated pulmonary metastases, who underwent exploration for surgical resection, were analyzed.(3,17)

Number of Metastases

The number of metastatic nodules on the preoperative
linear tomograms significantly correlated with postoperative

----

*The University of Texas System Cancer Center, M.D. Anderson
Hospital and Tumor Institute, Department of Thoracic
Surgery, 1515 Holcombe Boulevard, Houston, TX 77030.

J. R. Ryan and L. O. Baker (eds.), Recent Concepts in Sarcoma Treatment, 191–196.

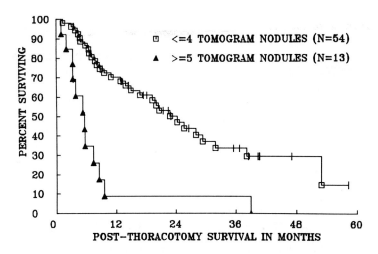

FIGURE 1: Post-thoracotomy survival in patients
with four or less nodules identified
on preoperative full-lung tomograms
compared to patients with five or more
nodules (p=0.001).

survival (Figure 1). Patients with four or fewer nodules had
a longer post-thoracotomy survival time (23 months median)
than patients with more than four nodules (6 months median).
The actual number of metastases present at exploration may be
two to four times the number on the preoperative radiographs
depending on the technique used.(18) This relationship was
observed for the documented number of metastases at surgery.
Patients with 15 or fewer metastases resected had a longer
post-thoracotomy survival (25 months median) than those
patients with 16 or more metastases (6 months median).

Disease-Free Interval

The disease-free interval (time from resection of the
primary tumor to appearance of pulmonary metastases) also
correlated with survival. Survival for patients with disease-
free interval of more than 12 months (30 months median) was
improved compared to patients with a disease-free interval of
12 months or less (10 months median).

Tumor Doubling Time

Because the time interval between a 1 cm diameter metastasis when the lesion is reproducibly visible on the roent-
genogram, and a 10 cm metastasis when the host is near death,
is relatively short in the total life history of a neoplasm,
the growth during this time may be approximated as linear.
The technique for measuring tumor doubling time has been
previously described.(16) In our series, patients with a
tumor doubling time of 20 days or more had a longer post-
thoracotomy survival (22 months median) than patients with a

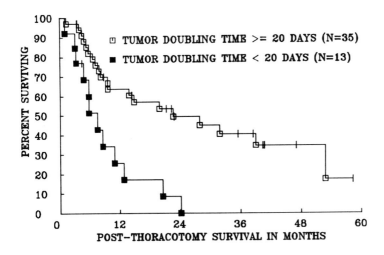

FIGURE 2: Post-thoracotomy survival in patients
with a tumor doubling time of $\geq$ 20 days
and < 20 days (p=0.003).

tumor doubling time of less than 20 days (6 months median)
(Figure 2).

Applicability to Other Histologies
        When the tumor doubling time, the number of metastases
on the preoperative tomograms, and the disease-free interval
were combined, there was a significant increase in the predictive ability of the model over either individual factor or
pair. Although all three criteria were useful in predicting
survival for patients with soft tissue sarcomas, they were
not equally useful for patients with osteogenic sarcoma. Only
the number of metastases visible on the preoperative tomogram
was predictive of survival for patients with osteogenic
sarcoma.(17) This occurred because the distribution of the
disease-free intervals and tumor doubling times were short
for the majority of osteogenic sarcoma patients, and thus
they were not distributed widely enough among patients with
varying prognoses. This is confirmed by a subsequent study
that also demonstrated a correlation of number of metastases
with survival, but showed no correlation for disease-free
interval.(15)

Indicators for Patients with an Isolated Pulmonary Recurrence
        Following the first resection of pulmonary metastases,
29 patients underwent a second resection for recurrence.(19)
Twenty patients had two subsequent procedures, seven had
three, and two had four. The number of metastases on
tomogram at first recurrence, but not the number seen at the
second recurrence, predicted survival. Although the interval
between resection of the primary and first lung recurrence
was not predictive of survival after the second resection,

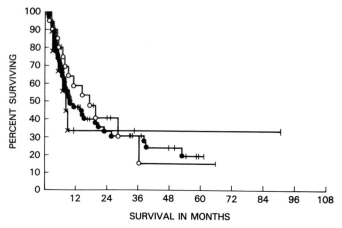

FIGURE 3: Survival from last resection by number of resections for pulmonary metastases.

the interval between the first pulmonary resection and the lung recurrence was predictive. The tumor doubling time of the initial metastases, but not of the subsequent metastases, predicted prognosis. The survival curves for patients who underwent one, two or greater than two procedures, were not statistically significantly different (Figure 3).

Conclusions

The number of metastases detected by preoperative tomography is the most readily obtainable and widely applicable of the prognostic indicators studied. Tumor doubling time correlates with prognosis for soft tissue sarcomas, but was not useful for osteogenic sarcomas. This measurement requires serial chest roentgenograms and is not easily determined in the clinic. None of the prognostic indicators are sufficiently accurate to exclude patients from surgical resection. However, they may be useful in the overall decision-making process, and can also serve to identify and stratify patients for investigational trials.

REFERENCES

1. Martini N, McCormack PM, Bains MS: Indications for surgery for intrathoracic metastases in testicular carcinoma. Sem Oncol 6:99-101, 1979.
2. Creagan ET, Fleming TR, Edmonson JH, Pairolero PC: Pulmonary resection for metastatic non-osteogenic

sarcoma. Cancer 44:1908-1912, 1979.

3. Putnam Jr. JB, Roth JA, Wesley MN, Johnston MR, Rosenberg SA: Analysis of prognostic factors in patients undergoing resection of pulmonary metastases from soft tissue sarcomas. J Thorac Cardiovasc Surg 87:260-267, 1984.

4. Burgers JMV, Breur K, Van Dobbenburgh OA, et al.: Role of metastasectomy without chemotherapy in the management of osteosarcoma in children. Cancer 45:1664-1668, 1980.

5. Putnam Jr. JB, Roth JA, Wesley MN, Johnston MR, Rosenberg SA: Survival following aggressive resection of pulmonary metastases from osteogenic sarcoma: Analysis of prognostic factors. Ann Thoracic Surg 38:516-523, 1983.

6. Cahan WG, Castro EB, Hajdu SI: The significance of a solitary lung shadow in patients with colon carcinoma. Cancer 33:414-421, 1974.

7. Cahan WG, Castro EB: Significance of a solitary lung shadow in patients with breast cancer. Ann Surg 181:131-143, 1975.

8. Morrow CE, Vassilopoulos P, Grage TB: Surgical resection for metastatic neoplasms of the lung. Cancer 45:2981-2985, 1980.

9. Takita H, Edgerton F, Karakousis C, Douglass HO, Vincent RG, Beckley S: Surgical management of metastases to the lung. Surg Gynecol Obstet 152:191-194, 1981.

10. Turney SZ, Haight C: Pulmonary resection for metastatic neoplasms. J. Thoracic Cardiovasc Surg 61:784-794, 1971.

11. Cahan WG, Castro B, Hajdu SI: Therapeutic pulmonary resection of colonic carcinoma metastatic to the lung. Dis Colon Rectum 17:302-309, 1974.

12. McCormack PM, Attiyeh FF: Resection of pulmonary metastases from colorectal cancer. Dis Colon Rectum 22:553-556, 1979.

13. Telander RL, Pairolero PC, Pritchard DJ, Sim FH, Gilchrist GS: Resection of pulmonary metastatic osteogenic sarcoma in children. Surgery 84:335-341, 1978.

14. Ishihara TK, Kikuchi K, Ikeda T, Yamazaki S: Metastatic pulmonary diseases: Biologic factors and modes of treatment. Chest 63:227-232, 1973.

15. Meyer WH, Schell MJ, Kumar APM, Rao BN, Green AA, Champion J, Pratt CB: Thoracotomy for pulmonary metastatic osteosarcoma: An analysis of prognostic indicators of survival. Cancer 59:374-379, 1987.

16. Joseph WL, Morton DL, Adkins PC: Prognostic significance of tumor doubling time in evaluating operability in pulmonary metastatic disease. J Thorac Cardiovasc Surg 61:23-32, 1971.

17. Roth JA, Putnam JB, Wesley MN, Rosenberg SA: Differing determinants of prognosis following resection of pulmonary metastases from osteogenic and soft tissue sarcoma patients. Cancer 55:1361-1366, 1985.

18. Pass HI, Dwyer A, Makuch R, Roth JA: Detection of pulmonary metastases in patients with osteogenic and soft-

tissue sarcomas: The superiority of CT scans compared with conventional linear tomograms using dynamic analysis. J Clin Oncol 3:1261-1265, 1985.

19. Rizzoni WE, Pass HI, Wesley MN, Rosenberg SA, Roth JA: Resection of recurrent pulmonary metastases in patients with adult soft tissue sarcomas. Arch Surg 121:1248-1252, 1986.

PULMONARY RESECTION IN SARCOMA METASTASES

Nael Martini, M.D.[1], and Patricia M. McCormack, M.D.[2]

The first pulmonary resection of a metastatic sarcoma to lung performed at Memorial Hospital was in 1940. For the ensuing 25 years, surgery was offered only to select patients with 1 or 2 metastases and a long disease-free interval after treatment of their primary tumor. Our early experience in treating systematically pulmonary metastases began in 1965 and was limited to osteogenic sarcoma. The initial 22 patients with resected metastases that we reported in 1971 have now been followed for 20 years and 6 of these (27%) are still alive and well.

From 1960 to 1983, pulmonary resection was carried out at our Center in 389 patients with metastases from a variety of soft tissue and bony sarcomas (Table 1).

The majority of patients (85%) had no symptoms at the time of diagnosis of their metastases. Only 15% were symptomatic due to pleural involvement or endobronchial invasion with secondary chest pain, cough or hemoptysis.

Since sarcomas have a particular predilection to metastasize to the lungs, taking chest roentgenograms has become an integral part of the workup and the follow-up in all patients with sarcoma. Once metastases are detected on the plain chest films, computerized chest tomography (CT) is now routinely done to determine the number and location of these lesions. Additional nodules are uniformly found on CT scans in patients presenting with multiple metastases on plain roentgenograms.

Since most pulmonary metastases are peripheral, bronchoscopy is generally unrewarding except in the rare instance of endobronchial involvement. In the presence of multiple lesions, a preoperative biopsy is usually not necessary. In the instance of a solitary lesion, differential diagnosis necessarily includes benign lesions of lung and a new lung primary tumor. Tissue diagnosis becomes essential in patients that will not be treated surgically. In those that are good operative risk, the correct histologic diagnosis is generally

---

[1]Chief, Thoracic Surgery Memorial Sloan-Kettering Cancer Center, 1275 York Avenue, New York, NY 10021; Professor of Surgery, Cornell University Medical College, New York, NY.
[2]Associate Attending Surgeon, Memorial Sloan-Kettering Cancer Center; Associate Professor of Surgery, Cornell University Medical College, New York, NY.

J. R. Ryan and L. O. Baker (eds.), Recent Concepts in Sarcoma Treatment, 197–200.
© 1988 by Kluwer Academic Publishers.

TABLE 1

ORIGIN OF THE PRIMARY TUMOR
(1960-1983)

Osteosarcoma		166
Chondrosarcoma		15
Soft tissue sarcoma		208
Synovial	38	
Leiomyo	38	
MFH	21	
Fibro	19	
Rhabdomyo	17	
Lipo	14	
Alveolar soft part	11	
Other	35	
Total		389

obtained at thoracotomy.

the surgical approach to pulmonary metastases varies with the state and treatment needs of the primary tumor and the timing of the appearance of the metastases. Surgical treatment of the metastases is offered to patients who are good operative risks and in whom the primary tumor is controlled, no extrathoracic metastases are present, and no effective nonoperative therapy is available. In simultaneous presentations, surgical treatment of the pulmonary metastases is recommended first, particularly if major ablative surgery is considered for the primary site. Once the lungs are cleared of tumor, the primary is then resected. The reverse sequence is entertained when resectability of the primary tumor is questionable and the pulmonary metastases are limited to 1 or 2 lesions in one lung.

The extent of resection depends on the location of the metastases. Small, peripheral lesions are easily removed by wedge excision, but a deep-seated tumor or central lesion may require a lobectomy or pneumonectomy. For the surgical treatment of pulmonary metastases to be effective and justified, two considerations are paramount. The first is removal of all gross tumor and the second is maximal conservation of functioning lung tissue. In general, most cases are treated by wedge resection, a few by lobectomy, and less than 5% by pneumonectomy. This latter procedure is done when metastases are solitary and central, and when complete resection can be effective with minimal risk. Enucleation is reserved for the small, deep-seated, multiple or solitary tumors in patients with impaired pulmonary reserve.

Since the majority of the patients with pulmonary metastases are asymptomatic, surgical treatment must be aimed for prolonged survival and cure. Palliative resection is limited to the symptomatic patients with an obstructing endobronchial lesion. For patients presenting with solitary or multiple pulmonary metastases, the posterolateral thoracotomy approach is preferred. Thus, access to all metastases is possible, and complete removal of all tumor is more certain. In patients with bilateral lung metastases, a median sternotomy is preferred by some, and staged lateral thoracotomy by others. A single operation is desirable whenever possible, but must be balanced against the need for complete removal of all tumor. Centrally placed lesions and those in the left lower lobe, particularly if multiple, are difficult to resect from a sternotomy approach. When the bilateral metastases are few, peripheral and anteriorly placed, a median sternotomy with split lung anesthesia is effective.

Extension of pulmonary metastases to mediastinum, chest wall or diaphragm, and effusion are poor prognostic signs, since neither adequate resection not prolonged survival are attained in this group of patients. In patients with solitary or central lesions found unresectable at thoracotomy, significant palliation can be achieved by interstitial irradiation with Iodine 125 permanent implant.

It is often necessary to consider resection in recurrent pulmonary metastases. So long as the risks are low and preservation of adequate lung tissue is possible, resection is offered if nonsurgical alternatives are not available.

The overall 5-year survival in resected metastases from all types of sarcoma is 25%, with little difference in survival among the various histologic types. More importantly, it has been our experience that in those accepted for thoracotomy, complete resection has been possible in over 90% of the patients. The overall morbidity is low and postoperative mortality remains around 1%.

Disease-free interval and tumor doubling time have not, in our experience, affected survival in patients where complete resection of all visible tumor was possible. The absolute number of metastases resectable is also variable. Many metastases are small and peripheral and are readily removed by multiple wedge resections without major sacrifice of lung tissue. In our experience, the specific number of metastases, per se, is no guideline for patient selection for surgical treatment, but complete resectability is. Setting the limit of resectability with potential cure to 4, as reported by some, is not in accord with our experience, where neither number nor disease-free interval have limited survival in the completely resected metastases.

Operation remains an important mode of treatment for lung metastases. This mode, however, is tempered by ongoing and improved systemic alternatives.

REFERENCES

1. Johnston MR: Median sternotomy for resection of pulmonary metastasis. J Thor Cardiovasc Surg 85:516, 1983.
2. Joseph WL, Morton EL, Aakins PC: Prognostic significance of tumor doubling time in evaluating operability in pulmonary metastatic disease. J Thor Cardiovasc Surg 61:23, 1971.

3. Martini N, et al.: Multiple pulmonary resections in the treatment of osteogenic sarcoma. Ann Thor Surg 12:271-280, 1971.
4. McCormack PM, Martini N: The changing role of surgery for pulmonary metastases. Ann Thor Surg 28:139, 1979.
5. Mountain CF, McMurtrey MJ, Hermes KE: Surgery for pulmonary metastasis: A 20-year experience. Ann Thor Surg 38:323-330, 1984.
6. Patterson GA, Todd TRH, Ilves R, et al.: Surgical Management of pulmonary metastases. Can J Surg 25:102, 1982.
7. Roth JA, Pass HI, Wesley MN, White D, Putnam JB, Seipp C: Comparison of median sternotomy and thoracotomy for resection of pulmonary metastases in patients with adult soft-tissue sarcomas. Ann Thor Surg 42:2, 134-138, 1986.
8. Takita H, Merrin C, Didalkar MS, et al.: The surgical management of multiple lung metastases. Ann Thor Surg 24:359, 1977.
9. Wilkins EW: The status of pulmonary resection of metastases: Experience at Massachusetts General Hospital. In Weiss L, Gilbert HA (eds.): Pulmonary Metastasis. Boston, Hall, pp.271-281, 1978.

TREATMENT OF GYNECOLOGIC SARCOMAS

George A. Omura, M.D.*

Introduction

The primary treatment of female pelvic sarcomas is surgical; the details of surgery are discussed elsewhere. The focus of this report will be on the chemotherapy of gyn sarcomas, and particularly on uterine sarcomas, in regard to both early stage high-risk disease and advanced disease. Some brief comments about pathology, etiology, staging and other modes of treatment are also included for comparison and contrast with the general group of soft tissue sarcomas.

Uterine Sarcomas

As with soft tissue sarcomas, the pathologic classification of the uterine sarcomas is complex.(1) The classification used by the Gynecologic Oncology (GOG) is based upon whether the derivation of the sarcoma is from uterine smooth muscle or from the glands and stroma. Leiomyosarcoma, endometrial stromal sarcoma and mixed mesodermal sarcoma are the major histologic types; the last is further subclassified as homologous (carcinosarcoma) if all the elements in the tumor have normal counterparts in the uterus, and heterologous if they do not (for example, cartilage or striated muscle). A variety of other sarcomas, such as rhabdomyosarcoma and lymphoma, have been reported with a much lower frequency. Leiomyosarcoma must be differentiated from cellular leiomyoma and bizarre leiomyoma (2), as well as the entity of benign metastasizing leiomyoma.(3) Endometrial stromal sarcoma must be distinguished from endolymphatic stromal myosis.(4) Sarcomas are said to comprise from 5 to 10% of corpus cancer; the frequency at UAB is 12%.(5) In one series, mixed mesodermal sarcomas comprised 60%, leiomyosarcoma 28%, endometrial stromal sarcoma 8%, and other cell types 4% of cases.(6) Mixed mesodermal sarcomas are equally divided between heterologous and homologous types. Some variation has been reported from other institutions.(7,8,9)

Previous therapeutic irradiation is mentioned as a causative factor in some cases (10,11), but most patients do not have such a history and not all studies agree.(12,13)

Vascular invasion and early spread to distant sites, especially the lungs, are common. One study indicated that

----

*Division of Hematology and Oncology, The University of Alabama at Birmingham, 223 Tumor Institute, University Hospital, Birmingham, AL 35233.

J. R. Ryan and L. O. Baker (eds.), Recent Concepts in Sarcoma Treatment, 201–209.
© 1988 by Kluwer Academic Publishers.

36% of mixed mesodermal tumors presented with involved pelvic nodes (14), although the frequency is lower in early stage cases. A prospective GOG study is further evaluating the local spread patterns of these tumors; so far, 16% of presumed Stage I and II mixed mesodermal tumors have had node metastases at diagnosis.(15) At least half of Stage I and II uterine sarcomas recur (16), with more initial pulmonary recurrences in the leiomyosarcoma group and more pelvic recurrences in the mixed mesodermal sarcoma category.

The staging system for uterine sarcomas is like that for endometrial carcinoma, but grade of tumor is not included in the criteria for Stage I (disease confined to the corpus). Stage II involves both cervix and corpus, while III and IV are more extensive.

When adjusted for stage, the prognosis for the different cell types is similar, with 5-year survival in Stage I of 50% for mixed mesodermal sarcomas, 56% for leiomyosarcoma, and 55% for stromal sarcomas; 11% of cases more advanced than Stage I survived 5 years, independent of cell type.(6)

Total abdominal hysterectomy and salpingoophorectomy are usually recommended unless the patient is medically inoperable or has obvious metastatic disease. The value of pelvic lymphadenectomy as a therapeutic procedure is unclear. Adjunctive pelvic irradiation may improve local control (7,14,17,18), but this has not been proven. A randomized trial of adjunctive radiation in early stage mixed mesodermal sarcomas is in progress, based on earlier GOG experience, which suggested that local control might be improved in this cell type.(16,19)

Chemotherapy. Over the past decade there have been a smattering of case reports and small series of chemotherapy trials published. There was 1 response (5%) of 17 patients treated with doxorubicin 90 mg. per M^2 every 3-4 weeks, but the cell types were not stated.(20) One patient with a stromal sarcoma had a partial response with doxorubicin and then prolonged survival after debulking and pelvic radiotherapy.(21) Stromal sarcomas, although rare, might be more responsive to chemotherapy than other cell types (22), but that is unclear. Complete response was reported in a leiomyosarcoma and a partial response in 1 of 3 stromal tumors, but no response in 5 previously untreated patients with mixed mesodermal sarcomas who received cyclophosphamide, vincristine, doxorubicin, and dacarbazine (CYVADIC).(23) Complete response was reported in 3 of 6 uterine leiomyosarcomas treated with vincristine, doxorubicin, and dacarbazine.(24) There was 1 CR (leiomyosarcoma) of 12 patients with uterine sarcomas treated with nitrosoureas.(25) Fluorouracil has not been systemically evaluated in recent years, but an old report included 5 temporary responses in 10 gyn sarcomas.(26) These reports were provocative but did not allow definitive conclusions.

In the early 1970's, the assumption was made that different types of uterine sarcomas probably had similar response rates to chemotherapy and that the information available from the general group of soft tissue sarcomas was relevant. At the same time there were unresolved questions about the activity of combination regimens. The GOG carried out 2 randomized trials in advanced or recurrent uterine sarcomas using doxorubicin combinations. The first (27) prospectively compared doxorubicin 60 mg. per M^2 every 3 weeks versus doxorubicin plus dacarbazine 250 mg. per M^2 times 5 every 3 weeks. Of 85 patients with measurable disease treated with doxorubicin alone, 5 had a complete response and 10 a partial response. Of 70 patients randomized to doxorubicin plus dacarbazine, 7 had a CR and 10 a PR. These results were not significantly different. When the individual cell types were examined, the response rate for leiomyosarcoma was 27% for 1 drug and 29% for both drugs. In homologous mixed mesodermal tumors, both regimens gave only a 9% response rate. In heterologous tumors doxorubicin alone produced a response in 2 of 22 patients, compared with 6 of 22 for the combination. These differences were not significant, but the combination regimen produced significantly more gastrointestinal and hematologic toxicity. The very poor result in mixed mesodermal tumors is notable; overall there were only 11/77 (14%) responses in mixed mesodermal sarcoma patients, none of whom had had prior chemotherapy.

Parenthetically, the combination of vincristine, actinomycin and cyclophosphamide (VAC) was evaluated in 41 patients with uterine sarcomas after failing doxorubicin with or without dacarbazine; there were no responses in those 41 patients.(27)

A second GOG trial (28) randomized doxorubicin 60 mg. per M^2 versus doxorubicin plus cyclophosphamide 500 mg. per M^2 every 3 weeks. The study was closed prematurely after 52 patients with measurable disease had been evaluated because the results (19% response rate in each arm) were no more promising than in the previous study.

Recently, several drugs have been systematically screened in uterine leiomyosarcoma and mixed mesodermal sarcoma. Piperazinedione had minimal activity in small numbers of patients.(29) VP-16 produced occasional responses, albeit in previously treated patients.(30) Doxorubicin had a 25% response rate in leiomyosarcomas, but less than a 10% response rate in mixed mesodermal sarcomas.(27,31) Cisplatin has had little activity in uterine leiomyosarcoma with 1 CR/19 in previously treated patients (32), and no better results in previously untreated patients.(33) In mixed mesodermal sarcomas, however, cisplatin produced 5/12 responses in one series (34) and definite, albeit less striking activity in the GOG experience as primary chemotherapy.(33) Even in previously treated patients, cisplatin had some activity (2 CR, 3PR/28) in mixed mesodermal sarcomas.(35) Preliminary information suggests that ifosfamide may also have activity in previously untreated mixed mesodermal sarcoma patients.(36)

Adjuvant Therapy in Early Stage High-Risk Patients

Stage I and II uterine sarcomas have a substantial risk of hematogenous spread as well as pelvic and intra-abdominal recurrence. As success was achieved in the adjuvant treatment of certain other types of cancer, "prophylactic" therapy of uterine sarcomas was applied on a small scale using regimens such as VAC or doxorubicin with inconclusive or negative results.(20,37,39)

The GOG conducted a prospective trial (16) in Stage I and II uterine sarcomas following definitive surgery. Patients were randomized to doxorubicin 60 mg/M^2 every 3 weeks X 8 doses or to no further treatment. At the time this study was started (1973), doxorubicin was thought to be highly active in advanced sarcomas of various types, and was expected to be even better in micrometastatic disease. In the leiomyosarcoma category, 11/25 (44%) recurred after doxorubicin compared with 14/23 (61%) on no adjuvant. With homologous tumors (carcinosarcoma), 10/25 (40%) recurred after doxorubicin compared with 12/23 (52%) without this treatment; 37% (7/19) of heterologous tumors failed after doxorubicin compared with 13/26 (50%) recurrences after no adjuvant drug. Unfortunately, although the numbers suggest benefit, they are not significantly different. Moreover, when progression-free interval and survival are examined, there was no statistically significant difference in any category, even after adjusting for any maldistribution of cases. Updated survival curves with an additional 2 years of follow-up continue to show no difference regarding adjuvant chemotherapy.(40)

Cervix. Sarcomas of the cervix are rare (41) comprising less than 1% of invasive cervix cancer (5); cell types such as leiomyosarcoma (42) can probably be considered with corpus lesions with respect to chemotherapy (see above). Embryonal rhabdomyosarcoma (43) is discussed below under vaginal sarcomas.

Vulvar sarcomas. These lesions comprise 1-2% of primary vulvar cancers.(5,44) The most common vulvar sarcoma is leiomyosarcoma (45); most of the other soft-tissue sarcoma types have been diagnosed in this location, including such lesions as alveolar soft part sarcoma (44) and epithelioid sarcoma.(46) One report included 12 patients with sarcoma of the vulva; two (1 leiomyosarcoma and 1 neurofibrosarcoma) were said to benefit from chemotherapy, but a specific protocol was not described.(47)

Vaginal sarcomas. These lesions represent about 2% of invasive vaginal cancers.(5) The major type in this location is embryonal rhabdomyosarcoma (sarcoma botryoides) which is apt to be seen in young children, but rarely has been reported in adults.(48) In contrast to the adult soft-tissue sarcomas, childhood embryonal rhabdomyosarcoma is relatively responsive to chemotherapy; a multimodality approach with curative intent is indicated.(49) VAC has been used in various dose schedules. CYVADIC was used in two patients with advanced disease without response.(23) Lesions arising in different anatomic sites seem to have similar responsiveness.(50,51)

Ovarian sarcomas. About 1% of ovarian malignancies are sarcomas.(5) The most common sarcoma cell type originating in this location is mixed mesodermal sarcoma.(52,53) A transient response with melphalan and 5-FU was reported, as well as one failure with VAC, and one patient given adjuvant doxorubicin with inconclusive results.(54) The Roswell Park Memorial Institute experience with mixed mesodermal sarcomas of the ovary has been reported with no consistently useful regimen; only 12% showing a temporary response to actinomycin or doxorubicin combinations.(55) The same group did observe a CR in a single case of ovarian angiosarcoma treated with CYVADIC.(23) The initial GOG experience (56) included one temporary complete response of 6 mixed mesodermal tumor patients treated with doxorubicin; VAC was not systematically tested but did not appear to be of predictable benefit. A recent GOG trial in ovarian sarcomas employed 75 mg/M^2 of doxorubicin; there was 1 PR/10; of 21 cases with nonmeasurable tumors, all but 4 progressed on study.(57) A high response rate (60%) was recently reported (58) in a group of 15 mixed mesodermal sarcomas using CYVADIC or cyclophosphamide, doxorubicin, and cisplatin; this needs to be confirmed in a larger trial.

Fallopian tube. Sarcomas of the tube, the rarest of the rare, are usually mixed mesodermal tumors. In one case, an involved inguinal node regressed on VAC and there was no evidence of disease for 20 months after resection of all resectable gross tumor, but then the patient progressed on doxorubicin.(59) One rhabdomyosarcoma of the tube was treated with CYVADIC and achieved a complete response.(23)

Summary

The treatment of gynecologic sarcomas has been briefly reviewed with emphasis on the chemotherapy of uterine sarcomas. Although not conclusive, the available evidence suggests a difference in drug sensitivity between leiomyosarcomas and mixed mesodermal sarcomas. To date, adjuvant chemotherapy has not been shown to improve outcome. The activity of currently available drugs is modest. Effective new agents are clearly needed. Information about the chemotherapy of other sites and cell types is fragmentary, with the exception of embryonal rhabdomyosarcoma, where a multimodality approach is indicated.

REFERENCES

1. Ober W: Uterine sarcomas: Histogenesis and taxonomy. Ann NY Acad Sci 75:568-585, 1959.
2. Christopherson W, Williamson E, Gray L: Leiomyosarcoma of the uterus. Cancer 115(29):1512-1517, 1972.
3. Banner A, Carrington C, Emory W, Kittle F, Leonard G, Ringus J, Taylor P, Addington W: Efficacy of oophorectomy in lymphangioleiomyomatosis and benign metastasizing leiomyoma. N Engl J Med 305:204-209, 1981.
4. Yoonessi M, Hart WR: Endometrial stromal sarcomas. Cancer 40:898-906, 1977.
5. Soong SJ: Personal communication, 1987.
6. Salazar O, Bonfiglio T, Patten S, Keller B, Fieldstein M, Dunne M, Rudolph J: Uterine sarcomas, natural history, treatment and prognosis. Cancer 42:1152-1160, 1978.

206

7. Badib A, Vongtama V, Kurohara S, Webster J: Radiotherapy in the treatment of sarcomas of the corpus uteri. Cancer 24:724-729, 1969.
8. Vongtama V, Karlen J, Piver S, Tsukada Y, Moore R: Treatment results and prognostic factors in stage I and II sarcomas of the corpus uteri. Am J Radiol 126:139-147, 1976.
9. Vardi J, Tovell H: Leiomyosarcoma of the uterus: Clinical pathologic study. Obstet Gynecol 56:428-434, 1980.
10. Meredith RF, Eisert DR, Kaka Z, Hodgson SE, Johnston GA, Boutselis JG: An excess of uterine sarcomas after pelvic irradiation. Cancer 58:2003-2007, 1986.
11. Norris H, Taylor H: Post-irradiation sarcomas of the uterus. Obstet Gynecol 26:689-694, 1965.
12. Silverberg S: Leiomyosarcoma of the uterus. A clinical pathologic study. Obstet Gynecol 38:613-627, 1971.
13. Messerschmidt G, Hoover R, Young R: Gynecologic cancer treatment: Risk factors for therapeutically induced neoplasia. Cancer 48:442-450, 1981.
14. DiSaia P, Castro J, Rutledge F: Mixed mesodermal sarcoma of the uterus. A.J.R. 117:632-636, 1973.
15. Major F, Silverberg S, Morrow P, Blessing J: A preliminary analysis of prognostic factors in uterine sarcoma. A Gynecologic Oncology Group Study. Proceedings f the Society of Gynecologic Oncologists (abstr.), 1987.
16. Omura GA, Blessing JA, Major F, Lifshitz S, Ehrlich CE, Mangan C, Beecham J, Park R, Silverberg S: A randomized clinical trial of adjuvant adriamycin in uterine sarcomas: A Gynecologic Oncology Group Study. J Clin Oncol 3:1240-1245, 1985.
17. Salazar O, Bonfiglio T, Patten S, Keller B, Fieldstein M, Dunne M, Rudolph J: Uterine sarcomas, analysis of failures with special emphasis on the use of adjuvant radiation therapy. Cancer 42:1161-1170, 1978.
18. Gilbert HA, Kagan AR, Lagasse L, Jacobs MR, Tawa K: The value of radiation therapy in uterine sarcoma. Obstet Gynecol 45:84-88, 1975.
19. Hornback NB, Omura G, Major FJ: Observations on the use of adjuvant radiation therapy in patients with stage I and II uterine sarcoma. Intl J Radiation Oncol Biol Phys 12:2127-2130, 1986.
20. Piver MS, Barlow JJ, Lele SB, Yazigi R: Adriamycin in localized and metastatic uterine sarcomas. J Surg Oncol 12:263-265, 1979.
21. Yazigi R, Piver MS, Barlow JJ: Stage III uterine sarcoma: Case report and literature review. Gynecol Oncol 8:92-96, 1979.
22. Lehrner LM, Mile PH, Enck RE: Complete remission of widely metastatic endometrial stromal sarcoma following combination chemotherapy. Cancer 43:1189-1194, 1979.
23. Piver MS, DeEulis TG, Lele SB, Barlow JJ: Cyclophosphamide, vincristine, adriamycin, and dimethyl-triazeno imidazole carboxamide (CYVADIC) for sarcomas of the female genital tract. Gynecol Oncol 14:319-323, 1982.
24. Azizi F, Bitran J, Javehari G, Herbst A: Remission of

uterine leiomyosarcomas treated with vincristine, adriamycin, and dimethyl-triazeno-imidazole carboximide. Am J Obstet Gynecol 133:379-381, 1979.

25. Omura GA, Shingleton HM, Creasman WT, Blessing JA, Boronow RC: Chemotherapy of gynecologic cancer with nitrosoureas: A randomized trial of CCNU and methyl-CCNU in cancers of the cervix, corpus, vagina, and vulva. Cancer Treat Rep 62:833-835, 1978.

26. Malkasian GD, Mussey E, Decker DG, Johnson CE: Chemotherapy of gynecologic sarcomas. Cancer Chemother Rep 51:507-516, 1967.

27. Omura GA, Major FJ, Blessing JA, Sedlacek TV, Thigpen JT, Creasman WT, Zaino RJ: A randomized study of adriamycin with and without dimethyl triazeno imidazole carboxamide in advanced uterine sarcomas. Cancer 52:626-632, 1983.

28. Muss HB, Bundy B, DiSaia P, Creasman W, Yordan P: Treatment of recurrent or advanced uterine sarcoma: A randomized trial of doxorubicin versus doxorubicin and cyclophosphamide: A Phase III trial of the Gynecologic Oncology Group. Cancer 55:1648-1653, 1985.

29. Thigpen JT, Blessing JA, Homesley HD, Hacker N, Curry SL: Phase II trial of piperazinedione in patients with advanced or recurrent uterine sarcoma: A Gynecologic Oncology Group Study. Am J Clin Oncol (CCT) 8:350-352, 1985.

30. Slayton RE, Blessing JA, DiSaia PJ, Christopherson WA: Phase II trial of etoposide in the management of advanced or recurrent mixed mesodermal sarcomas of the uterus: A Gynecologic Oncology Group Study. Cancer Treat Rep 71:661-662, 1987.

31. Gershenson DM, Kavanagh JJ, Copeland LJ, Edward CL, Freedman RS, Wharton JT: High-dose doxorubicin infusion therapy for disseminated mixed mesodermal sarcoma of the uterus. Cancer 59:1264-1267, 1987.

32. Thigpen JT, Blessing JA, Wilbanks GD: Cisplatin as second-line chemotherapy in the treatment of advanced or recurrent leiomyosarcoma of the uterus. Am J Clin Oncol (CCT) 9(1):18-20, 1986.

33. Thigpen JT: Personal communication, 1987.

34. Gershenson DM, Kavanagh JJ, Copeland LJ, Edwards CL, Stringer CA, Wharton JT: Cisplatin therapy for disseminated mixed mesodermal sarcoma of the uterus. J Clin Oncol 5:618-621, 1987.

35. Thigpen JT, Blessing JA, Orr Jr. JW, DiSaia PJ: Phase II trial of cisplatin in the treatment of patients with advanced or recurrent mixed mesodermal sarcomas of the uterus: A Gynecologic Oncology Group Study. Cancer Treat Rep 70:271-274, 1986.

36. Sutton G: Personal communication, 1987.

37. Buchsbaum HJ, Lifshitz S, Blythe JG: Prophylactic chemotherapy in stages I and II uterine sarcoma. Gynecol Oncol 8:346-348, 1979.

38. Van Nagel Jr. JR, Hanson MB, Donaldson ES, Gallion HH: Adjuvant vincristine, dactinomycin, and cyclophosphamide

208

therapy in stage I uterine sarcomas. Cancer 57:1451-
1454, 1986.
39. Hannigan EV, Freedman RS, Rutledge FN: Adjuvant chemotherapy in early uterine sarcoma. Gynecol Oncol 15:56-
64, 1983.
40. Omura GA, Blessing JA: unpublished observations, 1987.
41. Rotmensch J, Rosenshein N, Woodruff J: Cervical sarcoma:
A review. OB Gyn Survey 38:456-460, 1983.
42. Jawalekar KS, Zacharopoulou M, McCaffrey RM: Leiomyosarcoma of the cervix uteri. Southern Med J 74:510-511,
1981.
43. Montag T, D'Ablaing G, Schlaerth J, Gaddis O, Morrow CP:
Embryonal rhabdomyosarcoma of uterine corpus and cervix.
Gynecologic Oncology 25:171-194, 1986.
44. Shen JT, D'Ablaing G, Morrow CP: Alveolar soft part
sarcoma of the vulva: Report of first case and review of
literature. Gynecol Oncol 13:120-128, 1982.
45. Audet - LaPointe P, Pacquin F, Guerard MJ, Carbonneau A,
Methot F, Morand G: Case report: Leiomyosarcoma of the
vulva. Gynecol Oncol 10:350-355, 1980.
46. Hall DJ, Grimes MM, Goplerud DR: Epithelioid sarcoma of
the vulva. Gynecol Oncol 9:237-246, 1980.
47. DiSaia P, Rutledge F, Smith J: Sarcoma of the vulva.
Obstet Gynecol 38:180-184, 1971.
48. Lloyd RV, Hajdu SI, Knapper WH: Embryonal rhabdomyosarcoma in adults. Cancer 51:557-565, 1983.
49. Maurer HM, Moon T, Donaldson M, Fernandez C, Gehan EA,
Hammond D, Hays DM, Lawrence W, Newton W, Ragab A, Raney
B, Soule E, Sutow WW, Tefft M: The Intergroup Rhabdomyosarcoma Study: A preliminary report. Cancer 40:2015-
2026, 1977.
50. Hayes DM: Pelvic rhabdomyosarcomas in childhood: Diagnosis and concepts of management reviewed. Cancer 45:1810-
1814, 1980.
51. Ortner A, Weiser G, Haas H, Resch R, Dapunt O: Embryonal rhabdomyosarcoma (botryoid type) of the cervix: A
case report and review. Gynecol Oncol 13:115-119, 1982.
52. Barwick K, LiVolsi V: Malignant mixed mesodermal tumors
of the ovary. Am J Surg Pathol 4:37-42, 1980.
53. Anderson B, Turner D, Benda J: Ovarian sarcoma.
Gynecologic Oncology 26:183-192, 1987.
54. Hernandez W, DiSaia PJ, Morrow CP, Townsend DE: Mixed
mesodermal sarcoma of the ovary. Obstet Gynecol 49:59-
63, 1977.
55. Lele SB, Piver MS, Barlow JJ: Chemotherapy in management
of mixed mesodermal tumors of the ovary. Gynecol Oncol
10:298-302, 1980.
56. Morrow CP, D'Ablaing G, Bardy LW, Blessing JA,
Hreshchyshyn MM: A clinical and pathologic study of 30
cases of malignant mixed Mullerian epithelial and mesenchymal ovarian tumors: A Gynecologic Oncology Group
Study. Gynecologic Oncology 18:278-292, 1984.
57. Morrow CP, Bundy BN, Hoffman J, Sutton G, Homesley H:
Adriamycin chemotherapy for malignant mixed mesodermal
tumor of the ovary. Am J Clin Oncol (CCT) 9(1):24-26,

1986.
58. Moore M, Fine S, Sturgeon J: Malignant mixed mesodermal
    (MMM) tumors of the ovary: The Princess   Margaret
    Hospital (PMH) Experience. abstr. 444, 1986.
59. Hanjani P, Petersen RO, Bonnell SA: Malignant mixed
    Mullerian tumor of the fallopian tube: Report of a case
    and review of literature. Gynecol Oncol 9:381-393,
    1980.

THE CURRENT ROLE OF SURGICAL THERAPY IN EWING'S SARCOMA

James R. Neff, M.D.*

Introduction

The role of surgical therapy as an adjunct in the treatment of patients with Ewing's sarcoma of bone is becoming increasingly clear. Since Ewing's original description of the use of a radium pack in treating a patient with Ewing's sarcoma of the ulna, surgery has been reserved primarily for the management of bulky and destructive lesions or for amputation following local failures of radiation therapy. It was well recognized that radiation therapy could most often control the primary tumor; however, the majority of patients developed systemic disease and died within two years.

The advent of aggressive adjuvant chemotherapy programs in the 1970's was an attempt to control the late development of systemic disease. It soon became apparent that aggressive induction chemotherapy prior to local therapy commonly resulted in tumor regression.(4) Also, as more patients survived their disease, the issue of local control became more important.

Background

In 1975, Pritchard and his co-workers reported a retrospective review of 194 patients with nonmetastatic Ewing's sarcoma treated between 1912 and 1968. They concluded that patients' survival rates improved when the primary tumor presented in the extremities rather than in other sites. For patients whose primary lesion was in the extremity and who had surgical treatment, 44.7% survived five years; whereas, patients with primary extremity lesions in the extremities managed by nonsurgical means experienced a 13.1% survival. The most common method of surgical management was amputation. (10) The five- and ten-year survival rates for all patients who had surgery was approximately 30%, but only 10% in patients treated by nonsurgical methods.

These retrospective data can be compared to the IESS-I prospective data, where 57 patients in 334 randomized patients with Ewing's sarcoma had either a partial or complete surgical resection even though the protocol did not request surgical therapy. None of the lesions appeared to be

---

*Professor of Surgery, Section of Orthopaedics, Kansas University Surgery Association, Rainbow Boulevard at 39th St., Kansas City, KS 66103.

J. R. Ryan and L. O. Baker (eds.), Recent Concepts in Sarcoma Treatment, 210–217.
© 1988 by Kluwer Academic Publishers.

favorable for resection. There appeared to be a statistically significant advantage in prognosis in both time to relapse (p=0.03) and survival (p=0.01) in patients receiving surgery (either complete or incomplete resection) over those patients receiving radiation therapy. A later review of patients with primary rib lesions, however, suggested that the apparent prognostic advantage of those patients undergoing surgical excision of the ribs may have been explained by patient selection.(14)

In 1981, Rosen and co-workers published their ten-year experience of 67 consecutive patients with nonmetastatic Ewing's sarcoma. Of the 34 patients receiving radiation therapy as the only mode of local therapy, seven of 34 patients (21%) developed local recurrence. No local relapses were reported among patients having amputation alone (13 patients, primarily distal lesions) or surgery plus radiation therapy (20 patients). They concluded that surgical resection should be utilized where possible, and that the overall functional results were superior to those in patients managed by radiation therapy alone.(11)

Data reported from the Instituto Ortopedico Rizzoli on 124 patients with nonmetastatic Ewing's sarcoma also concluded that patients managed by surgery or surgery plus radiation therapy appeared to have a better overall outcome. For patients with primary lesions presenting within the pelvis, surgery did not appear to modify the local recurrence rate (43% with radiation therapy alone vs. 33% with surgery and radiation therapy). For lesions presenting within the extremities and/or other bones (axial skeleton), no local recurrences were observed in patients managed by surgery plus radiation therapy, as compared to 30% local recurrence in the extremities and 18% in other sites when receiving radiation therapy alone. They theorized that small foci of persistent tumor retained within the primary lesion after radiation therapy might be responsible for subsequent relapse.(1)

Analysis of 62 patients presenting with nonmetastatic Ewing's sarcoma of the pelvis, entered on IESS-I, showed that of 46 patients having biopsy alone, 13 (28%) developed local recurrence, while in 11 patients undergoing a complete resection, only two (18%) developed local recurrence. All patients received full-dose radiation therapy regardless of the completeness of resection. Although not significant, review of the individual patients suggested that those lesions resected were fairly evenly divided among primary tumors of the ilium, pubis, and sacrum. When considering only the ilium, eight out of 29 (28%) developed local recurrence after biopsy alone, while no patient undergoing complete resection developed local recurrence.

More recently, a retrospective analysis of 92 patients with nonmetastatic Ewing's sarcoma, studied from 1969 to 1982, was reported by Wilkins and others. Sixteen patients were managed by radiation therapy alone. Forty-nine patients were managed by radiation and chemotherapy, and 27 patients were managed by chemotherapy, complete surgical excision and radiation therapy. Only one of 27 patients managed by chemo-

therapy, complete surgical excision, and radiation therapy
developed local recurrence. The five-year survival rate of
those managed without surgery was 27%, whereas those managed
with chemotherapy, complete surgical excision and radiation
therapy was 74%.(16)
    Recent data from the Massachusetts General Hospital also
supports the efficacy of surgical therapy in the management
of Ewing's sarcoma. A retrospective analysis of 46 patients
with Ewing's sarcoma of bone and three with extraosseous
Ewing's sarcoma was performed. Twelve patients underwent
surgical resection of the primary tumor as part of the treatment plan. When all patients were considered, the five-year
actuarial survival was $.92 \pm .08$ vs. $.37 \pm .09$ for patients
receiving and not receiving surgical resections, respectively. Eight patients with local failure and ten additional
patients presenting with distant metastases within four
months of diagnosis were excluded to make the group more
comparable. After these exclusions, the presence or absence
of surgical resection had decreased significance: $.92 \pm .09$
vs. $.67 \pm .13$, respectively; p=.04 by Logrank, p=.22 by Cox.
They concluded that surgical resection has prognostic significance and may be related to a decrease in local failure
after resection.(12)

Functional Results

    The long-term functional results in patients treated
with radiation therapy appear to be related to multiple
factors. Certainly, the location of the primary tumor in the
upper extremity affects more favorable functional results in
that shortening, fibrosis, and atrophy are reasonably well-
tolerated in the upper extremity. The volume of tissue irradiated, the dose, whether or not a major joint is involved,
and the age of the patient are interrelated factors affecting
the overall functional result.(5) Lesions presenting in the
pelvis and weight-bearing lower extremities are frequently
larger, requiring a larger treatment volume, and commonly
involve a major growth epiphysis resulting in greater secondary effects of therapy. As more patients survive their
illnesses, the treatment-related late effects become more
apparent.

Secondary Malignancies

    In 1979, Chan and others reported four patients of 24
with primary Ewing's sarcoma arising within the pelvis and
surviving five years that developed secondary malignancies
within the irradiated fields and died. Three of the four patients also received intensive chemotherapy.(2) Also, Strong
and others reported an increased hazard of the development of
secondary malignancies in patients treated with radiation
therapy with a cumulative cancer risk over ten years at 35%.
The administration of intensive chemotherapy administered in
five or more courses appeared to exert an enhancing effect
increasing the rate of development of new tumors.(13) Li
also reported a 12% risk of developing a new cancer in 15 of
410 patients who survived childhood cancers.(6)

Most recently, Tucker and her co-workers estimated the subsequent risk of development of bone cancer in 9170 patients surviving two or more years. Data on treatment were evaluated on 64 patients in whom bone cancer developed after childhood cancer. Patients who had received radiation therapy had a 2.7 fold risk of development of secondary malignancies. There appeared to be a dose response reaching a 40 fold risk after doses to bone of more than 6000 rads. Similar numbers of patients were treated with orthovoltage and megavoltage, and the patterns of risk among categories of doses did not differ according to the type of voltage. Also, after adjusting for radiation therapy, treatment with alkylating agents also appeared to increase the subsequent risk of bone cancer.(15)

Current Concepts in Surgical Therapy

Almost all active multimodality Ewing's sarcoma protocols have made provisions for limited surgery in an effort to avoid the late effects of radiation therapy where possible. Most surgical procedures have been limited to resection of expendable bones, such as the rays of the hands and feet, the proximal four-fifths of the fibula, the pubis and wing of the ilium, ribs, distal four-fifths of the clavicle, the body of the scapula, and other small, well-localized lesions. The majority of these procedures do not require reconstruction because of the occasional need for additional radiation therapy and prolonged intensive adjunct chemotherapy.(8) It is now apparent, however, as induction chemotherapy becomes more effective in reducing tumor bulk and as more sophisticated and accurate imaging techniques improve, resections with clear margins (4-5 cm) followed by reconstructive techniques can be anticipated.

Surgical resection should be considered after induction chemotherapy in patients presenting with small primary lesions of the metacarpals or metatarsals where a ray amputation could render the patient free of disease with at least a 2 cm margin. Small midtarsal lesions and lesions within the os calcis can be treated with radiation therapy, but the majority of larger lesions may be better managed by an amputation or disarticulation. Lesions of the tibia should not be considered for resection except in rare instances where satisfactory tumor margins can be assured (4-5 cm), and when there is a high probability that postoperative radiation therapy will not be required. Commonly, the proximal four-fifths of the fibula can be resected with satisfactory margins, leaving at least 6 cm distally for satisfactory ankle function. A tibiofibular synostosis should be performed in skeletally immature patients to prevent proximal migration of the lateral malleolus. Lesions about the knee are amenable to local resection and prosthetic replacement where considerable destruction of bone by the tumor would likely lead to pathological fracture and possibly late amputation. Allograft or prosthetic ingrowth materials can also be used to reconstruct the shaft of the femur as an alternative to amputation; however, the majority of lesions will be managed by radiation therapy.

Destructive lesions about the proximal femur and acetabulum can be managed on occasion by resection and reconstruction where multiple pathological fractures would be anticipated. New modular titanium prostheses presently being developed or allograft/prosthetic combinations can be inserted for reconstruction where abduction function can be reliably retained.

Well-localized lesions presenting in the pelvis are resectable, primarily those confined to the wing of the ilium and small lesions in the pubis. Also, tumors arising in the lower portion of the sacrum and coccyx are amenable to resection. Careful consideration should be given, however, to the anticipated difficulty of resection and the resultant physical deficit prior to undertaking these technically demanding procedures.

Lesions arising within the vertebrae are rarely, if ever, amenable to resection because of the often associated involvement of the dura and associated neural structures. Decompressive laminectomy is often required for biopsy and to restore the often associated neurologic deficit.

Rib primaries, 3 cm or less, are commonly managed by excisional biopsy at the time of diagnosis. Incisional biopsy techniques should be used for larger lesions, reserving resection of the entire rib and surrounding soft tissue after completion of induction chemotherapy.

Primary tumors presenting in the infraspinous portion of the scapula, that do not invade the chest wall, can be resected without significant functional deficits. Lesions presenting in the region of the glenoid are usually best managed by radiation therapy. Small lesions in the acromion and scapular spine may also be excised.

The outer four-fifths of the clavicle can often be resected without significant physical impairment; however, the proximal one-fifth of the clavicle and the sternum are best managed by radiation therapy.

Resection of the proximal humerus is often associated with loss of active abduction and, therefore, should only be used on rare occasions. In general, functional deficits and limb-length inequalities are better tolerated in the upper extremity.

The Role of Amputation

Although the role of amputation in the management of patients with Ewing's sarcoma remains controversial, primary amputation or disarticulation may offer a clinical option superior to prolonged morbidity associated with pathological fracture or severe limb-length inequality, resulting in late or delayed amputation. Large destructive lesions in children under the age of ten years in males and eight years in females, may be managed best by primary amputation. Amputation should be considered when epiphysiodesis of the opposite limb does not provide a reasonable treatment option to approach equalization of limb lengths at skeletal maturity.

Innovative Local Therapy Techniques

With improving induction and maintenance chemotherapy, and with the appropriate use of improved imaging techniques (i.e., M.R.I., etc.), many patients not previously suitable for local resection are now potential candidates for local resection and reconstruction in carefully selected cases. As previously mentioned, resection of expendable bones usually does not require reconstruction. If the margins are judged unsatisfactory for adequate local control, postoperative radiation therapy can often be administered without significantly altering the overall functional result. Reconstruction techniques requiring incorporation of graft materials, however, may be inalterably affected by postoperative radiation therapy, resulting in loss of fixation and resorption of the graft with an overall poor clinical and functional result.

The present surgical experience and body of knowledge regarding the use and fixation of prosthetic devices and deep frozen allografts are increasing yearly. The source of information has been through experience gained by managing patients with other childhood tumors such as osteosarcoma. If the surgical margins of resection are appropriate for local control (i.e., intraosseous margin of 5 cm or greater and soft tissue margin of from 2-5 cm), then it is believed that these techniques can be utilized in the management of patients with Ewing's sarcoma of the extremities in well-selected patients.

The use of intraoperative radiation therapy at the time of local resection may also extend the reconstruction technique to include the use of autogenous tissues. Following resection of the primary lesion, if radiation therapy is required, the therapy needs could be tailored to the margins requiring treatment, thereby protecting other tissues and structures. Free or preferably vascularized fibular grafts could then be used to reconstruct the limb in which the vascular anastomosis could be performed in unirradiated tissues. Also, muscle pedicle flaps protected at the time of irradiation can be rotated into the operative field to provide additional blood supply and coverage to the free or vascularized graft materials. Experience gained using these techniques suggests that the grafts do revascularize and incorporate, but do so at a somewhat slower rate.(7)

Summary

The increasing role of surgical therapy in the local management of well-selected patients with Ewing's sarcoma appears to be beneficial with respect to overall survival and in reducing treatment-related late effects. It should be the common goal of all oncologists to optimize therapy wherever possible to provide the patient with the best overall clinical and functional result.

REFERENCES

1. Bacci G, Picci P, Gherlinzoni F, Capanna R, Calderoni P, Putti C, Mancini A, Campanacci M: Localized Ewing's sarcoma of bone: ten years' experience at the Instituto Ortopedico Rizzoli in 124 cases treated with multi-modality therapy. Eur J Can Clin Oncol 21:163-173, 1985.
2. Chan RC, Sutow WW, Lindberg RD, Samuels ML, Murray JA, Johnston DA: Management and results of localized Ewing's sarcoma. Cancer 43:1001-1006, 1979.
3. Evans R, Nesbit M, Askin F, Burgert O, Cangir A, Foulkes M, Gehan E, Gilula L, Kissane J, Makley J, Neff J, Perez C, Pritchard D, Tefft M, Thomas P, Vietti T: Local recurrence, rate and sites of metastases, and time to relapse as a function of treatment regimen, size of primary and surgical history in 62 patients presenting with nonmetastatic Ewing's sarcoma of the pelvic bones. Int J Radiat Oncol Biol Phys 11:129-136, 1985.
4. Hayes FA, Thompson EI, Hustu HO, Kumar M, Corburn T, Webber B: The response of Ewing's sarcoma to sequential cyclophosphamide and adriamycin induction therapy. J Clin Oncol 1:45-51, 1983.
5. Lewis RJ, Marcove RC, Rosen G: Ewing's sarcoma: functional effects of radiation therapy. J Bone Joint Surg 59A:325-331, 1977.
6. Li FP: Second malignant tumors after cancer in childhood. Cancer 40:1899-1902, 1977.
7. Metaizeau JP, Olive D, Bey P, Bordigoni P, Plenat F, Prévot J: Resection followed by vascularized bone autograft in patients with possible recurrence of malignant bone tumors after conservative treatment. J Ped Surg 19:116-120, 1984.
8. Neff JR: Nonmetastatic Ewing's sarcoma of bone: the role of surgical therapy. Clin Orthop & Rel Res 204:111-118, 1986.
9. Pritchard DJ: Surgical experience in the management of Ewing's sarcoma of bone. Natl Cancer Inst Mono 56:169-171, 1981.
10. Pritchard DJ, Dahlin DC, Dauphine RT, Taylor WF, Beabout JW: Ewing's sarcoma: a clinicopathological and statistical analysis of patients surviving five years or longer. J Bone Joint Surg 57A:10-16, 1975.
11. Rosen G, Caparros B, Nirenberg A, Marcove RC, Huvos AG, Kosloff C, Lane J, Murphy ML: Ewing's sarcoma: ten-year experience with adjuvant chemotherapy. Cancer 47:2204-2213, 1981.
12. Sailer SL, Harmon DC, Mankin HJ, Truman JT, Suit HD: Ewing's sarcoma: surgical resection as a prognostic factor. Presented at the 29th Annual Meeting of ASTRO, Mass Gen Hosp, 1987.
13. Strong LC, Herson J, Osborne BM, Sutow WW: Risk of radiation-related subsequent malignant tumors in survivors of Ewing's sarcoma. JNCI 62:1401-1406, 1979.
14. Thomas RPM, Perez CA, Neff JR, Nesbit ME, Evans RG: The

management of Ewing's sarcoma: role of radiotherapy in local tumor control. Can Treat Rep 68:703-710, 1984.

15. Tucker MA, D'Angio GJ, Boice JD Jr., Strong LC, Li FP, Stovall M, Stone BJ, Green DM, Lombardi F, Newton W, Hoover RN, Fraumeni JF Jr.: Bone sarcomas linked to radiotherapy and chemotherapy in children. N Engl J Med 317:588-593, 1987.

16. Wilkins RM, Pritchard DJ, Burgert EO Jr., Unni KK: Ewing's sarcoma of bone: experience with 140 patients. Cancer 58:2551-2555, 1986.

THE ROLE OF CHEMOTHERAPY IN THE MANAGEMENT OF EWING'S SARCOMA

Elizabeth I. Thompson, M.D.*

Introduction

Ewing's sarcoma (ES) is a rare malignancy of children and young adults which arises in bone but is not of osseous origin. Approximately 60% of primary lesions occur in long bones, and 40% in flat bones. Fifteen to 35% of patients have detectable metastatic disease at diagnosis, most frequently in the lungs and bones. The remainder have apparently localized disease but, without systemic treatment, rapidly develop visible metastases.

Until multiagent chemotherapy became available for Ewing's sarcoma, few patients survived. In spite of treatment with amputation, irradiation, or both, 24 of 26 patients in one series developed metastatic disease by 9 months from diagnosis.(15) In another series, only 8% of patients survived 5 years.(1) When nitrogen mustard, Vincristine (VCR), and Cyclophosphamide (Cyclo) became available to add to local therapy, the time to development of metastases was delayed and 20-30% of patients survived.(2) Cyclo, VCR, Dactinomycin (Dactino), and Adriamycin (Adria) have, until recently, been the 4 most active single agents against ES. Various combinations and schedules of these agents are given with radiation therapy or surgery. Currently, more than 50% of newly diagnosed patients with ES enter long-term remissions and may be cured.

Two recent developments may contribute significantly to future improvements in therapy. First, a combination of two new agents, Ifosfamide and VP-16, provided a 94% response rate in patients with relapsed ES.(3) These agents are now being tested in phase III studies. Secondly, retrospective evaluations in several studies suggest that patients with large primaries have the highest risk of failure and may be a subgroup requiring different or added therapy. Patients with overt metastases at diagnosis have always had a poorer prognosis.

Trials in Patients with Localized Disease at Diagnosis

The first Intergroup Ewing's Sarcoma Study (IESS-1)

----

*Department of Hematology/Oncology, St. Jude Children's Research Hospital, 332 North Lauderdale, P.O. Box 318, Memphis, TN 38101.
Division of Hematology-Oncology, Department of Pediatrics, University of Tennessee, Memphis, TN 38101.

J. R. Ryan and L. O. Baker (eds.), Recent Concepts in Sarcoma Treatment, 218–223.
© 1988 by Kluwer Academic Publishers.

demonstrated the contribution of multiagent chemotherapy to the control of disease locally (in the primary site) as well as systemically. With the same doses of irradiation to the primary site, local control varied according to chemotherapy given.

In IESS-1 (4), three groups of patients with localized ES at diagnosis all received Cyclo, VCR, and Dactino plus irradiation of 40-60 Gy to the primary site (Group 1). Group 2 patients received, in addition, 16-18 Gy to both lungs. Group 3 had Adria added to the other 3 drugs, but no lung irradiation. Shown in Table 1 is the 2-year freedom from relapse. The 4-drug group (3) had an increased disease-free survival, fewer pulmonary metastases, and a lower local recurrence rate (not shown).

TABLE 1

Therapy	% 2-yr. Freedom From Relapse	% Pulmonary Metastasis
1 - VAC	35	41
2 - VAC + Lung RT	58	20
3 - VAC + Adr	74	14

The improved results of therapy at 2 years in the 4-drug group were encouraging, but there was a large subgroup of patients who did not benefit - patients with pelvic or sacral primaries. These patients, most of whom had large bone and soft tissue tumors, had a 27% local recurrence rate and a 61% metastatic failure rate in all groups.(16) A new trial, the Pelvic and Sacral Arm of IESS-2, was developed to improve the results in this subgroup.

IESS-2 incorporated changes in both chemotherapy and other treatments used for local disease control: Cyclo, VCR, Dactino and Adria were given in higher doses and at more frequent intervals. Measures to improve local control included an option of surgery, careful definition of port dimensions and dosages for radiation therapy, and multi-institutional review for quality control. This study is still being analyzed, but preliminary results show a marked improvement in disease control, both local and metastatic; disease-free survival at 4 years is estimated to be 64%.(15)

Rosen and co-workers (5) added Methotrexate and Bleomycin to Cyclo, VCR, Dactino and Adria (T9 chemotherapy) for patients with localized disease. They reported an overall disease control of 79% (53/67). Looking at patients with axial primaries (which includes those with pelvic and sacral primaries), disease-free survival was 65% (15/23). In that study, radiation therapy or surgery were delayed to permit reduction of bulk disease and allow partial bone healing during the initial cycles of chemotherapy. While this approach may impact on late effects of therapy, the 2 additional agents did not seem to improve results over the projected results of IESS-2.

Trials in ES Patients with Metastases at Diagnosis

Patients with overt metastatic ES at diagnosis have fared less well than those with localized disease. In the first IESS trial for patients with metastases, Cyclo, VCR, Dactino and Adria were given with radiation therapy to all metastatic sites where possible. At a median of 84 months, only 30% of 44 patients survived.(6) In a second IESS study, the dose of Cyclo was increased, therapy given more frequently and 5-FU was added. Irradiation to metastatic sites was continued. At a median of 21 months, 60% of 49 patients were still disease-free, an improvement over the previous study. Rosen and co-workers (17) added BCNU, Methotrexate and Bleomycin with delayed irradiation to metastases, and also reported a disease-free survival of 60% (6/10 patients) at a median of 47 months. The results in this small series were encouraging, but toxicity was significant.

More recently, Hayes and co-workers (7) reported a 62% disease-free survival at a median of 47 months for 18 patients with ES metastatic at diagnosis. While these investigators gave Cyclo, Adria, VCR, and Dactino, the dose and schedule of the chemotherapy and timing of local therapy differed significantly from other studies. The 4 drugs were given in sequential drug pairs. Moderate dose daily Cyclo (150 mg/m^2 p.o. x 7) was followed by Adriamycin at 35 mg/m^2 IV on day 8. This 8-day course of therapy was repeated every 2-3 weeks for 5 courses in a chemotherapy alone induction phase. Patients were then reassessed and had either radiation therapy (30-35 Gy if resolution of the soft tissue mass occurred after induction treatment, or 50-55 Gy if residual soft tissue tumor remained) or surgery only for "expendable bones". Beginning simultaneously with irradiation (or after surgery), all patients received a 12-week course of weekly VCR and every other week, Dactino. All patients then received 6 additional courses of Cyclo, Adria. Patients with metastases at diagnosis received 12 more weeks of VCR and Dactino. Pulmonary radiation was not given if patients had complete resolution of lung metastases at 12 weeks. For fewer than 3 bone lesions, radiation therapy of 30-35 Gy was given to each lesion. This combination of therapy allows less extensive surgery in patients with potentially resectable bones, and a smaller radiation port in patients with extensive soft tissue masses at diagnosis.(8)

In this series of 18 patients, neither the primary site nor sites of metastases (lungs versus bones) related to disease-free survival. Surprisingly (given that these were patients with already overt metastases), the size of the primary did correlate with outcome. Only 1/6 patients with primary tumors less than 8 cm. in greatest dimension developed recurrent disease versus 7/12 with primary lesions larger than 8 cm.

Size of Primary

Following the observation that patients with localized pelvic or sacral primaries, who frequently have large tumors, fared poorly in IESS-1, Mendenhall and co-workers (9) observed that patients with large soft tissue extent of ES did less well than those with smaller lesions. Göbel and co-workers (10) estimated volumes of tumor in patients with localized disease and found that, at 36 months, 7/33 with volumes 100 cc. or less versus 20/27 with volumes greater than 100 cc. had developed recurrent disease. These patients had received cycles of VCR, Cyclo, Dactino and Adria at high doses and frequent intervals and 46-60 Gy irradiation to the primary site. The investigators found the estimate of volume to correlate better with outcome than greatest tumor diameter. However, in all 3 studies in which attempts at size estimations were carried out, 70-80% of patients with small primaries have done well, but only 20-40% of those with larger primaries remain disease-free. The introduction in current studies of significantly improved diagnostic imaging of ES by computerized tomography and MRI (magnetic resonance imaging) will require prospective corroboration of these observations. Large numbers of patients must be evaluated.

Future Directions

Ifosfamide, as a single agent, has produced both complete and partial transient responses in relapsed ES patients. Seeber and co-workers (11) tested Ifosfamide and cisplatinum; the combination was not superior, although responses achieved were longer lasting. As mentioned, Miser and co-workers (3) found the combination of Ifosfamide and etoposide produced a very high response rate - 95% in relapsed ES patients. These agents may improve both local and systemic control for ES patients. Still to be determined, is the optimal time for incorporating surgery and/or radiation therapy in patients. Sequential Cyclo and Adria, as utilized by Hayes and co-workers (8), permits a greater than 50% reduction in soft-tissue tumor volume at 12 weeks in 95% of patients. Most patients show signs of bone healing, and half of the biopsied residual masses show necrosis and fibrosis without identifiable soft-tissue tumor. The strategy of reduction of tumor by chemotherapy converts some patients with large tumors to surgical candidates and potentially decreases necrosis and hypoxic tumor areas prior to radiation therapy. Other investigators postulate that the addition of all modalities as quickly as possible would theoretically decrease emergence of resistant cells.

Both sequential half-body irradiation following chemotherapy (12) and autologous bone marrow transplantation following melphalan and high dose cyclophosphamide (13) have produced complete responses in small series of relapsed ES patients and may be integrated into future studies.

Other potential therapies for ES may become evident as basic knowledge of the ES tumor cell is increased. In one series, chromosome studies in 13 cases of ES patients showed a t(11;22) translocation in 9.(14) As with other malignant diseases, the abnormality was not found in every case. Further, this abnormality has also been observed in tumors of primitive neuro-ectodermal origin, raising questions of common ancestry. Whether or not specific chromosomal changes in Ewing's tumor cells activate proto-oncogenes and lead to malignant transformation is a subject of current intense interest and research activity.

Finally, the problem of late relapse, a relatively frequent event in Ewing's sarcoma, invites speculation that perhaps biologic response modifiers may someday be utilized to promote destruction or differentiation of tumor cells which may remain in small numbers following cessation of therapy. Specific monoclonal antibodies are being sought which may improve our ability to identify subclinical disease and/or aid in delivery of targeted therapy to the tumor.

REFERENCES

1. Pritchard DJ, Dahlin DC, Dauphine RT, Taylor WF, Beabont JW: Ewing's sarcoma: a clinicopathological and statistical analysis of patients surviving five years or longer. J Bone Joint Surg 57A:10-16, 1975.
2. Hustu HO, Holton C, James D, Pinkel D: Treatment of Ewing's sarcoma with concurrent radiotherapy and chemotherapy. J Pediatr 73(2):249-251, 1968.
3. Miser JS, Kinsella TJ, Triche TJ, Tsolios M, Jarosinski P, Forques R, Wesley R, Magrath I: Ifosfamide with mesna Uroprotection and etoposide: an effective regimen in the treatment of recurrent sarcomas and other tumors of children and young adults. J Clin Oncol 5(8):1191-1198, 1987.
4. Vietti TJ, Gehon EA, Nesbit M, Burgert EO, Pilepich M, Tefft M, Kissone J, Pritchard DJ: Multimodal therapy in Ewing's sarcoma: an Intergroup study. Natl Cancer Inst Monogr 56:279-284, 1980.
5. Rosen G, Caparros B, Nirenberg A, Marcone RC, Hunos A, Kosloff C, Lane J, Murphy ML: Ewing's sarcoma: ten year experience with adjuvant chemotherapy. Cancer 47:2204-2213, 1981.
6. Pilepich M, Vietti T, Nesbit M, Tefft M, et al.: Radiotherapy and combination chemotherapy in advanced Ewing's sarcoma - Intergroup study. Cancer 47:1930-1936, 1981.
7. Hayes FA, Thompson EI, Parvey L, Rao B, Kun L, Parham D, Hustu HO: Metastatic Ewing's sarcoma: remission induction and survival. J Clin Oncol 5(8):1199-1204, 1987.
8. Hayes FA, Thompson EI, Hustu HO, et al.: The response of Ewing's sarcoma to sequential cyclophosphamide and adriamycin induction therapy. J Clin Oncol 1:45-51, 1983.
9. Mendenhall GM, Marcus RB Jr., et al.: The prognostic significance of soft tissue extension in Ewing's sarcoma. Cancer 51:913-917, 1983.
10. Göbel V, Jürgens H, Etspüler G, Kemperdick H, Jungblut RM, Stienen V, Göbel V: Prognostic significance of tumor volume in localized Ewing's sarcoma of bone in children and adolescents. J Cancer Res Clin Oncol 113:187-191, 1987.
11. Seeber S, Nagel GA, Brade W: Ifosfamide in tumor therapy. München: Karger 1987 (in press).

12. Berry MP, Jenkins RDT, Harwood AR, Cummings BJ, Quirt IC, Sonley MJ, Rider WD: Ewing's sarcoma: a trial of adjuvant chemotherapy and sequential half-body irradiation. Int J Radiat Oncol Biol Phys 12:19-24, 1986.

13. Cornbleet MA, Corringham RET, Prentice HG, et al.: Treatment of Ewing's sarcoma with high dose melphalan and autogenous bone marrow transplantation. Cancer Treat Rep 65:241-244, 1982.

14. Douglass EC, Valentine M, Green AA, Hayes FA, Thompson EI: t(11;22) and other chromosomal rearrangements in Ewing's sarcoma. JNCI 77(6):1211-1213, 1986.

15. Personal Communication, TJ Vietti, 1987.

16. Evans R, Nesbit M, Askin F, Burgert O, et al.: Local recurrence, rate and sites of metastases, and time to relapse as a function of treatment regimen, size of primary and surgical history in 62 patients presenting with non-metastatic Ewing's sarcoma of the pelvic bones. Int J Rad Oncol Biol Phys 11:129-136, 1985.

17. Rosen G, Juergens H, Caparros B, Nirenberg A, Huvos AG, Marcove RC: Combination chemotherapy (T-6) in the multi-disciplinary treatment of Ewing's sarcoma. Natl Cancer Inst Monogr 56:289-299, 1981.

THE ROLE OF RADIATION THERAPY IN THE MANAGEMENT OF EWING'S SARCOMA

Richard G. Evans, Ph.D., M.D.*

The role of radiation therapy in the overall management of patients with Ewing's sarcoma is an evolving one. In this chapter, following some pertinent introductory comments, we will discuss the impact of modern staging techniques, prognostic factors that have emerged, importance of local control and how best this may be attained, complications and late effects and, finally, new approaches to treatment.

Introduction

Although Ewing's sarcoma is a relatively rare tumor (approximately 250 new cases/year in the United States), it occurs in adolescents and young adults and, therefore, any impact that can be made on the cure rate could potentially be reflected in many years of fruitful life. Prior to the 1960's, when surgery and radiation were the mainstays of treatment for Ewing's sarcoma, most patients were doomed to die from systemic spread of their disease, but with the introduction of multiple-agent chemotherapy, the last twenty years have seen significant improvements in both local control and eventual long-term survival. Although these benefits have been attained with some cost in terms of second primary tumors and functional defects, Ewing's sarcoma remains an excellent model for evaluating the efficacy of combined-modality treatment, since the tumor is not only radiosensitive but is also sensitive to chemotherapeutic agents and amenable to surgical resection in many cases. Physicians dealing with these patients now have the added responsibility of selecting treatment strategies appropriate to the different subpopulations of patients that should result in the best treatment gains with the least morbidity to the patient.

Staging

Although no staging system, as such, exists for Ewing's sarcoma, attempts have been made to divide patients up into low-risk and high-risk groups. The emergence of more refined imaging techniques, in particular in bone and CT scanning and, more recently, MR imaging, has provided us with more exact information on the local extent of the tumor, as well as a more accurate assessment of the sites involved with metastatic disease at presentation. The high local failure

---

*Professor and Chairman, Department of Radiation Oncology, University of Kansas Medical Center, 39th & Rainbow Blvd., Kansas City, KS 66103.

J. R. Ryan and L. O. Baker (eds.), Recent Concepts in Sarcoma Treatment, 224–230.
© 1988 by Kluwer Academic Publishers.

rate seen in many of the earlier studies reflected, in part, a failure of the radiographic studies to accurately assess the extension of tumor into soft tissues adjacent to bone. MR imaging appears to be emerging as superior to CT scanning with regard to involvement of bone marrow, soft-tissue tumor extent and the relationship of tumor to blood vessels.(1). These imaging techniques should allow us to more accurately identify patients at high risk, such as those with primaries in central locations (pelvis or spine), large soft-tissue components, extensive bone marrow involvement or metastatic disease at diagnosis, so that we might utilize more aggressive therapy tailored to these high-risk groups.

Prognostic Factors

Although many variables have been identified as being of prognostic significance, many have not emerged as independent variables when examined by multivariate analysis. However, the following are well recognized as having prognostic significance: systemic symptoms, metastatic disease at presentation, location of primary tumor (distal extremity, proximal extremity and central), size of primary and extent of soft-tissue disease and, more recently, degree of surgical resection of the primary. The recognition of these prognostic factors led the Intergroup Ewing's Sarcoma Study (IESS II) to divide patients up not only into those presenting with and without metastatic disease but also into those patients with primaries in pelvic and sacral bones compared to other sites, and to address these groups with different treatment strategies. Patients with primaries in the pelvis have historically responded less well to treatment and, although it is difficult to reason why location per se carries a poorer prognosis, the factors that might contribute to poorer outcome would include larger tumor bulk, a greater propensity for metastatic spread due to later diagnosis, failure to include all disease within the radiation beam and difficulties in obtaining an adequate degree of surgical resection in the pelvis due to constraints placed on the orthopedic surgeon. However, preliminary data from IESS II (nonmetastatic, sacral and pelvic primaries) suggests that better delineation of the soft-tissue extension of the disease and its inclusion within the radiation field, together with more intensive chemotherapy, can produce results comparable to those obtained for other sites. (These data are currently being updated.)

The more refined radiographic techniques brought to light the importance of tumor size and its soft-tissue extension. It appears that tumor volume, rather than maximal tumor extension, is a better measure of risk for local recurrence and subsequent survival and, in a recent German study, the three-year disease-free survival rate, according to life-table analysis, was 78% for tumors with a volume <100 ml, compared to 17% for tumors $\geq$100 ml.(4). Moreover, these results were independent of the site of the tumor, with the caveat that the larger tumors were primarily located in central and proximal extremity sites. These survival rates reflected a local recurrence rate of 74% noted in the larger tumors, compared to 21% in the smaller tumors. In IESS I, the local recurrence rate was only 8% in primaries with maximum dimensions <5 cm, as contrasted to 21% in patients whose tumors ranged from 10 to 15 cm.(3). Interestingly, in a recent study from Massachusetts General Hospital, tumor size (<500 ml versus >500 ml) was of prognostic significance by univariate analysis, but only primary site and surgical resection remained significant after multivariate analysis (9). Two other series, one from the University of Florida (7) and one unpublished from St. Jude's Research Hospital (11), also indicate that, when the size of the primary is >8 cm, there is an increased incidence of local failure compared to that of smaller primaries.

The prognostic significance of surgical resection is not as clear-cut but appears to be emerging as a positive prognostic factor, at least at some sites. Interpretation of data from various series is difficult because patients undergoing surgical resection tend to have smaller, more amenable tumors, often without distant metastases at presentation, and demonstrating high rates of response to induction chemotherapy. Investigators at the Mayo Clinic have proposed a larger role for surgical resection, and a recent publication from that institution demonstrated a five-year survival of 74% for the patients treated with surgery, compared to 27% for those not receiving a surgical resection (14). However, the data are confounded by the fact that the group of patients treated without a surgical resection tended to have primaries in less favorable sites with a larger tumor size, and also contained a significant number of patients treated without combination chemotherapy. In a review of IESS I patients with pelvic primaries only, no significant difference in local failure was noted in patients treated with a complete resection versus biopsy or incomplete resection (3). This observation is confirmed by the study from Germany (4), where, although radical surgery appeared to give better local control compared to radiation therapy only, when stratified for tumor volume, the differences in disease-free survival among the different local therapies were no longer significant in patients with small lesions, so that the better prognosis of patients following surgery may be explained, in part, by the smaller volume of tumors that were surgically removed. Moreover, in the study from Massachusetts General Hospital (9), if all patients were considered, the five-year actuarial survival was .92 versus .37 for patients receiving or not receiving surgical resection, but, when the two groups were made more comparable by removing the patients with local failure or presenting with distant metastases, the presence or absence of surgical resection lost its significance. It should be stressed, however, that this discussion is not meant to address any competition between radiation and surgery to obtain optimum local control, but that all factors need to be considered in tailoring the treatment to each individual situation and that, in some patients, both surgery and radiation may be indicated. This author is most sympathetic with the approach taken by investigators at St. Jude's Research Hospital who have modified the dose of radia-

tion to the primary site depending upon the response to
induction chemotherapy and post-induction surgical-pathologic
evaluation (5). Reducing the dose of irradiation to 30-35 Gy
may be appropriate for primaries <8 cm, but could lead to an
unacceptable local recurrence rate when used in larger primaries.

Local Control

One cannot sufficiently stress the importance of local
control in Ewing's sarcoma patients, as the prognosis of
those who recur following aggressive combined-modality therapy is dismal. Although it is virtually impossible to distinguish between true local failure and reseeding of the
primary site following systemic failure, it is clear that
primary control by whatever means will almost certainly
dictate the eventual outcome. Putting aside any questions of
the roles of chemotherapy and surgical resection in local
control, the disturbing frequency of second primaries (mostly
osteogenic sarcomas) within the radiation field, together
with functional defects, demands a rethinking of both the
volume and the dose of irradiation to be used. Traditionally,
radiation oncologists have included the entire bone in the
initial treatment field to 40-45 Gy, followed, using a
"shrinking field" technique, by a further 5-10 Gy (12). This
technique and total dose may only be necessary in the larger
tumors, especially if the response to induction chemotherapy
has been suboptimum. It is possible that MR imaging, with its
greater ability to delineate bone marrow involvement as
compared to CT scanning, will aid the radiation oncologist in
planning the extent of the initial field. As local failure
rarely occurs in parts of the bone outside the initial bulky
lesion, every consideration should be given to "tailored
port" (radiographic lesion plus 2 cm. margins) irradiation,
rather than conventional whole-bone irradiation. Unfortunately, the study initiated by the Pediatric Oncology Group (POG)
to address the question of "tailored port" irradiation
versus a more extensive radiation field had to be aborted
because of poor patient entry and the realization that the
completion of the objective to statistical certainty was
unlikely. However, to date, no differences in failure pattern
between the two arms have emerged, and a proposed POG study
contains "tailored port" irradiation only (2). Interestingly,
no reports to date have been able to demonstrate a radiation
dose response as far as local control is concerned and, as
the probability of an "in-field" second primary probably
increases as doses are taken above 60 Gy (13), it behooves
radiation oncologists to limit the radiation dose to 55 Gy or
less, at least on a routine basis, although large-volume
primaries, especially without the benefit of surgical resection, may justify the use of more aggressive doses. Certainly, avoidance of growth plates and careful attention to
treatment planning with sparing of tissue for lymphatic
drainage and limiting the dose to 55 Gy or less should keep
functional deficits following radiation therapy to acceptable
levels. When the primary involves expendable bones, in cases
of bulky destructive lesions and for skeletally immature

patients, amputation is the more appropriate choice for local
treatment. Attempts have been made to use twice daily fractionation techniques, and although the follow-up time is
short, results so far are encouraging in that long-term
complications such as fibrosis and pathological fractures
have been markedly reduced with no adverse effect on local
tumor control (7). It is clear that the local control rate
has risen with the advent of intensive chemotherapy, from
approximately 70% to about 90%, but is dependent, in part,
upon the size and the site of the primary lesion. There is a
danger, however, of losing this improved local control rate
if the radiation treatment is delayed by more than two to
three cycles of induction chemotherapy.

Complications and Late Effects of Treatment

The gratification derived from more effective treatment
of Ewing's sarcoma must be tempered by the morbidity of
treatment that emerges with longer follow-up on cured patients. We need to consider the effect of aggressive treatment on the incidence of fractures and delayed healing,
together with functional losses and, probably most importantly, the induction of second malignancies within the radiation
field.

Setting aside the cases where amputation was carried out
in very young patients and for patients with primaries in
expendable bones, the secondary effects of loss of function
and development of shortening and pathological fractures are
most evident in the weight-bearing bones. Unpublished data
from the IESS late effects study (8) noted that late changes
in the upper extremities were compatible with essentially a
normal life, but a significant limp, usually with stiffness,
was noted with patients treated for primaries in the pelvis.
Patients with presentation in the femur yielded the most
severe secondary effects, with two-thirds of patients developing shortening >2 cm. and with one-third developing pathological fractures. Although the development of fractures is
related to both radiation and chemotherapy, the use of
tailored radiation therapy ports, excluding the growth plates
whenever possible, should avoid, in most cases, the problem
of limb-shortening. By careful attention to radiotherapy
technique, fibrosis with subsequent edema can be avoided in
most cases.

Although one cannot rule out genetic predisposition to
second tumors in patients with Ewing's sarcoma, the second
malignancies noted in the irradiation field are almost certainly treatment-related effects. There is no doubt in this
observer's mind that the frequency of second malignancies is
radiation dose-related and increases with doses above 60 Gy.
Chemotherapy (alkylating agents in particular) appears to
exert an enhancing effect, not only increasing the rate of
development but also shortening the latent period following
completion of treatment (10). In some small series, incidence
of second primaries can be as high as 10% but, of 251 irradiated patients in IESS I, only three osteosarcomas have been
noted within the radiation therapy portals, though with
longer follow-up, it is possible that this may represent

underreporting (8). Radiation oncologists should encourage their surgical colleagues to debulk the tumor whenever feasible so that the lowest radiation dose may be used without sacrificing local control.

Evolving Treatment Approaches

Every effort must be made to identify patients at high risk of failure, such as those with metastatic disease, primaries at unfavorable sites and those with bulky disease at diagnosis. These patients should be treated with more intensive chemotherapeutic regimens and should be considered for bone marrow transplantation while in first remission. The National Cancer Institute (6) and the University of Florida (7) are two institutions with protocols in progress addressing these high-risk patients who, following complete remission by traditional approaches, are conditioned with total body irradiation and further intensive chemotherapy prior to autologous bone marrow transplantation. Results three years from cessation of all treatment in ten high-risk patients at the University of Florida show a relapse-free survival plateau of approximately 75%. Data from the NCI on 30 high-risk patients with Ewing's sarcoma, treated with intensive chemotherapy and consolidated with total body irradiation prior to autologous bone marrow transplantation, show a 50% freedom from adverse event (death from toxicity or relapse) at three years. The NCI investigators are recommending the use of more aggressive surgical resections in the hope of achieving a higher rate of complete remission. This author would like to propose the use of intraoperative radiation at the time of surgical debulking, which would add little extra morbidity to normal tissues but which might achieve an improved local control in those patients who present with bulky disease.

As the number of new Ewing's sarcoma cases per year is low, these patients should be entered, whenever feasible, on studies being carried out, either at large centers or within national groups. Through combined-modality approaches with continuing dialogue between pediatric and radiation oncologists and orthopedic surgeons, we can continue to build on the important advances that have been made in the treatment of Ewing's sarcoma over the last 20 years.

REFERENCES

1. Boyko OB, et al.: Am J Radiol 148:317-322, 1987.
2. Donaldson S: Personal communication, 1987.
3. Evans RG, et al.: Intl J Rad Oncol Biol Phys 11:129-136, 1985.
4. Gobel V, et al.: J Cancer Res Clin Oncol 113:187-191, 1987.
5. Hayes FA, et al.: J Clin Oncol 1:45-51, 1983.
6. Miser J, et al.: ASCO Proceedings #859, 1987.
7. Marcus RB, et al.: Intl J Rad Oncol Biol Phys 13:181-182, 1987.
8. Neff J: Personal communication, 1987.

230

9. Sailer SL, et al.: Intl J Rad Oncol Biol Phys (in press), 1987.
10. Strong LC, et al.: J Natl Cancer Inst 62:1401-1406, 1979.
11. Thompson EI: Personal communication, 1987.
12. Thomas PRM, et al.: Cancer Treat Rep 68:703-710, 1984.
13. Tucker MA, et al.: N. E. J. Med 317:588-593, 1987.
14. Wilkins RM, et al.: Cancer 58:2551-2555, 1986.

THE GERMAN PEDIATRIC ONCOLOGY (GPO) COOPERATIVE STUDY ON EWING'S SARCOMA

K. Winkler[1]   and H. Juergens[2]

In 1981, the GPO cooperative Ewing's Sarcoma study (CESS-81) was initiated (1). Patients under the age of 25, with histologically proven diagnosis and without evidence of metastases, received four 9-week cycles of 4-drug chemotherapy with vincristine, actinomycin D, cyclosphosphamide and adriamycin (VACA), administered as outlined in Figure 1. Local therapy was done after the first two cycles and consisted of either: 1) extracompartmental surgery, 2) wide resection followed by radiation, or 3) radiation therapy without surgery. The radiation dose was 60 Gy for the tumor bulk, including a 5 cm safety margin, and the dose for the remainder of the tumor bearing compartment as well as after non-radical surgery was 36 Gy. The decision for local therapy was individualized. A total of 93 eligible patients were registered on protocol from January 1, 1981 to February 28, 1985, from 54 participating institutions in West Germany, Austria, Switzerland and the Netherlands.

At a median observation time of 29 months, recurrent disease developed in 39/93 patients, the life table analysis of all patients showing a calculated DFS-rate of 60% at 36 months and 55% at 69 months (Figure 2). In 39 patients who developed recurrent disease, the site of relapse was local only in 12, systemic only in 18, and systemic as well as local in 9. The type of local treatment significantly influenced the local failure rate, which was found highest amongst patients with radiation only (15/32), lowest in patients with radical surgery (1/31), and intermediate after combined modality treatment (5/29). However, the rate of systemic metastases was higher in patients after radical surgery (10/31) as compared to radiation only or combined modality treatment (7/61). Since an interim survey had revealed an unusually high incidence of local failures in patients who had received radiotherapy, and since an analysis thereupon had given evidence of poor compliance to the radiation protocol (2,3), a radiation planning center was established in 1983 and centralized radiation planning based on radiographic

---

[1]Department of Pediatric Oncology of the University of Hamburg, Universitats-Krankenhaus Eppendorf, Martinistr. 52 2000 Hamburg 20.
[2]Department of Pediatric Oncology, University of Düsseldorf, W.Germany.

J. R. Ryan and L. O. Baker (eds.), Recent Concepts in Sarcoma Treatment, 231–234.

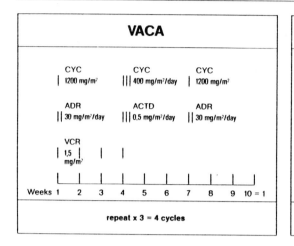

FIGURE 1: Outline of chemotherapy of the Ewing's sarcoma study CESS-81.

studies made at diagnosis was made mandatory. Thereafter only 1/16 as compared to 19/45 patients developed local failure following radiotherapy or combined modality local treatment. The period of observation, however, is shorter for the latter patients.

The tumor volume at diagnosis was found to be a significant prognostic factor (4). The calculated DFS-rate at three years was 81% for 51 patients with small tumors (<100 ml), as compared to 32% for 38 patients with larger tumors (p <0.001, Fig. 2). The histological response to preoperative chemotherapy was found to be another significant prognostic factor (3). Out of 45 available specimens, 38 were graded as good responders (< 10% vital tumor), and 16 as poor responders, the respective calculated DFS-rates at 3 years being 79% and 31% (p <0.001). The prognostic influence of tumor volume and of tumor site, besides the variables age, sex, histological subtype, serum LDH, clinical regression under initial chemotherapy and compliance to chemotherapy, were evaluated using a Cox-regression-analysis. Only tumor volume and histological response to initial chemotherapy appeared to be of statistical relevance.

The overall DFS of the CESS-81 trial compares favorably with the results of other cooperative studies (5-10), however, in comparison to the Intergroup Ewing's Sarcoma study, a comparatively low systemic failure rate is compromised by a

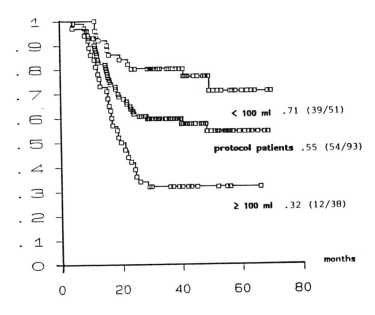

proportion
relapse-free

< 100 ml   .71 (39/51)

protocol patients   .55 (54/93)

≥ 100 ml   .32 (12/38)

months

FIGURE 2: Actuarial DFS-rate of all 93 patients with primary Ewing's sarcoma treated according to the CESS-82 study, and of the fraction of patients with small tumors (<100 ml) vs. the fraction with large tumors (≥ 100 ml).

relatively high local failure rate (11). The latter might be caused by an inadequate compliance to the radiation treatment as pointed out earlier. On the other hand, though delaying surgery may harbor some risk, preoperative chemotherapy, aimed at early eradication of subclinical systemic spread, seems to be a very effective strategy. Interruption of systemic chemotherapy for local treatment, in turn, has to be considered as disadvantageous for systemic control. In this conflict, simultaneous local treatment and systemic chemotherapy would appear most beneficial. The concomitant use of conventional radiotherapy and of radiosensitizing drugs like actinomycin D and DOX, however, would produce intolerable tissue damage. In a controlled trial, the ongoing study CESS-86 uses simultaneous chemo-radio-therapy vs. interposed radiotherapy. To minimize normal tissue damage, radiation is given as an accelerated hyperfractionated split course. In addition, chemotherapy is tailored to the risk of relapse. In high risk patients (central or large tumors), conventional dose cyclosphosphamide is replaced by high dose IFO, accounted for by the efficacy of high dose alkylating agents in Ewing's sarcoma (11,12).

REFERENCES

1. Jürgens H et al.: Klin Pädiatr 193:253-256, 1981.
2. Sauer R, Jürgens H et al.: Verh Dtsch Krebs Ges 5:801-804, 1984
3. Jürgens H, Gobel V et al.: Klin Pädiatr 197:225-232, 1985.
4. Göbel V, Jürgens H et al.: J Cancer Res Clin Oncol 113:187-191, 1987.
5. Nesbit ME, Perez CA et al.: Natl Cancer Inst Monogr 56:255-262, 1981.
6. Rosen G, Caparros B, Mosende C et al.: Cancer 41:888-899, 1978.
7. Gasparini M, et al.: Eur J Cancer Clin Oncol 17:1205-1209, 1981.
8. Zucker JM, Henry-Amar M, Sarrazin D et al.: Cancer 52:415-423, 1983.
9. Gnudi S, Picci P, Gherlinzoni F et al.: Proceedings of the 13th Intl Congress of Chemotherapy, Vienna, Austria, part 251:19-22, 1983.
10. Demeocq F, Carton P, Patte C et al.: Presse Med 13:717-721, 1984.
11. Göbel V et al.: J Cancer Res Clin Oncol 111 (Suppl):30, 1986.
12. Pinkerton CR et al.: Cancer Chemother Pharmacol 15:258-262, 1985.

NATURAL HISTORY OF OSTEOSARCOMA--HAS IT CHANGED?

Douglas J. Pritchard, M.D.*

Osteosarcoma is the most common primary bone sarcoma, accounting for approximately 20% of all bone sarcomas.(1) The variants of classic osteosarcoma are well recognized.(2) Because each of these variants may have its own distinctive clinical and biologic behavior, these must be taken into consideration when classifying and analyzing results of various clinical trials. For example, patients with parosteal osteosarcoma may be treated by surgery alone with the expectation that 90% will be cured. However, the osteosarcoma which arises in Paget's disease has a particularly poor prognosis.

In 1967, Dahlin and Coventry reported a study of 600 cases of osteosarcoma from the Mayo Clinic.(3) They found a 5-year survival rate of 20.3%. Other studies published at approximately that same time arrived at comparable survival rates. In 1970, Marcove et al. published results of the treatment of patients with osteosarcoma who were less than 21 years old.(4) Again, the 5-year survival rate was approximately 20%. Thus, 20% became a bench mark against which newer results were compared.

Subsequent to the report by Dahlin and Coventry, several clinical trials were carried out at the Mayo Clinic. In one, all patients underwent amputation for the primary tumor and then were randomized to receive either elective whole-lung irradiation or observation.(5) There was no apparent improvement in survival among patients treated by irradiation of the lung fields; however, both groups showed greatly improved survival compared with historical controls. In another study at the Mayo Clinic, patients were randomized to receive either a combination chemotherapy regimen (methotrexate, doxorubicin, adriamycin, and vincristine) or transfer factor as a form of immunotherapy.(6) There was no apparent advantage for either regimen; however, both regimens produced improved survival compared with historical controls.

In the early 1970's, there were several reports of the efficacy of adjuvant chemotherapy for osteosarcoma. In 1972, the group at the M.D. Anderson Hospital reported that use of a chemotherapy regimen--CONPADRI (cytoxan, vincristine, melphalan, adriamycin)--provided an overall 2-year survival

---

*Section of Orthopedic Oncology, Mayo Clinic and Mayo Foundation, Rochester, MN 55905.

J. R. Ryan and L. O. Baker (eds.), Recent Concepts in Sarcoma Treatment, 235–238.
© *1988 by Kluwer Academic Publishers.*

rate greater than 50%.(7) In 1974, there were two additional reports, one of a study using adriamycin as a single agent after primary amputation, and the other of a study using high-dose methotrexate therapy.(8,9) In both studies, the overall 2-year survival rate was greater than 60%. A number of subsequent reports from different institutions described improved disease-free and overall survival for patients receiving various types of chemotherapy regimens.

Thus, by the end of the 1970's, virtually all institutions were reporting improved survival for osteosarcoma patients with numerous different types of treatment regimens producing similar results. Some studies used a single agent and some used multiple agents. Some studies used relatively high doses of drugs and others used relatively low doses. Indeed, even interferon was used in conjunction with surgical treatment of the primary lesion and resulted in a survival rate greater than the 20% quoted in the past.(10)

In 1978, a group at the Mayo Clinic suggested that a change may have occurred in the natural history of osteosarcoma.(11) Patients treated between 1972 and 1974 without chemotherapy had an overall survival rate of approximately 50%. In addition, in 1980, Edmonson et al. reported on a randomized prospective trial comparing use of adjuvant high-dose methotrexate chemotherapy to no use of adjuvant chemotherapy; the survival rate was approximately 50% in both groups at 2 years.(12)

Certainly, factors independent of treatment might explain some of the improvement in survival of osteosarcoma patients. The clinical staging of patients has improved considerably in the last decade. Computed tomography undoubtedly detects occult metastatic pulmonary disease that would have been overlooked in the past, and these patients are automatically excluded from the analysis of patients with primary localized disease.

One factor that should not be overlooked is the general improvement of medical awareness on the part of both patients and referring physicians. Physicians at the Mayo Clinic have for many years exerted a major educational effort directed toward physicians within our referral area. We believe that patients are more likely to seek medical attention at an early stage, and physicians are much more willing to refer patients with suspect lesions to major institutions even before a biopsy is undertaken. Institutions that have a concentration of physicians with a special interest in the treatment of osteosarcoma can evaluate the patient, stage, and biopsy the lesion, and begin treatment within 48 hours from the time the patient arrives. In the past, the initial physician often obtained the biopsy specimen and then sent the histologic slides to several different institutions for interpretation. Thus, the patient was not referred for definitive treatment until after a delay of a month or more. While this delay may not have had any major effect in an individual case, overall it undoubtedly will have affected survival statistics.

In addition, actual survival undoubtedly is influenced

by the more common use of thoracotomy for resection of metastatic pulmonary disease.(13,14) Again, with the use of computed tomography to examine the lung fields, such nodules can be detected at an early stage when they can be resected readily. In the past, the philosophy in general was to observe such pulmonary nodules and only to offer thoracotomy if they remained solitary and relatively stable. This total change in surgical philosophy certainly has had a dramatic effect on the survival of patients with metastatic disease.

The role of various adjunctive treatment programs in the improvement in survival for patients with osteosarcoma is difficult to quantitate. Part of the problem is simply the rarity of this disease. In order to achieve sufficient numbers of patients for meaningful analysis of results, it may be necessary to perform cooperative studies such as those undertaken by the Children's Cancer Study Group (15) and the recent study reported by the Pediatric Oncology Group.(16) The results of the latter study, in combination with the recently reported study by Eilber et al. (17), have led most medical oncologists to believe that the role of adjuvant chemotherapy in the management of osteosarcoma is now well established.

There is no question that patients with osteosarcoma now have improved survival compared with patients with this disease treated 20 years ago. Most of us want to believe that it is our treatment that has effected this improvement. It is quite possible that other factors, including some change in the natural history of the disease, may be playing a role in this improvement.

REFERENCES

1. Osteosarcoma. In: Bone Tumors, Fourth Edition, Dahlin DC, Unni, KK (Eds.), Springfield, Illinois, Charles C. Thomas Publishers, pp.269-307, 1986.
2. Dahlin DC, Unni KK: Osteosarcoma of bone and its important recognizable varieties. Am J Surg 1:61-72, 1977.
3. Dahlin DC, Coventry MB: Osteogenic sarcoma: a study of six hundred cases. J Bone Joint Surg (Am) 49:101-110, 1967.
4. Marcove RC, Mike V, Hajek JV, Levin AG, Hutter RV: Osteogenic sarcoma under the age of twenty-one. J Bone Joint Surg (Am) 52:411-423, 1970.
5. Rab GT, Ivins JC, Childs DS Jr, Cupps, RE, Pritchard DJ: Elective Whole lung irradiation in the treatment of osteogenic sarcoma. Cancer 38:939-952, 1976.
6. Ritts RE Jr, Pritchard DJ, Gilchrist GS, Ivins JC, Taylor WF: Transfer factor versus combination chemotherapy: an interim report of a randomized postsurgical adjuvant study in osteogenic sarcoma. Prog Cancer Res Ther 6:293-198, 1978.
7. Sutow WW, Sullivan MP, Fernbach DJ, Cangir A, George SL: Adjuvant chemotherapy in primary treatment of osteogenic sarcoma: A Southwest Oncology Group Study. Cancer 36: 1598-1602, 1975.

8. Cortez EP, Holland JF, Wang JJ, Sinks LF, Blom J, Senn H, Bank A, Glidewall O: Amputation and adriamycin in primary osteosarcoma. N Engl J Med 291:998-1000, 1974.

9. Jaffe N, Frei E III, Traggis D, Bishop Y: Adjuvant methotrexate and citrovorum factor treatment of osteogenic sarcoma. N Engl J Med 291:994-997, 1974.

10. Strander H: The interferon system and its possible use in the treatment of neoplastic disease. Cancer Immunol Immunother 3:35, 1977.

11. Taylor WF, Ivins JC, Dahlin DC, Pritchard DJ: Osteogenic sarcoma experience at the Mayo Clinic, 1963-1974. Prog Cancer Res Ther 6:251-268, 1978.

12. Edmonson JH, Green SJ, Ivins JC, Gilchrist GS, Creagan ET, Burgert EO, Pritchard DJ, Hahn RG, Dahlin DC, Taylor WF: Post surgical treatment of primary osteosarcoma of bone: comparison of high dose methotrexate versus observation: preliminary report (abstract). Proc Am Assoc Cancer Res Am Soc Clin Oncol 21:476, 1980.

13. Martini N, McCormick PM, Bains MS, Beattie EJ Jr: Surgery for solitary and multiple pulmonary metastases. NY State J Med 78:1711-1714, 1978.

14. Telander RL, Pairolero PC, Pritchard DJ, Sim FH, Gilchrist GS: Resection of pulmonary metastatic osteogenic sarcoma in children. Surgery 84:335-341, 1978.

15. Krailo M, Ertel I, Makley J, Fryer CJ, Baum E, Weetman R, Yunis E, Barnes L, Bleyer WA, Hammond GD: A randomized study comparing high dose methotrexate with moderate-dose methotrexate as components of adjuvant chemotherapy in childhood nonmetastatic osteosarcoma: a report from the Children's Cancer Study Group. Med Pediatr Oncol 15:69-77, 1987.

16. Link MP, Goorin AM, Miser AW, Green AA, Pratt CB, Belasco JB, Pritchard DJ, Malpas JS, Baker AR, Kirkpatrick JA, et al.: The effect of adjuvant chemotherapy on relapse free survival in patients with osteosarcoma of the extremity. N Engl J Med 314:1600-1606, 1986.

17. Eilber F, Giuliano A, Eckardt J, Patterson K, Moseley S, Goodnight J: Adjuvant chemotherapy for osteosarcoma: a randomized prospective trial. J Clin Oncol 5:21-26, 1987.

LIMB SALVAGE FOR OSTEOSARCOMA

Michael A. Simon, M.D.*

Five issues need to be addressed when considering limb salvage instead of amputation for osteosarcoma of the extremities. Is there any decrease in survival with limb salvage when compared to amputation? What are the differences in the immediate morbidity between the two surgical procedures? What is the durability of the reconstructions and the delayed morbidity of each type of limb salvage surgical procedure? How does the salvaged limb function when compared to amputation at the homologous anatomic site? Lastly, are there any psychosocial benefits for patients who have limb salvage instead of amputation? I will only address the impact of limb salvage on the incidence and consequences of local recurrence, the length of the disease-free interval, and the rate of long-term survival for patients who have osteosarcoma of the extremities.

Recent single institutional studies have found that limb salvage, while possibly increasing the local recurrence rate to 10% (almost exclusively in femur tumors), does not seem to have an adverse impact on disease-free and long-term survival rates. These studies have the distinct disadvantage of observer bias, small patient accrual, variable anatomic sites and patient ages included in study, and significant patient selection. However, each institution had fairly consistent adjuvant or neoadjuvant chemotherapy regimens, pathologic support, and surgical strategy for limb salvage and thoracotomy.

One multi-institutional study also confirms data that limb salvage will also have about a 10% local recurrence rate for distal femur osteosarcomas. But, again, there is little, if any, compromise of disease-free or long-term survival rates compared to amputation. Again, although the study was nonrandomized, observer bias and patient selection were diluted by the inclusion of many institutions. In addition, when compared to single institutional studies, this study had the advantage of investigating, over a short period of time, a large number of patients who were under the age of 30 years, and who had tumors in only one anatomic site. The

---

*Professor and Chairman, Section of Orthopaedic Surgery and Rehabilitation Medicine, Department of Surgery, The University of Chicago, 5841 S. Maryland Avenue, Box 102, Chicago, IL 60637.

J. R. Ryan and L. O. Baker (eds.), Recent Concepts in Sarcoma Treatment, 239–240.

disadvantage of the study was the variability of the chemotherapy regimens administered, the lack of a central pathologic review, and the potential variability in the surgical technique and strategy for limb salvage and thoracotomy.

In spite of the potential drawbacks to the above studies, it appears that limb salvage, when performed by experienced surgeons with wide surgical margins in an adjuvant or neoadjuvant chemotherapy setting, does not cause a significantly increased rate of death. Therefore, unless there are significant factors which preclude the achievement of wide surgical margins, such as an extensive tumor, anatomic locations that have significant technical problems (i.e., distal tibia), or markedly displaced pathologic fractures, most patients are candidates for limb salvage if they and their families understand the ambiguities of the other four issues.

PELVIC RESECTION IN BONE SARCOMAS*

R. Capanna[1], N. Guernelli[2], A. Briccoli[2], G. Bacci[1],
P. Picci[1], R. Biagini[1], R. De Cristofaro[1], C. Martelli[1],
M. Campanacci[1]

Between 1968 and 1986, 77 pelvic resections were performed at the Istituto Ortopedico Rizzoli for the treatment
of primary bone tumors. There were 73 malignant tumors: 35
were low grade (all chondrosarcomas) and 38 high grade (13
chondrosarcomas, 14 Ewing's sarcomas, 5 osteosarcomas, 3
M.F.H., 2 fibrosarcomas and 1 angiosarcoma). Four cases were
benign but aggressive (stage 3) lesions (1 chondromyxoid
fibroma, 1 aneurysmal bone cyst, 1 giant cell tumor and 1
hidatid cyst).

Resection Types, Reconstructions and Outcome

Pelvic resections were divided into three major types,
according to Enneking's classification: iliac wing resections
(type A = 27 cases), periacetabular resections (type B = 36
cases) and anterior arch resections (type C = 14 cases).

On the basis of the extension of the resection, a type A
procedure was subdivided into four classes: A_1 if a wedge
resection of the iliac wing was performed without interruption of the pelvic ring (14 cases), A_2 if a resection of the
whole thickness of the ilium was performed with interruption
of the pelvic ring (7 cases), A_3 when a complete resection of
the iliac wing with the sacroiliac joint was performed (4
cases), A_4 when half sacrum was resected en bloc with the
sacroiliac joint (2 cases). No reconstruction of the pelvic
ring was required in A_1 resections, while it was not possible
in type A_4 resections. Reconstruction of the continuity of
the pelvic ring with autogenous grafts was attempted and
obtained in 5 out of 11 cases having an A_2 or A_3 resection.
The functional results were improved when the iliac wing was
reconstructed.

Type B procedures were also subdivided into four
classes: B_1 if a partial resection of the acetabulum was
performed (1 case); B_2 or B_3 when the entire acetabulum was
resected together with the iliac wing (9 cases) or the anter-
anterior arch (23 cases); B_4 when an extra-articular

----
[1] Bone Tumor Center, Istituto Ortopedico Rizzoli, Bologna
  40136 Italy.
[2] Surgical Department, University of Modena, Modena, Italy.
----
* Supported by Grant No. 86.02679.44, Special Project
  "Oncology", Italian National Research Council.

J. R. Ryan and L. O. Baker (eds.), Recent Concepts in Sarcoma Treatment, 241–244.
© 1988 by Kluwer Academic Publishers.

resection of the proximal femur was performed (3 cases). Among 36 periacetabular resections, 27 were intra-articular and 9 extra-articular. A successful reconstruction of the acetabulum with autogenous grafts was performed in B_1 resections. In B_2 resections, the attempted reconstruction was: ischiofemoral arthrodesis with screws (5 cases), ischiofemoral coaptation with metallic wires (3 cases), and a flail hip (1 case). The attempted ischiofemoral arthrodesis was always obtained, while the coaptation with metallic wires was unsuccessful, a flail hip developing in most instances. In B_3 resections, the attempted reconstruction was: iliofemoral coaptation with wires (18 cases), iliofemoral arthrodesis with Cobra plate (5 cases). A fusion was obtained in 30% of the patients having an iliofemoral coaptation with wires, and in 43% of the patients having a rigid internal fixation with plate. A pseudarthrosis developed in the remaining patients. No significant differences in functional results were observed between an iliofemoral pseudarthrosis or arthrodesis. In type B_4 resections, a successful reconstruction with intercalary allografts (2) or prosthesis (1) was performed.

A type C procedure was also subdivided into three classes: C_1 when the resection of the anterior arch included the inferomedial part of the acetabulum (9); C_2 when a monolateral resection of the anterior arch was performed (3); C_3 when a bilateral resection of the anterior arch was performed (2). Reconstruction of the pelvic ring was attempted only in 1 case.

Complications

Complications in pelvic resections are frequent. Infections were more frequent in A_{2-3-4} and in B_3 resection where the surgical incision is near to perianal and perigenital regions. Vascular and visceral damages were more frequent in anterior arch resections; neurological damage in iliac wing resections, and mechanical complications in periacetabular resections. Only one patient (a periacetabular resection, B_2 type) had to be amputated because of a complication (vascular thrombosis of the iliac artery in the postoperative period) (Table 1).

	A_1	$A_{2/4}$	$B_{1/2/4}$	B_3	$C_{1/2/3/}$	TOTAL
INFECTION	7%	38%	23%	31%	21%	25%
NERVOUS	7%	23%	7%	13%	7%	10%
VASCULAR	-	-	7%	17%	-	7%
OSTEOART.	-	7%	7%	17%	28%	14%
UROGENITAL	-	-	-	-	21%	4%
ABD. HERNIA	-	7%	7%	9%	7%	6%
GENERAL	-	-	7%	13%	-	5%

TABLE 1: COMPLICATIONS

Functional Results

Functional results were usually excellent in type C and A_1 resections. They were usually fair in periacetabular

resections or in resections of the iliac wing when the interrupted ring was not reconstructed or it was complicated by
neurological damage (Table 2).

TABLE 2: FUNCTIONAL RESULTS

FUNCTIONAL RESULTS	ILIUM NO INTERRUPT.	ILIUM INTERRUPT.	ACETAB.	ANT. ARCH
Excellent	73%	-	6%	64%
Good	18%	40%	24%	9%
Fair	9%*	60%*	59%	18%
Poor	-	-	11%	9%

*Patients who had neurological damage.

Oncological Results

The follow-up ranged from 1 to 14 years (mean, 6 years).
The oncological results were far better in benign or low
grade tumors (100% and 86% disease-free patients) than in
high-grade tumors (44% disease-free patients) or Ewing's
sarcoma (23%) (Table 3).

TABLE 3: ONCOLOGICAL RESULTS

	NED I	NED II	ALIVE WITH DISEASE	DEAD
Benign (4)	100%	-	-	-
Low (35)	78%	8%	8%	6%
High (25)	36%	8%	20%	36%
Ewing (13)	23%	-	15%	62%

The local recurrence was frequent (23/77, 30%). The
local recurrence rate was 37% in type A, 28% in type B and
22% in type C resections. The local control was strictly
dependent on the achieved surgical margins. The local recurrence rate was 12% (4/34) after wide resection, 35% (9/26)
after wide/marginal or wide/contaminated procedures, 57%
(4/7) after marginal resections, and 60% (6/10) after intralesional resections. With the same surgical margins, high
grade tumors relapsed twice as much as low grade tumors
(Table 4).

Conclusions

Most pelvic resections represent a complex procedure.
The main indications are low grade malignancies of the pelvic
bone, and particularly chondrosarcomas.

In addition, with appropriate preoperative chemotherapy,
it may also be possible to consider limb-sparing resections
in high grade tumors such as osteosarcoma or malignant
fibrous histiocytoma. There is also some evidence that
Ewing's sarcoma may have a better prognosis after local
resection, rather than reliance on radiotherapy alone.

TABLE 4: LOCAL RECURRENCES

	BENIGN	LOW GRADE	HIGH GRADE
Wide	0%	6%	19%
Wide/Marginal or Wide contaminated	0%	28%	45%
Marginal	0%	60%	64%
Intralesional	0%	-	

The incidence of local tumor recurrence is closely related to the tumor grade and the achieved surgical margins and in high grade lesions, the probability of success is low. These operations require extensive preoperative study (NMR, CT scan, bone scan, angiography, cystography), specific surgical experience, team work with general (vascular, urology) surgeon, intensive care facilities.

Complications are frequent and this procedure is not indicated in metastatic tumors, in very bad local or general conditions, or severe obesity.

REFERENCES

1. Enneking WF, Durham WK: Resection and reconstruction for primary neoplasms involving the innominate bone. J Bone Joint Surg 60A:731-746, 1978.

EN BLOC SURGERY FOR OSTEOGENIC SARCOMA: ANALYSIS AND REVIEW OF 180 CASES

Ralph C. Marcove, M.D.[1], Andrew G. Huvos, M.D.[2],
Paul A. Meyers, M.D.[3], Brenda Caparros-Sison, M.D.[4],
Gerald Rosen, M.D.[5]

This paper describes our experience in limb-salvage procedures for fully malignant sarcomas done by one surgeon at Memorial Hospital. Historically, the limb salvage rate for even the lowest grade of osteogenic sarcoma (usually juxta-cortical, Grade I and Grade II) in the past have been dismal for both the knee (78% local failure rate) and the upper extremity (100% failure).(1,8,12) Symes, in an early publication, found a very high local recurrence rate when amputating through a joint adjacent to a fully malignant tumor. Specific operative techniques were not described in these early papers, but obviously surgery at the pseudocapsule layer is most probably doomed to failure and removing the adjacent joint for epiphyseal lesions would be helpful!

Materials and Methods

Eighty-eight patients with distal femoral involvement are included in this study. Twenty-three proximal femur osteogenic sarcomas were treated. Twenty-six have upper tibial involvement and 33 have fully malignant central osteogenic sarcomas involving the upper humerus. One patient had scapular and one proximal fibula involvement. Four pelvic cases are also analyzed (Tables 1-4). Four have other sites involved. The total number of patients involved is 180.

Technique

A preoperative arteriogram to evaluate the proximity of the neurovascular bundle is often done. Almost all of our patients had adjacent soft tissue masses (2A lesions). At presentation, two already had pulmonary metastases.(5,10) Some had fractured limbs which healed on preliminary chemotherapy.(9,10) This was a finding that H. L. Jaffe felt was almost uniformly fatal prior to the modern chemotherapy

---

[1]Associate Attending Surgeon, Department of Orthopedics, Memorial Hospital, 517 East 71st. Street, New York, NY 10021.

[2]Attending, Department of Pathology, Memorial Hospital, New York, NY.

[3]Assistant Attending Pediatrician, Memorial Hospital, New York, NY.

[4]Clinical Assistant Attending Pediatrician, Memorial Hospital, New York, NY.

[5]Medical Director, Comprehensive Cancer Center, Beverly Hills, CA.

J. R. Ryan and L. O. Baker (eds.), Recent Concepts in Sarcoma Treatment, 245–249.
© 1988 by Kluwer Academic Publishers.

246

TABLE 1. SUMMARY OF TOTAL PATIENTS TREATED - 180 PATIENTS

36	total femur replacement /distal femur lesions
34	Tikhoff-Linberg procedures/one scapula + 33 Upper humeral lesions
52	long stem Guepar knee replacements/distal femur lesions
23	proximal femur replacement/proximal femur lesions
27	total knee replacements/upper tibia + one fibula lesions
4	pelvic replacements
4	other sites

180 patients

TABLE 2. SUMMARY OF ALL PATIENTS TREATED WHO HAD A SECOND LIMB
INVOLVEMENT - 180 PATIENTS TOTAL

| 2 | total femur replacements/later developed opposite distal femoral lesions |
| 1 | Tikhoff-Linberg procedure/for upper humeral primary, later an iliac metastasis secondary. This patient did well with local excision and cryosurgery. |

3/180 = 1.6%

evaluation.

Most, but not all, had pre-resection chemotherapy.(9) The basic surgical technique removed the entire adjacent joint. At first, all of the involved bone was resected (first 35 patients with distal femoral disease) for fear of intraosseous skip areas.(2,6) As specimens were further studied, it was decided to remove only a radical portion of the local femoral bone involved with a 2 to 3.0 inch margin away from the osseous edge of the tumor. No intraosseous skin areas have been found in this series (although they can certainly occur). The 36th total femur had frank tumor at both ends and appears to be successfully resected.

The operation consists of a dissection through only normal tissue (the pseudocapsule is never seen), and the first effort often is to free the neurovascular bundle from the tumor area. This is usually done from distal to proximal. The adjacent artery is dissected close to the main stem along its adventitia and the small vessels feeding the tumor are tied as close to the main stem as possible; it can quickly be decided that the neurovascular bundle can be successfully freed from tumor. All muscles are cut at a distance away from the pseudocapsule so that this latter area is never seen during the dissection. Cut ends of marrow are confirmed as free from tumor by frozen section diagnosis. As mentioned, the nearby adjacent joint is usually removed.

TABLE 3.   SUMMARY OF ALL PATIENTS TREATED WHO HAD SKIP LESIONS
            ACROSS THE JOINT-180 PATIENTS TOTAL

2 distal femur lesions to ipsilateral ilium secondary (both died)
1 Tikhoff-Linberg procedure for upper humeral lesion 2° to upper end
  of scapula (died)
1 fibula skip to ajacent tibia (survived)

4/180 = 2.2%   1/4 survived

TABLE 4.   LOCAL RECURRENCE IN 180 PATIENTS

6 distal femur lesions/treatment was total femoral resection
1 upper tibia lesions/treatment was total knee resection
1 upper femur location/treatment was local resection of upper femur (died)
2 pelvic sites/treatment was local resections (both have local recurrence
                                              unresectable)

10/180 = 5.5%

Pathologic examination is carefully done. The edges are
stained with dye and the margins of resection away from the
tumor are analyzed. At times, one may be only 0.25 to 0.5 cm
from the tumor. If the surgeon sees pseudocapsule, or if the
pathologist advises that we have been at that level, prompt
amputation is performed. In the last 5 years this has been
quite unusual, as preoperative evaluation and clinical judge-
ment improves. In the knee, the quadriceps mechanism is
usually extremely weakened. At the shoulder, even the deltoid
may be removed for margin so that only elbow and hand function can be expected. If the length of the humerus is markedly shortened, it has been found that a Kuntscher nail-bone
prolongation, sutured to the residual muscles at the shoulder
area, facilitates elbow flexion and strength. The upper end
of the nail caused irritation in a third of the cases, but
few needed specific local treatment. Patients are warned that
a weakened leg or arm will result, but distal sensation is
usually good. Only one patient, early in this series, com-
plained of extreme numbness in his lower extremity and re-
quested amputation. He is pleased with his amputation and we
have, therefore, learned to try to save more sensory nerves.
    To repair the knee, we modified existing Guepar knee
prostheses to make their stems longer and stronger. The 5°
valgus has been eliminated, therefore, eliminating the need
for right and left sides. Intraoperative choice for various
resection lengths are kept available. In my experience, the
need for an expanding prosthesis is quite rare since these
children are usually quite tall. Lengthening has been
successfully performed several ways from prosthetic changing

to Wagner limb traction. This is a relatively minor problem. The diameter of the knee axis is kept small because of the necessity to remove much quadriceps tissue with the excision. Skin closure is, therefore, facilitated. The patient is also told that metal can fatigue, eventually break and may need replacement. We found that a prosthetic stem 10 mm in diameter was too weak and that loosening, bending, or breakage often followed, but this has been largely eliminated with the use of stems tapering from 14 to 12 mm width (Dow Corning Wright). Stress also may be reduced using ischial weight-bearing braces. Some, however, choose not to use it. The enlarged stem prosthesis difficulties are largely (but not always) overcome.

Results

Six local recurrences occurred before December 1978 in the total femur group. One upper tibia locally recurred in 1975. One upper femur recurred locally in 1986, and two pelvic cases locally recurred this same year. One successful pelvic resection was aided by cryosurgery in 1980.

Conclusions

With experience and better selection, only 3 proven local recurrences have occurred within the past 7 years (one proximal femur and two pelvic). There was skip across the local joint in 4 patients, but one patient's leg could still be salvaged and she is doing well. A second bone involvement occurred in 3 patients, one of which could be saved with a limb-sparing iliac bone removal (in 1980) after the primary Tikhoff-Linberg procedure. Two patients presented with pulmonary metastasis, one of whom is still alive and well now 8 years and 5 months later. The other patient was free of disease 5 years and later died of intracardiac metastasis. The rate of pulmonary metastasis after en bloc resection is 34% and the survival after attempting multiple pulmonary resections is 32%, with an average pulmonary surgery follow-up time of 96 months. In addition, as more drug agents were added, the overall survival rate seems to be improving for all but the most chondrosarcomatous types of osteogenic sarcoma.(9-11) Even chondrosarcomatous types of osteogenic sarcoma, as well as frank dedifferentiated chondrosarcomas, have an improved rate of survival on high-dose chemotherapy.

Summary

This is the largest series and largest follow-up of patients with limb operations done by one surgeon. Other subsequent reports from Memorial Hospital involve a group of other surgeons; however, the survival rates are largely comparable. This series demonstrates that local recurrences (5.5%) probably can be reduced with more experience. This has also been shown in Vienna by Salzer, whose early local recurrence rate was 30% and, with experience, was later lowered to 15%.(12) The early experience of the Mayo Clinic is 24% local recurrence rate for tumors with soft tissue masses (2A type). The early series done by Dr. Francis had an overall survival of not over 25%, but these cases had less radical surgery and no chemotherapy. In our series, most - but not all, had chemotherapy (some patients refused). These figures document that en bloc procedures can have good overall survival and tend to improve with more radical local surgery. They also demonstrate that the rate of local recurrence decreases with experience and that these operations should not be undertaken by the `occasional' tumor surgeon, as many others have so correctly emphasized. The use of a local expander is almost always unnecessary in these usually tall children, and one must instead look at the author's published survival rates and not the type of prosthesis used. If a medical center cure rate is not published, the referring physician should avoid directing a patient for "limb-sparing surgery" merely because of highly-touted type of prosthesis. All prostheses are available to anyone, but the overriding statistic must be the survival rate of the patients reflecting the surgeon's ability to remove the tumor successfully.

REFERENCES

1. Ahuja SC, Villacin AB, Smith J, et al.: Juxtacortical osteogenic sarcoma. J Bone Joint Surg 59A:632-649, 1977.
2. Marcove RC, Mike V, Hajek JV, et al.: Osteogenic sarcoma under the age of twenty-one. A review of 145 operative cases. J Bone Joint Surg 52A:411-423, 1970.
3. Marcove RC: En bloc resection of osteogenic sarcoma. Cancer 45:3040-3044, 1980.
4. Marcove RC: En bloc resection for osteogenic sarcoma. Bull NY Acad Med 55:744-750, 1979.
5. Marcove RC, Martini N, Rosen G: The treatment of pulmonary metastasis in osteogenic sarcoma. Clin Orthop 111:65-70, 1975.
6. Marcove RC: The Surgery of Tumors of Bone and Cartilage. New York, Grune and Stratton, 1981.
7. Martini N, Huvos AG, Mike V, Marcove RC, Beattie EE Jr: Multiple pulmonary resections in the treatment of osteogenic sarcoma. Ann Thorac Surg 12:271, 1971.
8. McKenna RJ, Schwinn CP, Soong KY, et al.: Sarcomata of the osteogenic series. Analysis of 552 cases. J Bone Joint Surg 48:1-26, 1966.
9. Rosen G, Marcove RC, Caparros B, et al.: Primary osteogenic sarcoma. The rationale for preoperative chemotherapy and delayed surgery. Cancer 43:2163-2177, 1979.
10. Rosen G, Huvos AG, Mosende C, et al.: Chemotherapy and thoracotomy for metastatic osteogenic sarcoma. Cancer 41:841-849, 1978.
11. Rosen G, Capparos B, Huvos AG, et al.: Preoperative chemotherapy for osteogenic sarcoma: selection of postoperative adjuvant chemotherapy based on the response of the primary tumor to preoperative chemotherapy. Cancer 1221-1230, 1982.
12. Salzer M, Salzer-Kuntschik M: Vergleichende rontgenologisch-pathologische-anatomische Untersuchungen von Osteosarkomen in Hindblick auf die Amputationshohe. Arch Orthop. Fall-Chir 65:322-326, 1969.

THE USE OF BONE ALLOGRAFT TRANSPLANTS IN THE MANAGEMENT OF BONE TUMORS[*]

Mark C. Gebhardt, M.D.[1], and Henry J. Mankin, M.D.[1]

Introduction

The use of allograft skeletal parts in the management of patients with segmental bone loss as a result of tumor or trauma, has been a procedure of considerable interest to a number of investigators.(18,19,29,30,31,39) In consideration of the theoretical immunological issues and the known high complication rate (22,38), allografting ought to be considered as, perhaps, a less than optimal solution for the patient with massive bone loss. Despite these problems, however, the system has become an increasingly popular method of dealing with major skeletal defects as created by trauma or resection for musculoskeletal tumors. Furthermore, in recent years, allografting has become an important part of the armamentarium of the total joint surgeon who finds the technique useful in the treatment of loss of bone stock as a result of failure of metallic devices. Part of the explanation of this seeming paradox requires that one review the current alternatives available for the treatment of major skeletal loss. Implantation of avascular, or more recently, vascularized autografts, is the time-honored solution; and clearly the best tolerated, most predictable and durable substitute to fill a defect in a patient's skeleton is a segment of autogeneic bone.(3,9,10,16,40-44) The difficulties with this solution are self-evident, however: the amount of autograft is limited in quantity, size and shape, donor site morbidity can be a significant problem to a patient who is often already severely impaired by the disease and/or the surgery, and it is obviously impossible to reconstruct an articular surface. Following the early successes of metallic and plastic implants in the treatment of joint disease, numerous custom and, more recently, modular artificial devices, have been proposed for use in the treatment of massive defects of the skeleton, and reports describing the devices and the short-term results of their implantation have begun to appear with increasing frequency.(6,8,26,32,33)

---

[1]Orthopaedic Oncology Service, Massachusetts General
Hospital, Boston, MA 02114.

---

[*]Supported in part by National Institutes of Health Grants
AM 21896 and CA 32968.

J. R. Ryan and L. O. Baker (eds.), Recent Concepts in Sarcoma Treatment, 250–260.
© 1988 by Kluwer Academic Publishers.

Real concern has been expressed by some of the more thought-ful proponents of this system of skeletal reconstruction, however, particularly for the treatment of bone tumors in which the average age of the patients in most series is below 30. Since the failure rate for the standard hip prosthetic devices has been climbing rapidly and is now believed to be over 20% at 10 years (1,35,36), (and as has been suggested by Chandler et al. (4), these values are even greater in younger patients) the threat of failure in young tumor patients, who have been treated in many cases with less than optimal custom devices, must be considered a significant future problem if the patient survives.

For the past 15 years, the Orthopaedic Oncology Service at the Massachusetts General Hospital has been investigating the use of bone allografts to reconstruct massive bone loss, primarily due to tumor, and the current results will be presented herein.

Technical Aspects of the Operative Procedure

A bone bank has been in operation at the Massachusetts General Hospital for over 10 years and the procedures, stan-dards, precautions and logistics (including the costs) have been the subject of several recent reports.(7,37) In gener-al, we maintain standards identical to, and in full agreement with, the Guidelines promulgated by the American Association of Tissue Banks (12,13) and retain membership in the New England Organ Bank, an organization that is responsible for the living donor program in Massachusetts and surrounding regions. Selection of donors is for the most part dependent on the living organ harvest and almost all bone procurements follow such procedures. To satisfy our (and most other organ-izational) criteria, the donors should be between 15 and 45 years of age, free of overt infectious (bacterial, but es-pecially viral such as hepatitis or AIDS) or neoplastic disease, and dead usually no longer than 12-15 hours. The technical aspects of the procurement and operative procedure have been previously described.(23,24)

The surgical procedure in which the alloimplant is utilized is really two quite distinct operations. The first is a marginal or wide resection of the tumor, including a cuff of normal soft tissue surrounding the bone from which the tumor has arisen, as well as the tract of previous sur-gery or biopsy. The second, often equally arduous, is the implantation and fixation of the graft. Planning for the reconstruction should obviously be included in the overall approach to the surgical procedure, but should never take precedence over the safety of the resection and insuring adequacy of the surgical margins. Finally, it should be pointed out that in evaluating the results of the surgery in an attempt to determine the success or failure of the allo-graft reconstruction, one should take cognizance of the fact that many of the patients have had a long and bloody opera-tion with considerable trauma to or loss of soft tissue as part of the resective procedure and may also have already or will receive radiation therapy or chemotherapy. Comparison of the results in these patients with others who have had a lesser surgical resection, or even a standard total joint replacement, may be inappropriate.

The reconstructive part of the procedure and insertion of the graft is usually not as difficult as the resection, but careful attention to detail is essential to achieve a successful outcome. We employ fresh, frozen bone segments, the articular surfaces of which have been cryopreserved with 8% DMSO and are stored at -80° C. Matching of the graft with the host is currently not an "exact" science and, particularly for osteoarticular units, it is sometimes essential to have grafts of several sizes available if at all possible. Since the graft is easily infected, it should be carefully handled and maintenance of wound sterility is essential. Following thawing of the part, it is cut to size using a saw and fit into the defect. The capsular structures, ligaments and tendinous structures are sutured using stout nonabsorbable sutures, and the bone held in place using compression plates or, less commonly, intramedullary devices. If at all possible, neither the allograft bone or the hardware should lie immediately beneath the skin and subcutaneous tissue, and the use of muscle flaps is often extraordinarily valuable in avoiding a skin slough. Antibiotics should be administered intraoperatively and intravenously postoperatively for from 4 days to a week; and in addition, we have been in the practice of administering oral antibiotics for several months during the convalescent period. The limb is immobilized to allow the reconstructed ligaments and tendons to heal and, following removal of the casts, a supervised active and passive exercise program is begun and a cast type brace is employed until the joints are considered stable and the host donor junction sites are healed.

The Clinical Series

Between November 1971 and April 1987, the orthopaedic oncology unit at the Massachusetts General Hospital has performed 363 orthotopic fresh frozen cadaveric allograft transplantations, mostly for tumors of the extremities, but also for a small number of non-neoplastic conditions (Table 1).

Although a number of the lesions were benign or low grade, a significant number fell among the higher grade tumors and, hence, required greater concern regarding the threat of local recurrence or distant metastasis in their operative and postoperative management. One hundred and sixty-three males comprised 44.9% of the patients, and 200 females represented a slightly larger percentage (55.1%). The mean age for the group was 32.5 years, with a range from 11 to 79, but the vast majority of the patients were tightly clustered in the second to the fifth decades. The length of follow-up ranged from 1 to 186 months, with a mean duration of 55.9 months.

The types of grafts and the sites of implantation are shown in Table I and, as can be noted, four types of procedures were performed: osteoarticular, in which an entire or portion of an articular joint was included with the bony replacement part (221 cases); intercalary, in which the

TABLE 1

Allograft Transplantation Diagnosis in 363 Patients

TUMORS:

```
Giant cell tumor..............102
Chondrosarcoma.................60
Central osteosarcoma...........55
Parosteal osteosarcoma.........20
Fibrosarcoma or MFH............13
Adamantinoma....................9
Osteoblastoma...................8
Chondroblastoma.................6
Metastatic carcinoma............7
Ewing's sarcoma.................4
Desmoplastic fibroma............3
Lymphoma........................3
Chondromyxoid fibroma...........2
Angiosarcoma....................3
Aneurysmal bone cyst............2
Liposarcoma.....................2
Myeloma.........................2
Ossifying fibroma...............1
```

NON-TUMOROUS CONDITIONS:

```
Failed allo or TJR.............28
Traumatic loss.................11
Massive osteonecrosis..........10
Gaucher's disease...............4
Fibrous dysplasia...............4
Villonodular synovitis..........2
Paget's disease.................1
Eosinophilic granuloma..........1
```

SITES FOR 363 TRANSPLANTS

OSTEOARTICULAR (221):

```
Distal femur...................92
Proximal tibia.................55
Proximal humerus...............23
Proximal femur.................21
Distal radius..................17
Distal humerus..................8
Proximal ulna...................3
Distal tibia....................2
```

INTERCALARY (64):

```
Femur..........................26
Tibia..........................20
Humerus........................14
Radius..........................3
Ulna............................1
```

ALLOGRAFT PLUS PROSTHESIS (44):

```
Proximal femur.................35
Distal femur....................8
```

ALLOGRAFT ARTHRODESIS (34):

```
Proximal humerus...............13
Distal femur...................14
Proximal tibia..................3
Proximal femur..................2
Distal tibia....................2
```

graft consisted of a portion of the shaft of a long bone without an articular surface (64 cases); <u>allograft plus prosthesis</u>, in which the bony graft is coupled with a conventional prosthetic implant to replace the excised joint (44 cases); and <u>allograft-arthrodesis</u>, in which the graft was used to span an excised joint (glenohumeral, hip, knee or ankle) (34 cases).

Results

In the analysis of any operative procedure, the results can be assessed according to a large number of different parameters, and although we have tried a variety of systems, the one which appears to be most valid is that originally introduced in 1978 (17,23), and although somewhat subjective, is dependent on survival, tumor status, pain and function. We have graded as <u>excellent</u> those patients who have no evident disease, are pain free and have essentially "normal" function of the part (with the exception of high performance athletics). Patients are classified as <u>good</u> if they also enjoy freedom from disease and pain but have some degree of impairment of function which materially limits their recreational but not occupational activities. Patients are classified as <u>fair</u> if they have sufficient pain or disability to require aids or supports (crutches, canes, braces, etc.) and/or are unable to return to an appropriate work status; and those patients who require removal of the graft or an amputation as a result of complications, or die as a result of failure of local control of the tumor, are considered as <u>failures</u>.

Table 2 shows the overall result for 269 patients followed for from 2 to 15 years with the allograft implants (mean figure of over 7 years) and as can be noted there is considerable variation by type of graft. For the 182 osteoarticular grafts, only 70.3% of the patients were rated as good or excellent, 4.4% as fair and 25.3% as failures. The results for the intercalary grafts were considerably better with 89.1% of the patients being classified as good or excellent, and for the 19 with allografts and prostheses, almost equally as good with satisfactory results in over 84%. The 22 allograft arthrodesis fared less well with 5/22 classified as failures. The overall values for the series are seen to be almost 75% satisfactory (excellent and good) but if the 19 tumor failures are deleted (in order to assess the worth of the allograft procedure alone without the complications of tumor failure), the value for satisfactory results rises to almost 80%.

By appropriate analysis of these data, it is possible to assess the effect of various factors on outcome. The first and clearly the most important of these are the various complications of the procedure, which are shown in Table 2. As can be readily noted, of the 269 patients, almost half had an uneventful course and developed neither tumor nor allograft complications. Of the 68 patients with high-grade tumors (and, therefore, at risk for metastasis, local recurrence of death), 38 (55.9%) remained continuously disease free. Of the remaining 30 patients with tumor complications, 22 patients (32.4%) of the entire group died of their disease, 29 (42.7%) developed pulmonary metastases and 6 (8.8%) had a local recurrence.

Allograft complications accounted for the bulk of the problems of the patients in the series. In all, 113/269 (42.0%) developed some problem with the alloimplant. These ranged from unstable joint (6.3%), and non- or delayed union (13.0%), to more serious complications of fractures (19.7%) and infection, an extraordinarily high value of over 12%. The effect of these complications on end result are apparent in that if no complications arose (199 patients), the results fall into the satisfactory (excellent or good) category for 98.6% of the patients. If infection occurs, the likelihood of

TABLE 2

ALLOGRAFT TRANSPLANTATION

Results by Type of Graft for 269 Patients Followed for Two or More Years

RESULT AND PERCENT TYPE	EXCELLENT	GOOD	FAIR	FAILURE
OSTEOARTICULAR (182)	68 (37.9%)	59 (32.4%)	8 (4.4%)	46 (25.3%)
INTERCALARY (46)	34 (73.9%)	7 (15.2%)	1 (2.2%)	4 (8.7%)
ALLOGRAFT + PROS (19)	12 (63.2%)	4 (21.1%)	1 (5.3%)	2 (10.5%)
ALLO-ARTHRODESIS (22)	1 (4.6%)	15 (68.2%)	1 (4.6%)	5 (22.7%)
TOTALS (269)	116 (43.1%)	85 (31.6%)	11 (4.1%)	57 (21.2%)

PERCENT `SATISFACTORY'............74.7%

IF 19 TUMOR FAILURES ARE DELETED:

TOTALS (250)	116 (46.4%)	83 (33.2%)	11 (4.4%)	40 (16.0%)

PERCENT `SATISFACTORY'............79.6%

LATE COMPLICATIONS IN 269 PATIENTS FOLLOWED FOR TWO OR MORE YEARS

TUMOR COMPLICATIONS IN 68 PATIENTS WITH HIGH GRADE TUMORS:

     DEATHS...................22 (32.4%)
     METASTASES...............29 (42.7%)
     LOCAL RECURRENCE..........6 (8.8%)

ALLOGRAFT COMPLICATIONS IN ALL 269 PATIENTS:

     INFECTION................33 (12.3%)
     FRACTURE.................53 (19.7%)
     NON-UNION................35 (13.0%)
     UNSTABLE JOINT..........17 (6.3%)

N.B. BECAUSE MANY OF THE PATIENTS HAD MORE THAN ONE COMPLICATION, THE NUMBERS SHOWN ABOVE CAN NOT BE ADDED: IN ALL, 128 "WINNERS" (47.6%) HAD NEITHER TUMOR NOR ALLOGRAFT COMPLICATIONS.

failure rises to 84.8%, and if fracture supervenes, the effect is less severe, but still a problem in that only 51.2% of the patients end with a satisfactory result. Both nonunion and unstable joints also take their toll in that for both the excellent or good results drop below the 70% figure.

When the results for distal femoral and proximal tibial allografts, in which the entire joint surface was replaced (`total') is compared with surgery, in which only a portion of the surface was included (`hemi'), it was considerably better than for the totals, and that the complications were fewer with the lesser surgery. Although this observation suggests that patients who have the lesser operation fare better than those with more extensive replacement, it should be clearly noted that the `hemi's' are almost all performed for giant cell tumor while the `totals' included most of the parosteal osteosarcomas, some of the chondrosarcomas and a relatively high number of central osteosarcomas. A more appropriate interpretation of the data may be that they suggest that the results are poorer for more malignant lesions in which more extensive surgery and adjunctive chemotherapy are considered to be necessary to achieve a cure.(14) Analysis of data for the distribution of percentages of good and excellent results according to stage (11) support this contention. For 37 patients with Stage 0 disease, the success rate for the procedure was 86.5%. One hundred twenty-nine of 164 patients (78.7%) with Stage 1 (1A or 1B) neoplasms had excellent or good results when followed for two or more years. On the other hand, an evaluation of the status of 68 patients with higher grade lesions (Stages 2A, 2B or 3) showed that only 58.8% had achieved what was considered to be an excellent or good result at two to 14 years after the surgery.

Finally, it is important to consider the success rate for the procedure in terms of length of follow-up. The data for all 250 patients in the series (satisfactory results in over 79%) suggest that once the peak periods for infection (almost all manifest by 12 months (17,20,23-25)), and fracture (almost all occur by 3 years (2,20,23-25)) have passed, the patients stabilize and remain in the excellent or good category for up to at least the 14 years of follow-up represented by the first patient in this series.

Discussion

The data reported in this study strongly support the hypothesis that allograft transplantation can be a useful adjunct in the management of patients with massive skeletal defects of the extremities as a result of tumor, trauma or bone disease of various sorts. The tabular information provided in this review provides evidence that despite the rigors of dealing with the initial neoplastic problem, the results of the procedure fall at the rather respectable level of almost 80% good and excellent for a large series of patients followed for from 2 to over 15 years. In our setting, with careful attention to technical aspects of the procedure, the operation seems to be a very satisfactory method for reconstructing a limb.

Although the results for patients with high grade tumors are less satisfactory than for low-grade tumors (see above), the method seems to have clearly defined advantages over the metal and plastic implants. The principal advantage of the allograft parts lies in the biological nature of the system, which implies and, in fact, has been demonstrated to include vascularization and ultimate incorporation of the implant into the body. A second and significant advantage lies in the ability to restore, by suture resected and severed ligaments, tendons and capsular structures to the graft, thus improving the likelihood of a reasonably normal function of joints. Perhaps equally important in such operative procedures is the fact that when grafts fail, especially by fracture (21) but also for some which develop an infection (20), they can be treated by conventional means and rarely require a solution which threatens the limb or seriously disables the patient.

The principal disadvantage of the operation lies in what seems to be a high primary failure rate, (it should be clearly evident that if almost 80% of the patients are excellent and good, then slightly more than 20% are only fair or are failures), which correlates closely and is almost entirely accounted for by the extraordinary rate of complications. An infection rate of over 12%, fracture and nonunion rates of almost 20% and 13%, respectively, are obviously sources of concern to us, and should be to any surgeon considering the procedure as a method of treating bone lesions of any sort. Although the data suggest that these complications are part of the technical problems of the surgical management of the neoplastic process (and to some extent they may be in that the incidence of serious complications appears to correlate with the stage of the tumor, the extent of the resective surgery and the use of adjunctive chemotherapy and radiation (14)), it is also highly probable that they represent some subtle forms of a "rejection" phenomenon.

Although the current results of this and other series seem to be "acceptable" and certainly equivalent or perhaps even more suitable than many other methods used in the management of these types of patients, it is evident that the system could be materially improved by continued investigation. Allograft implantation, although still an imperfect system, represents a biological solution to the problems raised by massive defects in the skeleton. Experience is growing and a number of large series have been reported with results which exceed or are comparable to those of the other systems.(5,15,17,21,23-25,27,28,34) Allograft material, despite the immune response, is generally well tolerated and nontoxic, and the supply is theoretically unlimited. The shape of the material is usually anatomically correct for the host, especially if sufficient tissues are available in the bank so that a close match can be achieved. Grafts are likely to have appropriate mechanical properties and the structure is relatively easily shaped and implanted. Perhaps the most important issue, however, is a biological one. Allograft bone is eventually invaded by host tissues and, over time, is incorporated, perhaps not completely, but sufficiently to be considered a living tissue. This means that if successful, an allogeneic segment represents a permanent implant rather than a temporary spacer, such as the metallic devices.

REFERENCES

1. Beckenhaugh RD, Ilstrup DM: Total hip arthroplast: a review of three hundred and thirty-three cases with long term followup. J Bone Joint Surg 60A:306-313, 1978.
2. Berrey BH, Mankin HJ, Gebhardt MC: Allograft fractures: frequency, treatment and end result (in manuscript).
3. Campanacci M, Costa P: Total resection of the distal femur or proximal tibia for bone tumours: autogenous

bone grafts and arthrodesis in twenty-six cases. J Bone Joint Surg 61B:455-463, 1979.

4. Chandler HP, Reineck FT, Wixon RL, McCarthy JC: Total hip replacement in patients younger than 30 years old: a five year follow-up study. J Bone Joint Surg 63A:1426-1434, 1981.

5. Dick HM, Malinin TI, Mnaymneh WH: Massive allograft implantation following radical resection of high grade tumors requiring adjuvant chemotherapy treatment. Clin Orthop 197:88-95, 1985.

6. Dobbs HS, Scales JT, Wilson JN: Endoprosthetic replacement of the proximal femur and acetabulum. J Bone Joint Surg 63B:219-224, 1981.

7. Doppelt SH, Tomford WW, Lucas AD, Mankin HJ: Operational and financial aspects of a hospital based bone bank. J Bone Joint Surg 63A:244-248, 1981.

8. Eckardt JJ, Eilber RF, Grant TT, et al.: Management of Stage IIB osteogenic sarcoma: experience at the University of California. Cancer Treat Symp 3:117-130, 1985.

9. Enneking WF, Eady JL, Burchardt H: Autogenous cortical bone grafts in the reconstruction of segmental skeletal defects. J Bone Joint Surg 62A:1039-1058, 1980.

10. Enneking WF, Shirley PD: Resection-arthrodesis for malignant and potentially malignant lesions about the knee using an intramedullary rod and local bone grafts. J Bone Joint Surg 59A:223-236, 1977.

11. Enneking WF, Spanier SS, Goodman MA: A system for the surgical staging of musculoskeletal sarcoma. Clin Orthop 153:106-120, 1980.

12. Friedlaender GE: Current concepts review: bone banking. J Bone Joint Surg 64A:307-311, 1982.

13. Friedlaender GE, Mankin HJ: Guidelines for the banking of musculoskeletal tissues. Newsletter, American Association Tissue Banks 3:2-7, 1979.

14. Gebhardt MC, Lord CF, Friedlaender GE, Mankin HJ: The effect of chemotherapy on the clinical results of allograft transplantation in the treatment of malignant tumors of bone (in press).

15. Gross AE, McKee NH, Langer F, Pritzker K: Surgical techniques and clinical experience with articular allografts at the knee. In Osteochondral Allografts. Friedlaender GE, Mankin HJ, Sell KW (Eds.), Boston, Little, Brown and Co pp.289-300, 1983.

16. Heiple KG, Chase SW, Herndon CH: A comparative study of the healing process following different types of bone transplantation. J Bone Joint Surg 45A:1593-1616, 1963.

17. Hiki Y, Mankin HJ: Radical resection and allograft replacement in the treatment of bone tumors. J Japan Orthop Assoc 54:475-500, 1980.

18. Lexer E: Joint transplantation and arthroplasty. Surg Gynecol and Obstet 40:782-809, 1925.

19. Lexer E: Die Verwendung der freien Knochenplastik nebst versuchen uber gelenkversteifung und gelenktransplantation. Arch f Klin Chir 86:939-954, 1908.

20. Lord CF, Gebhardt MC, Mankin HJ: The incidence, epidemiology and treatment of infection in allograft transplantation (in manuscript).
21. Makely JT: The use of allografts to reconstruct intercalary defects of long bones. Clin Orthop 197:58-75, 1985.
22. Mankin HJ: Complications of allograft surgery. In Osteochondral Allografts, Friedlaender GE, Mankin HJ, Sell KW (Eds.), Boston, Little, Brown and Co pp.259-274, 1983.
23. Mankin HJ, Doppelt SH, Sullivan TR, Tomford WW: Osteoarticular and intercalary allograft transplantation in the management of malignant tumors of bone. Cancer 50:613-630, 1982.
24. Mankin HJ, Doppelt SH, Tomford WW: Clinical experience with allograft implantation: the first 200 cases. Clin Orthop 174:69-86, 1983.
25. Mankin HJ, Fogelson FS, Thrasher AZ, Jaffer E: Massive resection and allograft replacement in the treatment of malignant bone tumors. N Engl J Med 294:1247-1255, 1976.
26. Marcove RC, Rosen G: En bloc resections for osteogenic sarcoma. Cancer 45:3040-3044, 1978.
27. McDermott AGP, Langer F, Pritzker KPH, Gross AE: Fresh small-fragment osteochondral allografts: long term follow-up study on first 100 cases. Clin Orthop 197:96-102, 1985.
28. Mnaymneh W, Malinin TI, Makely JT, Dick HM: Massive osteoarticular allografts in the reconstruction of extremities following resection of tumors not requiring chemotherapy and radiation. Clin Orthop 9:666-677, 1986.
29. Ottolenghi CE, Muscolo DL, Maenza R: Bone defect reconstruction by massive allograft: technique and results of 51 cases followed for 5 to 32 years. In Clinical Trends in Orthopaedics, Straub LR, Wilson PD Jr, (Eds.), New York, Thieme-Stratton Inc pp.171-183, 1982.
30. Ottolenghi CE: Massive osteo and osteoarticular bone grafts: technique and results. Clin Orthop 87:156-164, 1972.
31. Parrish FF: Allograft replacement of all or part of the end of a long bone following excision of a tumor: report of twenty-one cases. J Bone Joint Surg 55A:1-22, 1973.
32. Sim FH, Chao EY-S: Segmental prosthetic replacement of the hip and knee. In Tumor Prostheses for Bone and Joint Reconstruction. Chao EY-S, Ivins JC (Eds.), Thieme-Stratton Co pp.247-266, 1983.
33. Sim FH, Ivins JC, Taylor WF, Chao EY-S: Limb-sparing surgery of osteosarcoma: Mayo Clinic experience. Cancer Treat Symp 3:139-154, 1985.
34. Smith RJ, Mankin HJ: Allograft replacement of the distal radius for giant cell tumor. J Hand Surg 2:299-309, 1977.
35. Stauffer RN: Ten year followup study of total hip replacement: with particular reference to roentgenographic loosening of the components. J Bone Joint Surg 64A:983-

990, 1982.

36. Sutherland CJ, Wilde AH, Borden LS, Marks KE: A ten year follow-up of one hundred consecutive Muller curved-stem total hip replacement arthroplasties. J Bone Joint Surg 64A:970-982, 1982.

37. Tomford WW, Doppelt SH, Friedlaender GE: 1983 bone bank procedure. Clin Orthop 174:15-21, 1983.

38. Tomford WW, Mankin HJ: Investigational approaches to articular cartilage preservation. Clin Orthop 174:22-27, 1983.

39. Volkov, M: Allotransplantation of joints. J Bone Joint Surg 52B:49-53, 1970.

40. Watari S, Ikuta Y, Adachi N, et al: Vascular pedicle fibular transplantation as treatment for bone tumors. Clin Orthop. 133:158-164, 1978.

41. Weiland AJ, Daniel RK: Microvascular anastomosis for bone grafts in the treatment of massive defects in bone. J Bone Joint Surg 61A:98-104, 1979.

42. Wilson PD Jr: Biomechanical behavior of massive bone transplants. Clin Orthop 87:81-109, 1972.

43. Wilson PD Jr, Lance EM: Surgical reconstruction of the skeleton following segmental resection for bone tumors. J Bone Joint Surg 47A:1629-1656, 1975.

44. Wood MB, Cooney WP, Irons GB: Skeletal reconstruction by vascularized bone transfer: indications and results. Mayo Clinic Proc 60:729-734, 1985.

SURGICAL ALTERNATIVES TO STANDARD ENDOPROSTHETIC REPLACEMENT AND ALLOGRAFT RECONSTRUCTION FOR MALIGNANT TUMORS OF THE MUSCULOSKELETAL SYSTEM

Jeffrey J. Eckardt, M.D.[1], Frederick R. Eilber, M.D.[2], Michael H. Kody, M.D.[1], Gerald Rosen, M.D.[3]

Introduction

The advent of adjuvant chemotherapy modalities and limb sparing surgical techniques has permitted oncological surgeons and their patients with musculoskeletal tumors to consider a variety of limb salvage reconstructions.(1-11) The diminished role of primary amputation is illustrated by a recent analysis of 160 malignant bone tumors treated at UCLA between January 1981 and September 1986. During that period, only 23 patients (14.4%) underwent primary amputation for local control of the tumor. Tumor size alone was considered to be the indication for amputation in 13 patients, age less than 11 years with lack of skeletal maturity was considered to be the indication in 6 patients, and location in the tibia was the sole indication in 4. The remaining 137 patients (85.6%) underwent primary limb salvage procedures, with endoprosthetic reconstruction in 103 patients (64%), internal hemipelvectomy resections in 20 (12.5%), and excision alone in an additional 14 patients (8.8%). In 1983, Dubousset described the medial gastrocnemic transfer for coverage of proximal tibial replacements, and in 1984, Lewis introduced the expandable endoprosthesis.(12,13) Since then we have not utilized amputation for primary control of proximal tibial lesions or lesions in the skeletally immature. Although allograft reconstructions are used by many, they have not been used at UCLA for reconstruction following malignant tumor resection since 1979.(4,8) Alternative methods of extremity reconstruction, following excision of aggressive benign and malignant bone tumors, include the traditional resection arthrodesis and newer techniques: intercalary allograft arthrodesis, intercalary endoprosthesis arthrodesis, composite allograft with total or hemi-joint replacement, the rotationplasty and expandable endoprosthesis.

Resection Arthrodesis

The historical approach to tumors about the distal femur and proximal tibia has been resection arthrodesis. This pro-

---

[1]Division of Orthopaedic Surgery, UCLA School of Medicine, Room A6-164/CHS Bldg., Los Angeles, CA 90024-1749.

[2]Division of Surgical Oncology, UCLA Medical Center, Los Angeles, CA.

[3]Department of Pediatrics, UCLA Medical Center, Los Angeles, CA.

J. R. Ryan and L. O. Baker (eds.), Recent Concepts in Sarcoma Treatment, 261–268.
© *1988 by Kluwer Academic Publishers.*

cedure was first carried out by Lexer in 1907 and subsequently popularized by Merle D'Aubigne (1958), Wilson and Lance
(1965), Enneking and Shirley (1977), and Campanacci, et al.
(1987).(14-18) Recent authors have combined specially designed intramedullary rods with either ipsilateral tibial,
femoral, or sometimes fibular bone grafts. Enneking's multi-
institutional review of 82 knee arthrodesis patients revealed
good to excellent results in 83%. In spite of the ultimate
high success rate, they noted that the procedure is technically difficult. Deep infection in 5 cases, nonunion problems
in 4, and a local recurrence rate of 5% leading to amputation
in 4 cases, contributed to an 18% major complication rate and
an unsatisfactory outcome in 17%. In addition, 20% of the
patients stated an emotional dislike for the procedure because of the stiff knee.(19) Sim has reported that the preferred technique of knee arthrodesis at the Mayo Clinic is
the hemicylindrical ipsilateral sliding tibial or femoral
graft, in conjunction with an intramedullary rod and
additional internal fixation. They recommend it for patients
who can emotionally accept the fused knee and who tend to be
younger, active, overweight, and who have aggressive benign
lesions. In spite of a 48% complication rate and a 26% subjective lack of enthusiasm with the technique secondary to
the rigid knee, they ultimately achieved a stable result in
78% and a pain-free knee in 85%. The resultant extremities
were both useful for strenuous walking and recreational
activities.(20)

Interposition of an intercalary allograft over an intramedullary rod with supplemental internal fixation is an
alternative method of achieving a resection arthrodesis of
the knee. Reports by Sim, et al., Gebhardt, et al., and
McDermott and Gross all indicate that this procedure is technically easier than the resection arthrodesis which utilizes
ipsilateral sliding tibial or femoral grafts, and that the
initial results were promising in spite of the introduction
of the added variable of allograft bone.(20,21,22) Gebhardt,
et al. utilized this technique for resection arthrodesis
about the shoulder and felt that the reconstruction was
superior to that of other reconstruction techniques when the
deltoid has to be sacrificed. In spite of the short follow-
up, they had only a 6% nonunion rate.(21) Arthrodesis remains a standard technique for reconstruction of both
aggressive benign and malignant tumors. Though complicated to
perform, and in spite of a high incidence of complications,
once healed, they result in a stable, enduring, and functional extremity.

Composite Allograft with Joint Arthroplasty

Intercalary allografts, in combination with hemi- or
whole joint replacements, have been reported in the proximal
humerus by Rock, and the hip and knee by Gitelis.(23,24)
They have the advantages of anatomic restoration and the
opportunity for soft tissue ingrowth into the allograft bone.
They overcome the osteochondral allograft problems of early
instability and late arthritic changes. These procedures
combine the advantages of allograft and endoprosthesis recon-

struction which appear to improve the functional results over osteochondral allograft alone.(24)

The Growing Child

Conventional allograft and endoprosthetic reconstruction for malignant tumors can not be done in the child with significant growth potential. Here, the alternatives remain amputation, rotationplasty and expandable endoprosthesis. Rotationplasty was first described by Borggreve in 1930 and later by Van Nes in 1948 and 1950 for reconstruction, both of patients with congenital and post-traumatic and post-infection femoral defects.(25-27) In 1974, it was first used as an alternative to amputation for osteosarcoma by Saltzer.(28) Reports by the Vienna group continue to confirm their enthusiasm with this procedure because of the low local recurrence rate and improved functional results over amputation.(29,30) They have observed that all nonunions and fractures go on to heal following the completion of chemotherapy or with additional orthopaedic procedures. Vascular resection carries with it a 15% risk of thrombosis, resulting in amputation. The advantage to providing a knee joint clearly adds to the functional result, so that properly selected patients achieve a 68% excellent and 28% good overall result. It has further been their finding that the survival of patients with rotationplasty is equivalent to that of their amputation series (80%), an improvement over the survival in their resection-endoprosthesis patient group (60%).(31) This survival disadvantage for resection-endoprosthesis patients has not been found where oncological margins are, by necessity, closer than with the rotationplasty in the setting of appropriate pre- and postoperative neoadjuvant therapy.(3)

An informal survey of 7 members of the Musculoskeletal Tumor Society, known to have performed rotationplasties for patients with malignant bone tumors of the distal femur, revealed experience in 30 cases: Drs. Frank Sim (4), Martin Malawar (1), Paul Jacobs (2), Norman Jaffe (6), Joseph Lane (13), and Dempsey Springfield (4).(32) Twenty-four additional cases have been reported by Krajbich from Toronto's Hospital for Sick Children.(33) In this combined group of 54 patients, only one patient ultimately underwent amputation because of psychological problems (Malawar, personal communication). All treating physicians and surgeons indicated that patient selection was critical and that once performed, the patients and their parents became the greatest advocates of the technique. Done mostly, but not exclusively, for patients with significant residual growth potential, a number of these younger children went on to participate actively in elementary and high school athletics. In spite of the fact that they do not think of themselves as amputees because the foot is retained, a major disadvantage is that the patients do require a prosthesis, and parental acceptance is generally more difficult to achieve preoperatively.

An alternative to amputation or rotationplasty is the use of the expandable prosthesis. First described by Lewis in 1986, this expandable and adjustable prosthesis has been utilized now in over 30 skeletally immature patients.(13,34)

Reoperation for expansion is necessary, but not difficult.

Our own experience with expandable endoprostheses at UCLA consists of 10 patients. At the time of their surgery, the 5 males and 5 females ranged in age from 4 to 13 years, with an average of 8.8 years. Osteosarcoma Stage IIB was the diagnosis in 6, osteosarcoma IIA in one, and Ewing's sarcoma in 3. Six underwent distal femoral replacement, and in single instances an expandable total humerus, total femur, proximal humerus and proximal femoral replacement were implanted (Figure 1). All patients received preoperative adjuvant treatment, either the T-10 protocol for osteosarcoma or combination chemotherapy and radiation therapy for the Ewing's sarcoma patients. All resections were considered to be wide and all components were cemented in place. Immediate motion was used for the knee replacements, abduction braces utilized for the total femur and proximal femur replacements, and a supportive sling was used for the two upper extremity replacements. Follow-up on this group of patients is short, ranging from one to 33.5 months, with an average of 12.8 months. Eight of the prostheses were expandable adjustable prostheses (Dow Corning Wright), and two were prostheses designed for expansion through the joint (Techmedica, Inc.). Four prostheses have been successfully expanded to equalize extremity lengths. Two patients died prior to acquiring expansion and were ambulatory with distal femoral replacements prior to death. One patient has acquired skeletal maturity without requiring expansion and has equal leg lengths. Three patients have less than a three-month follow-up and have not yet been considered for expansion.

The functional results are typical of endoprosthetic replacements elsewhere, with lack of active shoulder motion for the proximal humeral replacement and total humeral replacement, and a positive Trendelenberg gait for the proximal femoral replacement. In contrast to conventional distal femoral replacements, where average active knee range of motion is in excess of 100 degrees (35), the average active range was 60 degrees. For these 10 patients, the MSTS functional result, though early on for some, was excellent in one, good in 5, fair in 4, and poor in none.(36) These young patients were quick to develop knee flexion and extension contractures because of their unwillingness or inability to cooperate with rehabilitation efforts in the immediate postoperative period. In spite of the fact that an improved range of motion may be obtained at the time of expansion with pseudocapsulotomy and muscle releases, this is a potential disadvantage of this technique. Although patients with the expandable distal femoral replacement retain the extremity and become ambulatory, they can not participate in athletics to the degree that most rotationplasty patients and certain amputees can achieve. On the other hand, they do not require a prosthesis and do have the psychological advantage of their own extremity, an important point for patients who refuse rotationplasty or amputation. A rotationplasty can always be done as a subsequent salvage procedure, perhaps with better patient acceptance.(29)

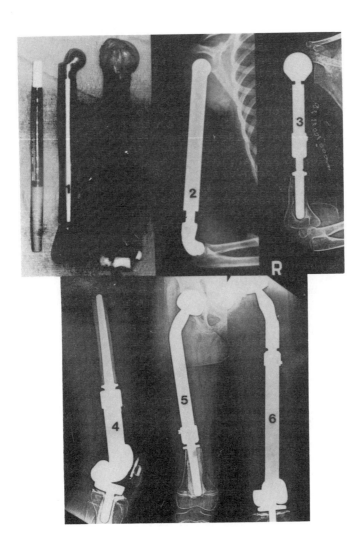

FIGURE 1: Expandable endoprostheses. (1) and (2)
a total humeral replacement for a 4 year old
with Ewing's sarcoma, Techmedica, Inc.; (3)
a proximal humeral replacement following expansion for a 5 year old with IIB osteosarcoma; (4) a distal femoral replacement for an
11 year old with IIB osteosarcoma; (5) a proximal femoral replacement for an 8 year old with
Ewing's sarcoma; and (6) a total femoral replacement for an 11 year old with Ewing's sarcoma. Prostheses 3, 4, 5 and 6 -- Dow Corning
Wright.

These young patients with expandable prostheses will need to be carefully and continually evaluated. Expandable prostheses are preferable to amputation for upper extremity and proximal femoral lesions in the skeletally immature patient where a rotationplasty is not applicable. For those patients who refuse amputation or rotationplasty, an expandable prosthesis is an alternative choice and may be important for a patient who still faces a considerable risk of early death in spite of adjuvant protocols.

Conclusion

The oncological musculoskeletal surgeon now has a variety of reconstruction techniques in lieu of amputation: resection arthrodesis, allograft or endoprosthesis reconstruction, composite allograft with total or hemi-joint replacement, intercalary endoprostheses, and for the skeletally immature, rotationplasty or expandable endoprosthesis. Careful patient selection and longitudinal follow-up of the oncological outcome and the reconstructive result will be necessary in order to determine the best indications for each technique. At the present time, it appears that limb salvage programs can be done safely with no additional risk of local recurrence or progression of disease than amputation when done with appropriate preoperative adjuvant protocols and postoperative chemotherapy.(3,5)

REFERENCES

1. Chao EYS, Ivins JC (eds.): Tumor Prostheses for Bone and Joint Reconstruction: The Design and Application. New York, Thieme-Stratton, 1983.
2. Dick H, Malinin TI, Mnaymneh WA: Massive allograft implantation following radical resection of high-grade tumors requiring adjuvant chemotherapy Treatment. Clin Orthop 197:88, 1985.
3. Eckardt JJ, Eilber FR, Grant TT, et al.: The UCLA experience in the management of Stage IIB osteogenic sarcoma. Cancer Treat Symposia 3:117, 1985.
4. Eckardt JJ, Eilber FR, Dorey FJ, et al.: The UCLA experience in limb salvage surgery for malignant tumors. Orthopedics 8:612, 1985.
5. Eilber F, Guiliano A, Eckardt J, et al.: Adjuvant chemotherapy for osteosarcoma: A randomized prospective trial. J Clin Oncol 5:21, 1987.
6. Eilber FR, Morton DL, Eckardt JJ, et al.: Limb salvage for skeletal and soft tissue sarcomas. Multidisciplinary preoperative therapy. Cancer 53:2579, 1984.
7. Enneking WF (ed.): Limb salvage in musculoskeletal oncology. New York, Churchill Livingstone, 1987.
8. Mankin HJ, Doppelt SH, Sullivan TR, et al.: Osteoarticular and intercalary allograft transplantation in the management of malignant tumors of bone. Cancer 50:613, 1982.
9. Marcove RC, Rosen G: En bloc resections for osteogenic sarcoma. Cancer 45:3040, 1980.

10. Sim FC, Bowman WE Jr, and Chao EY-S: Limb salvage for primary malignant bone tumors. In Kotz R (ed.): Proceedings of the Second International Workshop on the Design and Application of Tumor Prostheses for Bone and Joint Reconstruction. Egermann Druckereigesellschaft, Vienna, p.153, 1983.

11. Rosen G, Caparros B, Huvos AG, et al.: Preoperative chemotherapy for osteogenic sarcoma: Selection of post-operative adjuvant chemotherapy based on the response of the primary tumor to preoperative chemotherapy. Cancer 49:1221, 1982.

12. Dubousset J: Gastrocnemic flap and proximal tibial replacement. In Kotz R (ed.): Proceedings of the Second International Workshop on the Design and Application of Tumor Prostheses for Bone and Joint Reconstruction. Egermann Druckereigesellschaft, Vienna, 1983.

13. Lewis MM: The use of an expandable and adjustable prosthesis in the treatment of childhood malignant bone tumors of the extremity. Cancer 57:499, 1986.

14. Lexer E: Joint transplantations and arthroplasty. Surg Gynecol Obstet 40:782, 1925.

15. Merle D'Aubigne R, Dejouany JP: Diaphysoepiphyseal resection for bone tumor at the knee. With report of nine cases. J Bone and Joint Surg 40B:385, 1958.

16. Wilson PD, Lance EM: Surgical reconstruction of the skeleton following segmental resection for bone tumors. J Bone and Joint Surg 47A:1629, 1965.

17. Enneking WF, Shirley PD: Resection-arthrodesis for malignant and potentially malignant lesions about the knee using an intramedullary rod and local bone grafts. J Bone and Joint Surg 59A:223, 1977.

18. Campanacci M, Cervellati L, Guerra A, et al.: Knee resection-arthrodesis. In Enneking WF (ed.): Limb Salvage in Musculoskeletal Oncology, New York, Churchill Livingstone, p.364, 1987.

19. Enneking WF, Springfield DS, Present DA: Functional evaluation of resection-arthrodesis for lesions about the knee. In Enneking WF (ed.): Limb Salvage in Musculo-skeletal Oncology, New York, Churchill Livingstone, p.389, 1987.

20. Sim FH, Beauchamp CP, Chao EYS: Reconstruction of musculoskeletal defects about the knee for tumor. Clin Orthop 221:188, 1987.

21. Gebhardt MC, McGuire MH, Mankin HJ: Resection and allograft arthrodesis for malignant tumor of the extremity. In Enneking WF (ed.): Limb Salvage in Musculoskeletal Oncology. New York, Churchill Livingstone, p.567, 1987.

22. McDermott AGP, Gross AE: Use of allograft and a new locking intramedullary nail for limb salvage procedures. In Enneking WF (ed.): Limb Salvage in Musculoskeletal Oncology. New York, Churchill Livingstone, p.583, 1987.

23. Rock M: Intercalary allografts and custom Neer prosthesis after en bloc resection of the proximal humerus. In Enneking WF (ed.): Limb Salvage in Musculoskeletal Oncology. New York, Churchill Livingstone, p.586, 1987.

268

24. Heligman D, Gitelis S, Quill G, et al.: The use of large allografts for tumor reconstruction and salvage of the failed total hip arthroplasty. Clin Orthop (in press).

25. Borggreve: Kniegelenkersatz durch das in der Beinlangsachase um 180 gedrehte fussgelenk. Arch Orthop, Unfallchir, 28:175, 1930.

26. Van Nes CP: Transplantation of the tibia and fibula to replace the femur following resection. J Bone and Joint Surg 30A:854, 1948.

27. Van Nes CP: Rotationplasty in the treatment of congenital defects of the femur. J Bone and Joint Surg 32B: 12, 1950.

28. Kotz R, Salzer M: Rotation-plasty for childhood osteosarcoma of the distal part of the femur. J Bone and Joint Surg 64A:959, 1982

29. Knahr K, Kotz R, Kristen H, et al: Clinical evaluation of patients with Rotationplasty. In Enneking WF (ed.): Limb Salvage in Musculoskeletal Oncology. New York, Churchill Livingstone, New York, p.429, 1987.

30. Knahr K, Kristen H, Ritschl P, et al.: Prosthetic Management and functional evaluation of patients with resection of the distal femur and rotationplasty. Orthopedics 10:1241, 1987.

31. Winkler K, Beron G, Kotz R, et al.: Einfluss des lokalchirurgischen vorgehens auf die inzidenz von metastasen nach neoadjuvanter chemotherapie das osteosarkroms. Z Orthop 124:22, 1986.

32. Sim F, Malawar M, Jacobs P, Jaffe N, Lane J, Springfield D: Personal communications, 1987.

33. Krajbich JI: Personal communication, 1987.

34. Lewis MM, Spires WP Jr, Bloom N: Expandable prosthesis: An alternative to amputation. In Enneking WF (ed.):Limb Salvage in Musculoskeletal Oncology. New York, Churchill Livingstone, New York, p.606, 1987.

35. Eckardt JJ, Eilber FR, Kabo JM, et al.: The kinematic rotating hinge knee - distal femoral replacement for tumor of the distal femur. In Enneking WF (ed.): The International Symposium on Limb Salvage in Musculoskeletal Oncology, New York, Churchill Livingstone, p.392, 1987.

36. Enneking WF: Modification of the system for functional evaluation of surgical management of musculoskeletal tumors. In Enneking WF (ed.):Limb Salvage in Musculoskeletal Oncology. New York, Churchill Livingstone, New York, p.626, 1987.

ARTERIAL INFUSION IN THE TREATMENT OF OSTEOSARCOMA

R.S. Benjamin, M.D.[1], S.P. Chawla, M.D., C. Carrasco, M.D.
A.K. Raymond, M.D., T. Fanning, M.D., S. Wallace, M.D.
A.G. Ayala, M.D., J. Murray, M.D.

Intra-arterial cis-platinum was introduced into the treatment of human cancer in 1977 in a patient with intransit metastases of malignant melanoma.(1) After an impressive response in that patient, a broad Phase II study was initiated.(2) One of the earliest patients on that study had an extensive malignant fibrous histiocytoma of the pubis with a soft-tissue mass which filled more than half the pelvis. The tumor had progressed in size despite therapy with radiation, 70 Gray, plus weekly systemic adriamycin. When she presented to us, she had extensive peripheral edema and was considered inoperable for a hemipelvectomy. We reasoned that since cis-platinum had some reported activity against osteosarcoma, malignant fibrous histiocytoma of bone might respond in a similar way, and that since the tumor was localized to the pelvis, the intra-arterial route would be optimal. The patient was treated, returned home to California, and called two weeks later to report the development of a new mass. Despite our efforts to convince her that it was too early to tell whether any beneficial effect of the therapy had occurred, and that she could not be retreated so soon after initial therapy, she was on the next plane to Houston and was seen the following morning in our clinic. The "new mass" was actually her anterior iliac crest, which had not been palpable for several months. The peripheral edema and the pelvic mass had largely disappeared, and at the end of 3 courses of chemotherapy, there was no evidence of residual soft-tissue tumor by computerized tomography. At that time, the patient underwent a limited resection of the pubis with limb salvage and went on to live another 5 years without local tumor recurrence, although she did die of metastatic disease after cumulative toxicity prevented further cis-platinum administration.

Intra-arterial infusion increases drug delivery to a local area of tumor involvement, and since patients die of disseminated rather than local disease, many oncologists wonder whether there is any advantage to intra-arterial chemotherapy. We have measured the concentrations of platinum in the draining vein from the infused extremity and in the

---

*Department of Medical Oncology, The University of Texas System Cancer Center, M.D. Anderson Hospital & Tumor Institute, Box 77, 1515 Holcombe, Houston, TX 77030.

J. R. Ryan and L. O. Baker (eds.), Recent Concepts in Sarcoma Treatment, 269–274.
© 1988 by Kluwer Academic Publishers.

systemic circulation.(3) Tumor uptake of the drug is small relative to total body distribution and does not significantly alter the systemic concentration; therefore, essentially the same dose of cis-platinum reaches the lungs whether it is given intravenously or intra-arterially. In contrast, the concentration in the draining vein is 1.5-4 times higher after intra-arterial drug administration. Thus, intra-arterial infusion allows full-dose, systemic chemotherapy, while at the same time delivering an increased drug dose to the primary tumor. The net result is an extremely rapid response in the primary tumor without a sacrifice of systemic efficacy.

The safe administration of cis-platinum at a dose of 120 mg/m^2 requires vigorous hydration.(4) We administer 6 liters per day of 5% dextrose and half normal saline with 20-30 meq/liter of KCL and 4 meq Mg SO_4 until 24 hours after the end of the chemotherapy infusion and until the patient can tolerate forced oral fluids to continue hydration without the necessity of an intravenous infusion. We also utilize hypertonic saline and mannitol diuresis at the time of cis-platinum infusion to further decrease nephrotoxicity. Doses up to 120 mg/m^2 are infused over 2 hours through percutaneously placed intra-arterial catheters with a pulsatile infusion pump to decrease laminar flow and local toxicity. Doses above 120 mg/m^2 are administered over 24 hours to prevent dose-limiting ototoxicity. The intra-arterial catheter is inserted percutaneously by the interventional radiologist using the Seldinger technique. A subtraction arteriogram is then performed, which provides the best estimate of response to chemotherapy in patients with primary bone tumors.(5) The drug is infused, and the catheter is removed.

Initially, we treated 14 patients who had osteosarcoma with intra-arterial cis-platinum as a single agent. Approximately 60% responded clinically.(6) The majority of the patients had recurrent, or locally advanced, unresectable disease; however, after drug activity was noted, 4 patients with primary, operable osteosarcoma of the extremities were included. Despite good clinical response, only one of these patients achieved pathologic complete remission. Therefore, in our subsequent therapeutic programs we elected to add adriamycin to the primary therapy.

Adriamycin was given systemically to avoid dose-limiting local toxicity while delivering a full therapeutic dose to the lungs. The drug was administered as a 96-hour, continuous intravenous infusion through a central venous catheter to decrease cardiac toxicity.(7) Adriamycin was given on days 1-4 as an outpatient infusion in a dose of 90 mg/m^2 course. On day 5, the infusion was disconnected, and the patient was admitted to the hospital for hydration, prior to an arteriogram and the intra-arterial infusion of cis-platinum at a dose of 120 mg/m^2 on day 6. Drug doses were decreased only for significant morbidity, not for severe neutropenia. Adriamycin and cis-platinum were continued intravenously after surgery until cumulative-dose-limiting neuropathy or ototoxicity necessitated discontinuation of the cis-platinum.

At that point it was replaced by DTIC.

Thirty-seven patients with primary osteosarcoma of the extremities were treated between 1979 and 1982. Except for a lower age limit of 16 years, the patients were typical of those with osteosarcoma, with the majority in their second and third decades. Most of the tumors were localized around the knee, and males outnumbered females.

Antitumor activity was determined definitively by the pathologist by measurement of the percentage of tumor necrosis in the surgical specimen.(8) Twenty-four percent of the patients had no detectable tumor on pathologic examination, 35% had 90-99% tumor necrosis, 24% had 60-89% tumor necrosis, and 16% had less than 60% tumor necrosis. Five-year continuous disease-free survival is 53%, and overall survival is 62% in this mature series.

A prognostic-factor analysis utilizing a Cox regression identified 4 significant pretreatment prognostic variables: primary site in the lower extremity; dedifferentiated, small-cell, or high-grade surface-tumor histology; soft tissue mass >1 cm; and male sex. The p value for the regression was 0.003.(4) In addition, we identified telangiectatic osteosarcoma, traditionally a highly incurable disease (9), as a particularly responsive sub-type (10) that was not detected in our regression analysis because of the small number of patients involved and the prevalence of proximal humeral primaries in the initial series.

When complete remission, defined as $\geq$90% tumor necrosis, was added to our prognostic-factor analysis as an independent variable, it essentially displaced all pretreatment prognostic factors from the equation. The p value for the difference between those with $\geq$90% tumor necrosis, and those with <90% tumor necrosis was 1×10^{-6}. Thus, this single prognostic factor, response to chemotherapy, was more than 1000 times more important than the combination of all known pretreatment prognostic variables. When analyzed as disease-free survival from the time of surgery, according to the landmark method of Anderson et al. (11), complete responders had a 5-year disease-free survival of 84% compared with 14% for those with lesser response. The disease-free survival of the nonresponding patients was similar to that of patients in our historical control series; thus, the advantage of response to the responding patients was not achieved at the detriment of the nonresponding patients and cannot be explained by selection of those with inherently good prognosis.

Based on the analysis of this initial set of patients, we modified our chemotherapy regimen in 1983 and have treated an additional 37 patients. The majority of patients with osteosarcoma are males with primary tumors in the leg and soft tissue masses >1 cm; thus, they already have 3 of the 4 poor pretreatment prognostic factors. All patients with $\geq$3 poor prognostic factors treated since 1983 have received an intensified chemotherapy regimen. In addition, any patient treated initially with our standard regimen, who did not have a good arteriographic response, also received intensification chemotherapy.

The intensification consisted of increase in the cis-platinum dose from 120 mg/m^2 to 160-200 mg/m^2. This dose had to be given as a 24-hour infusion to avoid severe ototoxicity. (In a few patients, the cis-platinum dose was divided on days 1 and 8, before and after the systemic adriamycin.) In addition, patients who did not attain $\geq$90% tumor necrosis received an alternating postoperative chemotherapy regimen consisting of high-dose methotrexate, adriamycin-DTIC, and a modified bleomycin, cyclophosphamide, actinomycin-D regimen.

Twenty-five percent of the patients achieved 100% tumor cell destruction at the time of surgery, 44% of the patients had 90-99% tumor cell destruction, and 28% had 60-89% tumor necrosis. Only a single patient, representing 3% of the group, who had an initial clinical response to treatment but relapsed during the preoperative phase of his chemotherapy before surgery, had <60% tumor necrosis. Thus, the major effect of cis-platinum intensification was an increase in the number of patients with $\geq$90% tumor necrosis from 59% in the first group to 69% in the second group, with an accompanying decrease in those with very poor response from 16% in the initial group, to 3% in the second group. The overall disease-free survival was 70% at 3 years despite the fact that 10% of patients relapsed prior to surgery and were never disease free.

When patients with $\geq$90% tumor necrosis and those with <90% tumor necrosis were analyzed by the landmark method, a significant advantage favoring those with $\geq$90% tumor necrosis was still found; however, the difference is less striking than in the earlier series (p = 0.01). Patients with $\geq$90% tumor necrosis did equally well in both groups, but those with <90% tumor necrosis fared significantly better in the second group, with a 3-year continuous disease-free survival of 57% versus 14% in the original group. Patients in the second series received more courses of chemotherapy preoperatively, received a more intensive cis-platinum dose, and had a higher percentage of tumor necrosis. In addition, their postoperative therapy was altered to include an immediate switch to a high-dose-methotrexate-containing regimen. The treatment strategy was designed to increase disease-free survival rather than to determine which factors contributed most significantly to that increase. Nevertheless, in view of the very poor disease-free survival in patients with 60-89% tumor necrosis in our first series, we believe that the addition of high-dose methotrexate to the postoperative treatment regimen for such patients is an important contributing factor to our improved results.

The goal of therapy in each case is a cured, intact patient. While it is premature to predict the cure rate in our most recent group, 3-year continuous relapse-free survival has improved from 20% in our historical control series to 50% in an adriamycin-based adjuvant chemotherapy series, to 60% in our first adriamycin-cis-platinum series, and to 70% in the current group. This increase has come despite the fact

that all patients in the initial two series underwent amputation, whereas 60% of the patients in our first adriamycin-
cis-platinum series, and almost 90% in our second, have had
limb-salvage surgery. In fact, the continuous disease-free
survival of patients undergoing limb-salvage surgery in our
patients is significantly superior to those undergoing amputation.(12) This observation is, of course, logical since
the worst patients are candidates only for amputation.

Only 8% of patients in each of our two groups were
considered candidates for limb-salvage surgery in the absence
of chemotherapy, based on the size and location of their
primary tumors and the absence of a significant soft-tissue
mass. The fact that 60% of the patients in the first group
and 87% of the patients in the second group actually underwent limb-salvage surgery is directly attributable to their
responses to chemotherapy, which essentially downstaged the
tumors from 2B lesions to 2A lesions and allowed adequate
tumor resection with a margin of normal tissue in all but two
cases.

The therapy of osteosarcoma continues to improve; however, at least 30% of patients continue to relapse. We have
observed impressive responses to ifosfamide, even in patients
resistant to multiple other chemotherapeutic agents.(13,14).
Others have observed the activity of ifosfamide against
osteosarcoma as well.(15-17) We, therefore, plan to incorporate ifosfamide into primary therapy in our next series of
patients.

REFERENCES

1. Pritchard JD, Mavligit GM, Wallace S, Benjamin RS,
    McBride CM: Regression of regionally advanced melanoma
    after arterial infusion with cis-platinum and actino-
    mycin-D. Clin Oncol 5:179-182, 1979.
2. Calvo DB, Patt YZ, Wallace S, Chuang VP, Benjamin RS,
    Pritchard JD, Hersh EM, Bodey GP, Mavligit GM: Phase I-
    II trial of percutaneous intra-arterial cis-DDP (II) for
    regionally confined malignancy. Cancer 45:1278-1283,
    1980.
3. Stewart DJ, Benjamin RS, Zimmerman S, Caprioli RM,
    Wallace S, Chuang V, Calvo D, Samuels M, Bonura J, Loo
    TL: Clinical pharmacology of intra-arterial cis-DDP
    (II). Cancer Res 43:917-920, 1983.
4. Benjamin RS, Murray JA, Carrasco CH, Raymond AK, Chawla
    SP, Wallace S, Ayala A, Papadopoulos NEJ, Plager C,
    Romsdahl MM: Preoperative chemotherapy for osteosarcoma:
    A treatment approach facilitating limb salvage with
    major prognostic implications. In Adjuvant Therapy of
    Cancer IV, Jones SE, Salmon SE (eds.), New York, Grune &
    Stratton, pp.601-610, 1984.
5. Carrasco CH, Chawla SP, Benjamin RS, et al.: Arterio-
    graphic prediction of tumor necrosis after primary
    treatment of osteosarcoma in adults. Proc Am Soc Clin
    Oncol 6:126, 1987.

6. Chuang VP, Wallace S, Benjamin RS, Jaffe N, Ayala A, Murray J, Zornoza J, Patt J, Mavligit G, Charnsangavej C, and Soo CS: The therapy of osteosarcoma by intra-arterial cis-platinum and limb preservation. Cardiovasc Intervent Radiol 4:229-235, 1981.

7. Legha SS, Benjamin RS, Mackay B, Ewer MS, Wallace S, Valdivieso M, Rasmussen SL, Blumenschien GR, Freireich EJ: Reduction of doxorubicin cardiotoxicity by prolonged continuous intravenous infusion. Ann of Intern Med 96:133-139, 1982.

8. Raymond AK, Chawla SP, Carrasco CH, et al.: Osteosarcoma chemotherapy effect: a prognostic factor. Seminars in Diagnostic Pathology 4:212-236, 1987.

9. Matsuno T, Unni KK, McLeod RA, et al.: Telangiectatic osteogenic sarcoma. Cancer 38:2538-2547, 1976.

10. Chawla SP, Raymond AK, Carrasco CH, Papadopoulos NEJ, Plager C, Romsdahl MM, Ayala AG, Wallace S, Murray JA, Bodey GP, Benjamin RS: High rates of complete remission, limb salvage and prolonged survival in telangiectatic osteosarcoma after preoperative chemotherapy with intra-arterial cisplatinum and systemic adriamycin. Am Soc Clin Oncol 4:152, 1985.

11. Anderson JR, Cain KC, Gelber RD: Analysis of survival by tumor response. J Clin Oncol 1:710-719, 1983.

12. Chawla SP, Benjamin RS, Jaffe N, Carrasco CH, Raymond AK, Ayala AG, Wallace S, Armen T, Papadopoulos NEJ, Plager C, Murray JA: Preoperative intra-arterial cis-platin and limb-salvage surgery for patients with high-grade osteosarcoma of the extremities. In Adjuvant Therapy of Cancer V, Salmon SE (ed.), New York, Grune & Stratton, pp.701-710, 1987.

13. Plager C, Papadopoulos NEJ, Chawla SP, Sandberg S, Legha SS, Benjamin RS: Ifosfamide (IFF) therapy for progressive pretreated metastatic sarcoma via compassionate IND. Proc Am Soc Clin Oncol (abstract 503) 6:128, 1987.

14. Legha S, Fitz K, Papadopoulos N, Chawla S, Plager C, Benjamin R: Evaluation of intravenous (IV) N-acetylcys-teine (NAC) as a uroprotector against ifosfamide (IFF) toxicity in patients (PTS) with advanced sarcomas. Proc. Am Soc Clin Oncol (Abstract 505) 6:129, 1987.

15. Marti C, Steiner R, Viollier AF: Hochdosierte ifosfamid-therapie: systemischer einsatz eines mukolytikums zur verminderung der urotoxizitat. Schweiz Med Wschr 109: 1885, 1979.

16. Seeber S, Meiderle N, Osieka R, Schutte J, Dimitriadis K, Schmidt CG: Experimentalle und klinische untersuchungen zur wirksamkeit von ifosfamide bei refraktaren neoplasien. Tumor Diagn & Therapie 5:39, 1984.

17. Bowman LC, Meyer WH, Douglass EC, Pratt CB: Activity of ifosfamide in metastatic and unresectable osteosarcoma. Proc Am Clin Oncol (Abstract 844) 6:214, 1987.

INTRA-ARTERIAL CIS-DIAMMINEDICHLOROPLATINUM-II IN PEDIATRIC OSTEOSARCOMA: RELATIONSHIP OF EFFECT ON PRIMARY TUMOR TO SURVIVAL

Norman Jaffe, MD[1], A. Kevin Raymond, MD[2], Alberto Ayala, MD[2], Humberto Carrasco, M.D.[3], Kuniaki Sesaki, M.D.[1], Sidney Wallace, MD[3], John Murray, MD[4], Resa Robertson, RN, PNP[1], Alexander Wang, PhD[1]

The therapeutic efficacy of intra-arterial cis-Diamminedichloroplatinum-II on the primary tumor was assessed in relationship to survival. Patients with a combined complete and partial response (over 60% necrosis) had a 64% metastases-free survival, and those with no response (under 60% necrosis) a 34% survival.

Introduction

Therapeutic research in osteosarcoma has demonstrated that intra-arterial cis-Diamminedichloroplatinum-II (CDP) is an effective modality for treatment of the primary tumor.(1) It is superior to high-dose methotrexate with citrovorum factor "rescue" (MTX-CF) (2), enhances the safety of the surgical approach for limb salvage (3), and induces healing of pathologic fractures.(4) This report examines the relationship of the effect of CDP on the primary tumor and survival.

Materials and Methods

From January 1979 to June 1985, the primary tumors in 35 consecutive pediatric patients entered into a specific protocol (TIOS-I)* were treated with intra-arterial CDP followed by surgical extirpation. Except for one patient treated with MTX-CF, no patient had received prior chemotherapy. The therapeutic efficacy of CDP was determined by clinical and radiologic studies and ultimately by pathologic examination of the surgical specimen.(1-4) Responses were defined as complete (CR) with 90 to 100% necrosis, partial (PR) with 60 to 90%, and none (NR) under 60%. Responding patients were treated with intravenous CDP, Adriamycin (ADR) and MTX-CF (Regimen A) (Figure 1). In contrast, patients demonstrating resistance to MTX-CF and responding to intra-arterial CDP

---

*Treatment and Investigation of Osteosarcoma.

---

[1]Department of Pediatrics, The University of Texas System Cancer Center, M.D. Anderson Hospital and Tumor Institute, 1515 Holcombe Blvd., Houston, TX 77030.

[2]Division of Pathology
[3]Division of Diagnostic Radiology
[4]Division of Surgery (Orthopedics)
The University of Texas System Cancer Center, M.D. Anderson Hospital and Tumor Institute, Houston, TX 77030.

J. R. Ryan and L. O. Baker (eds.), Recent Concepts in Sarcoma Treatment, 275–282.

were treated with intravenous CDP and ADR (Regimen B). Finally, patients who failed intra-arterial CDP and had not previously been exposed to MTX-CF, were treated with MTX-CF and ADR (Regimen C).

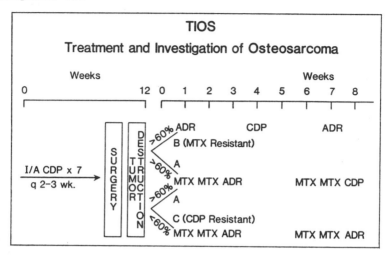

FIGURE 1: Treatment of primary tumor with intra-arterial cis-Diamminedichloroplatinum-II and selection of postoperative adjuvant therapy based upon response. (See References 1-3.)
CDP = Cis-Diamminedichloroplatinum-II 150 mg/M^2.
MTX = High-dose methotrexate (12.5 gm/M^2 over 6 hrs) with citrovorum factor, 15-100 mg q3h IV.
ADR = Adriamycin (25 mg/M^2/d x 3). Maximum cumulative dose 450 mg/M^2).
Duration of adjuvant therapy: 12 months
Occasional patients who did not tolerate intra-arterial CDP, or who failed initial treatment with intra-arterial CDP, were treated with MTX-CF.

All patients had high-grade osteosarcoma, were under 16 years of age and had no evidence of metastatic disease. Pretreatment evaluation included chest radiographs, computerized axial tomography of the lungs and a radionuclide bone scan. In the ensuing 2 years, radiographic examination of the chest was obtained at monthly intervals and computerized axial tomography of the chest, a radionuclide bone scan and radiographic examination of the stump or resected bone at 6 monthly intervals. After 2 years, the intervals between examinations were extended and by the fifth year, follow-up evaluation was restricted to annual radiographic examination of the chest and affected limb.

The mode of treatment with CDP by the intra-arterial route has previously been described.(1-4) Initially, one to 4 courses were administered and with experience, treatment was extended to 7 courses. Eligibility for limb salvage has also previously been documented.(3) Relapse was defined as the appearance of pulmonary and/or extra-pulmonary metastases. Metastases-free survival curves were calculated from date of diagnosis to relapse according to the method of Kaplan and Meier.(5) Overall survival (in some patients, recurrent disease was extirpated) was calculated from the date of diagnosis to last follow-up. Statistical significance was determined by a modified Wilcoxon test.(6)

Results

The anatomic sites of tumors and surgical procedures are outlined in Table 1. Tumor size was comparable in patients undergoing amputation and limb salvage. Patients were relegated to amputation as a consequence of skeletal immaturity rather than operability for limb salvage. Osteoblastic osteosarcoma, the most common tumor subtype, was equally distributed. The duration of preoperative treatment varied from 2 to 7 months (average 3).

	TABLE 1		
	ANATOMIC SITE AND SURGICAL PROCEDURE		
SITE	AMPUTATION	LIMB SALVAGE	TOTAL
FEMUR	15	5	20
TIBIA	3	6	9
HUMERUS	2	2	4
PELVIS	1		1
FIBULA		1	1
	21	14	35

Twenty-four patients received 4 to 7 courses of CDP, 10 patients 2 to 4 courses, and one patient one course. Variations in the number of courses were a consequence of Phase I studies, times to accommodate vicissitudes in the manufacture of custom made prostheses, tumor escape, occasional noncompliance, temporary renal insufficiency and convulsions accompanying the first course of therapy necessitating a change to MTX-CF. Twenty-four of 35 patients responded (69%). This includes healing in 3 of 4 with pathologic fractures.(4) An outline of the response in different histologic subcategories is presented in Table 2.

Amputation was performed in 21 patients. There were 13 responses (5 complete and 8 partial) followed by treatment with Regimen A (Table 3). Two patients who failed to respond, at their request, were also treated with Regimen A. No patient was treated with Regimen B; 5 received Regimen C. The last patient who failed to respond initially to intra-arterial CDP, and subsequently also to MTX-CF, was treated with the Compadri Regimen.(7)

	TABLE 2	
SUBTYPE	NO	RESPONSE
CHRONDROBLASTIC	4	1
OSTEOBLASTIC	26	20
FIBROBLASTIC	1	1
TELANGIECTATIC	2	1
MIXED	1	0
OTHER*	1	1
	35	24 (69%)

* Malignant Fibrous Histiocytoma

Ten of 21 patients developed metastases. One patient developed acute myelogenous leukemia at 32 months and died. Since she was continually free of osteosarcoma until this time, she was scored as living at 32 months. One patient with pulmonary metastases was later rendered disease-free by metastasectomy.

Limb salvage was performed in 14 patients initially considered eligible for this procedure. All received multiple courses of intra-arterial CDP except one who developed a convulsion with the first course, after which treatment was altered to MTX-CF. Eleven patients demonstrated responses (9 complete and 2 partial). Ten of these patients were treated with Regimen A. The eleventh had previously failed treatment with MTX-CF; she and the patient who developed convulsions with the first CDP course (vide supra) and, subsequently, also failed MTX-CF, were treated with Regimen B. Only one patient was treated with Regimen C. The last patient with a mixed osteoblastic-fibroblastic tumor achieved a response only in the osteoblastic component, and was also treated with Regimen A.

Five patients developed pulmonary metastases (2 nonresponders and 3 responders); 3 died and 2 were rendered disease-free by metastasectomy. Three patients developed local recurrences; 2 are included in the patients who developed and died of pulmonary metastases. The third patient did not develop pulmonary metastases and was rendered disease-free by amputation.

Lifetable analysis revealed a 52% metastases-free survival for amputation and 64% for limb salvage (Figure 2). The difference was not related to tumor size (vide infra) and was not statistically significant (p=0.44). Survival for the combined group was 56%. Lifetable analysis, as a function of CR, PR and NR, was 72%, 58% and 36%, respectively (Figure 3). Survival for CR and PR combined was 66% and, compared to NR (36%), approached statistical significance (p=0.06). Overall

TABLE 3

AMPUTATION

PATHOLOGIC RESULT (See Text)			ADJUVANT THERAPY (See Text)				METASTASES	SURVIVAL	
NR	PR	CR	A	B	C	O•		CMF^x	OVERALL
5					5		3	2	2
		5	5				1	4*	3°
2			2				2	0	1+
	8		8				4	4	4
1						1	1	1	1
—	—	—	—	—			—	—	—
8	8	5	15	5	1		10	11	11

LIMB SALVAGE

NR	PR	CR	A	B	C	O•	METASTASES	CMF^x	OVERALL
3			1	1	1		2	1	2+
	2		2				2	2	2
		9	8	1			3	6	7+
—	—	—	—	—	—		—	—	—
3	2	9	11	2	1		5	9	11

x Continuous Metastases Free

* Two patients extra-pulmonary metastases

° One patient died of myelogenous leukemia

+ One patient rendered disease free by metastasectomy

• COMPADRI REGIMEN

survival following extirpation of recurrent disease was 10 to 20% in excess of metastases-free survival.

Discussion

Survival in limb salvage was better, but not statistically superior to amputation. The preponderance of amputation (as opposed to limb salvage) was a consequence of skeletal immaturity rather than tumor size, which was comparable in both groups. The slight difference in survival, therefore, cannot be attributed to the surgical procedure or tumor bulk. Histology, also, did not influence the results since osteoblastic osteosarcoma, the most responsive subtype was equally distributed between amputation and limb salvage. Finally, no adverse effect emerged with pre-scheduled delays in initiation of surgery for amputation or limb salvage; analysis reveals that survival is comparable to other published reports.(8-11).

Tumor necrosis is the final arbiter of the cytotoxic capability of chemotherapy. Utilizing the primary tumor to

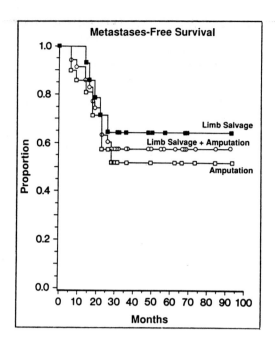

FIGURE 2: Metastases-free survival for amputation and limb salvage.

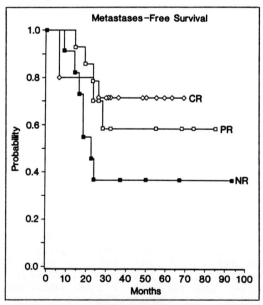

FIGURE 3: Metastases-free survival for complete response (over 90% necrosis), partial response (60-90% necrosis), and no response (under 60% necrosis).

evaluate response, a correlation between treatment and survival was observed; survival was poor in nonresponders (36%), and superior in responders (66%). This correlation assumes the existence of pulmonary micrometastases in over 80% of newly diagnosed patients with an innate drug sensitivity similar to that of the primary tumor.(12) This assumption also acknowledges treatment with a variety of postoperative regimens dictated by the cytocidal effects of CDP. Thus, intra-arterial CDP produces a major effect on the primary tumor (overall response 69%) and can be exploited to induce a reciprocal effect on survival.

REFERENCES

1. Jaffe N, Knapp J, Chuang VP, et al.: Osteosarcoma: intra-arterial treatment of the primary tumor with cis-Diamminedichloroplatinum-II (CDP): angiographic, pathologic and pharmacologic studies. Cancer 51:402-407, 1983.
2. Jaffe N, Robertson R, Ayala A, et al.: Comparison of intra-arterial cis-Diamminedichloroplatinum-II with high dose methotrexate and citrovorum factor rescue in the treatment of primary osteosarcoma. J Clin Oncol 3:1101-1104, 1985.
3. Jaffe N, Murray JA, Ayala A, et al.: Osteosarcoma limb salvage with preoperative chemotherapy. In The Design and Application of Tumor Prostheses for Bone and Joint Reconstruction. Chao EY-S, Iving JC (Eds.), New York, Thieme-Stratton Inc, New York Georg Thieme, Verlag Stuttgart, pp.69-77, 1983.
4. Jaffe N, Spears R, Eftekhari F, et al.: Pathologic fracture in osteosarcoma: impact of chemotherapy on primary tumor and survival. Cancer 59:0027-0035, 1987.
5. Kaplan EL, Meier R: Nonparametric estimation from incomplete observation. J Am Stat Assoc 53:457-481, 1958.
6. Gehan EA: A generalized Wilcoxon test for comparing arbitrarily singly - censored samples. Biometrika 52:203-223, 1965.
7. Sutow WW, Gehan EA, Vietti TJ, et al.: Multi-drug chemotherapy in primary treatment of osteosarcoma. J Bone Joint Surg 58A:629-633, 1976.
8. Weiner MA, Harris MB, Lewis M, et al.: Neoadjuvant high dose methotrexate, cisplatin and doxorubicin for the management of patients with non-metastatic osteosarcoma. Cancer Treat Rep 70:1431-1432, 1986.
9. Goorin AM, Perez-Atayde A, Gebhardt M, et al.: Weekly high dose methotrexate and doxorubicin for osteosarcoma: The Dana Farber Cancer Center Institute/The Children's Hospital Study III. J Clin Oncol 5:1178-1184, 1984.
10. Link MP, Goorin AM, Miser AW, et al.: The effect of adjuvant chemotherapy on relapse free survival in patients with osteosarcoma of the extremity. N Engl J Med 314:1600-1606, 1986.

11. Rosen G, Caparros B, Nirenberg A, et al.: Preoperative chemotherapy for osteogenic sarcoma: selection of post-operative adjuvant chemotherapy based on the response of the primary tumor to preoperative chemotherapy. Cancer 49:1221-1230, 1982.
12. Jaffe N: Chemotherapy in Osteosarcoma: Advances and controversies. In Experimental and Clinical Progress in Cancer Chemotherapy. Muggia FM (Ed.), Boston, Martinus Nijhoff, pp.223-233, 1985.

ADJUVANT CHEMOTHERAPY IN THE TREATMENT OF OSTEOSARCOMA:
RESULTS OF THE MULTI-INSTITUTIONAL OSTEOSARCOMA STUDY*

Michael P. Link, M.D.[1], Jonathan J. Shuster, Ph.D.[2],
Allen M. Goorin, M.D.[3], Angela Miser, M.D.[4],
W. H. Meyer, M.D.[5], Judith E. Kingston, F.R.C.P.[6],
Jean Belasco, M.D.[7], Alan R. Baker, M.D.[8],
Alberto G. Ayala, M.D.[9], Teresa Vietti, M.D.[10]

The prognosis for children with osteosarcoma has improved dramatically over the past 15 years. Prior to 1970,
fewer than 20% of patients with osteosarcoma treated only
with surgery of the primary tumor survived 5 years (1,2), and
it was inferred from the experience at multiple institutions
that at least 80% of patients presenting without overt metastatic disease, in fact, had microscopic subclinical metastases at the time of diagnosis. Today, projected 5-year
survivals of 60-80% are reported from a number of treatment
centers. This improvement in prognosis for more recently
diagnosed patients with osteosarcoma had been attributed to
the administration of adjuvant chemotherapy after surgery
which apparently was effective in eradicating micrometastatic
disease. However, the contribution of adjuvant chemotherapy
to the improvement in outcome for children with osteosarcoma
was challenged by results of studies from the Mayo Clinic and
elsewhere (2-4), which demonstrated that more recently diagnosed patients were less likely to have subclinical metastases, and that as many as 40% of patients with osteosarcoma
treated only with surgery of the primary tumor would survive
free of recurrence. A randomized controlled study of high
dose methotrexate conducted at the Mayo Clinic (5) demonstrated no benefit for patients receiving adjuvant chemother-

[1]Division of Hematology/Oncology, Children's Hospital at
 Stanford, 520 Sand Hill Road, Palo Alto, CA 94304-2099.
[2]Statistical Office of the Pediatric Oncology Group,
 St. Louis, MO.
[3]Dana-Farber Cancer Institute and Children's Hospital,
 Boston, MA.
[4]Pediatric Oncology, National Cancer Institute, Bethesda, MD
[5]St. Jude Children's Research Hospital, Memphis, TN.
[6]St. Bartholomew's Hospital, London, England.
[7]Children's Hospital of Philadelphia, Philadelphia, PA.
[8]Surgery Branch, National Cancer Institute, Bethesda, MD.
[9]M.D. Anderson Hospital and Tumor Institute, Houston, TX.
[10]Operations Office of the Pediatric Oncology Group, St.
 Louis, MO.

*Supported in part by grants from the National Cancer
 Institute, National Institutes of Health, No. CA33603[1],
 CA29139[2], CA31566[5], CA03713[9] and CA30969[10].

J. R. Ryan and L. O. Baker (eds.), Recent Concepts in Sarcoma Treatment, 283–290.
© 1988 by Kluwer Academic Publishers.

apy. Moreover, the relapse-free survival of patients in the control group of the Mayo Clinic trial was projected to be 44% at 5 years -- more than twice what was expected based on historical controls prior to 1970. These results disputed the apparent benefit of adjuvant chemotherapy that had been demonstrated in uncontrolled adjuvant trials of the 1970's.

To resolve the controversy over the role of adjuvant chemotherapy in the treatment of osteosarcoma, the Multi-Institutional Osteosarcoma Study (MIOS), a randomized controlled trial, was initiated in June 1982. The objective of this trial was to determine whether the administration of intensive multi-agent chemotherapy as adjuvant treatment after definitive surgery of the primary tumor would significantly improve disease-free survival and survival among patients with nonmetastatic osteosarcoma of the extremity, as compared with concurrent controls treated only with surgery without adjuvant therapy. Preliminary results of this study have been published.(2,6) This report will update the results of this trial and will focus on the outcome of patients treated with adjuvant chemotherapy.

Methods

Patients and randomization. Patients were entered from the majority of the institutions of the Pediatric Oncology Group (POG), from the Dana-Farber Cancer Institute, from the Pediatric and Surgical Branches of the National Cancer Institute, from the Children's Hospital of Philadelphia, and from the London Solid Tumor Group. Eligibility requirements included: 1) age less than 30 years, 2) histologic confirmation of high grade osteosarcoma, 3) no evidence of metastases as determined by radionuclide bone scan and thoracic CT scan, 4) primary tumor in an extremity, 5) complete surgical excision of tumor by amputation or resection with pathological confirmation that margins were tumor-free, 6) an interval of less than 6 weeks since biopsy and less than 4 weeks since definitive surgery, 7) no prior history of cancer, and 8) no previous therapy other than surgery of the primary tumor.

After eligible patients had given informed consent, they were randomly assigned to treatment through the POG Statistical Office. Eligible patients who declined randomization, but who accepted treatment according to one of the two study regimens, were followed in the same way as patients who accepted randomization.

Patients were randomized onto study between June 1982 and August 1984, at which time analysis of the study indicated a significant event-free survival advantage for patients receiving immediate adjuvant chemotherapy, and the randomization was closed. Thereafter, eligible patients were all treated with adjuvant chemotherapy as prescribed in the protocol. The study was closed to patient entry in October 1986.

Therapy and follow-up procedures. After definitive surgery of the primary tumor, patients were randomly assigned to a group receiving immediate intensive adjuvant chemotherapy or to a control group treated without adjuvant therapy. The chemotherapy regimen (Figure 1) utilized in this study is

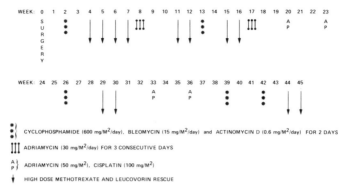

CYCLOPHOSPHAMIDE (600 mg/M²/day), BLEOMYCIN (15 mg/M²/day) and ACTINOMYCIN D (0.6 mg/M²/day) FOR 2 DAYS

III ADRIAMYCIN (30 mg/M²/day) FOR 3 CONSECUTIVE DAYS

A ADRIAMYCIN (50 mg/M²), CISPLATIN (100 mg/M²)
P

HIGH DOSE METHOTREXATE AND LEUCOVORIN RESCUE

FIGURE 1: Chemotherapy regimen of the Multi-Institutional Osteosarcoma Study.

described in detail elsewhere.(6) Chemotherapy was instituted 2 weeks after surgery of the primary for patients assigned to this treatment. Follow-up of patients in both adjuvant chemotherapy and control groups was identical and included monthly chest radiographs, thoracic CT scanning every 4 months, and radionuclide bone scanning every 6 months for two years after surgery. Relapse was defined as recurrence of tumor at any site.

Statistical considerations. The statistical considerations of this study are discussed in detail elsewhere.(6) All eligible patients were evaluated according to assigned treatment. For study of prognostic factors, all patients assigned to chemotherapy (by randomization, by choice, and those entered after the randomization was closed) were analyzed together. Study endpoint was event-free survival. Treatments were compared by the log rank test (7), and life tables were constructed according to the method of Kaplan and Meier.(8)

Results

Between June 1982 and August 1984, 113 eligible patients were entered onto study. The characteristics of the patients have been described previously.(6) Thirty-six patients accepted randomization: 18 were assigned to immediate adjuvant chemotherapy and 18 to observation alone. An additional 77 eligible patients declined randomization but were followed according to one of the treatment groups of this study; 59 of these patients elected immediate adjuvant chemotherapy and 18 elected observation alone. After the randomization was closed in August 1984, an additional 88 eligible patients were entered on study until the study was closed to patient entry in October 1986. These 88 patients were all treated with immediate adjuvant chemotherapy. Thus, a total of 165 patients were treated with immediate adjuvant chemotherapy on this study. There were 91 males and 74 females including 103 patients older than 12 years of age. Primary tumor sites

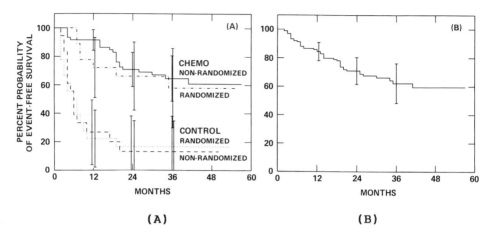

FIGURE 2: (A) Life tables for event-free survival for patients accepting and declining randomization according to assigned treatment. (B) Life table for event-free survival for all 165 patients treated with adjuvant chemotherapy on the MIOS.

among patients treated with immediate adjuvant chemotherapy included: distal femur 83 (50%), proximal tibia 46 (28%), humerus 13 (8%), distal tibia 9 (5%), proximal femur 7 (4%), mid femur 4 (2%), and other limb sites 3 (2%). Among patients receiving immediate adjuvant chemotherapy, 38 underwent resection of their primary tumor (limb-sparing surgery) and 127 underwent amputation.

The outcome of treatment is shown in Figure 2. Among 36 patients assigned to observation alone (by randomization or by choice), 30 have relapsed (including 15 of 18 randomized patients). Among 165 patients assigned to immediate adjuvant chemotherapy, 45 have relapsed and 2 patients have died without evidence of recurrent tumor (1 death attributed to complications of chemotherapy and 1 death of causes unrelated to osteosarcoma or treatment). Thus, 118 patients treated with immediate adjuvant chemotherapy remain alive without evidence of recurrent disease. By life table analysis, 60% of all eligible patients treated with intensive adjuvant chemotherapy after surgery are projected to remain alive and free of recurrent disease almost five years following definitive surgery (Figure 2B). By contrast, fewer than 20% of patients treated only with surgery of the primary tumor and without adjuvant chemotherapy survive without recurrent disease beyond two years (Figure 2A).

For analysis of prognostic factors, data from all 165 patients assigned to immediate adjuvant chemotherapy were pooled. Again, all eligible patients were included, although for some factors analyzed, data were not available for all patients. Neither age, sex, type of surgery (amputation

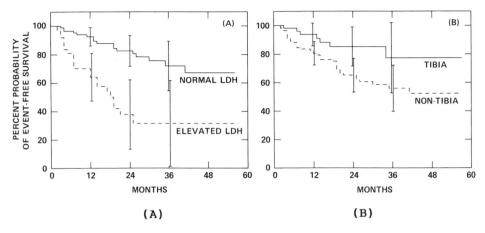

FIGURE 3: (A) Life tables of event-free survival for patients with normal vs. elevated LDH at diagnosis. (B) Life tables of event-free survival for patients with tibia vs. non-tibia primary tumors.

versus resection) or level of serum alkaline phosphatase at diagnosis predicted for event-free survival (data not shown). By contrast, level of serum lactic dehydrogenase (LDH) at diagnosis proved to be the single most important prognostic factor. One hundred twenty-five patients had serum LDH measurements at diagnosis. Eighty-six (69%) had serum LDH levels in the normal range, whereas 39 (31%) had LDH levels which were abnormally elevated. Patients with elevated LDH had a significantly worse outcome than patients with normal LDH (p <0.001) (Figure 3A). Similarly, site of primary tumor also proved to be predictive of outcome, since patients with tibia primaries fared significantly better than those with tumors at other sites (p <0.05) (Figure 3B). Tibia primary confirmed a superior outcome even after correction for LDH Level.

Discussion

From results of the MIOS, the favorable impact of adjuvant chemotherapy on event-free survival in patients with osteosarcoma appears incontrovertible. In the initial reported results of this trial (6), the outcome for patients treated with immediate adjuvant chemotherapy was significantly better than for patients in the control group treated only with surgery of the primary tumor. Further follow-up of these patients has not changed the result (Figure 2A). Life tables of event-free survival for patients treated without adjuvant chemotherapy in the MIOS confirm the historical experience prior to 1970. Fifty percent of the patients suffered a relapse within 6 months of diagnosis, and, overall, more than 80% of these patients developed recurrent disease. This result was also confirmed in another study (9). Thus, it is apparent that the natural history of osteosarcoma has not changed in the past two decades, since fewer than 20% of patients treated only with surgery of the primary tumor will survive without recurrence.

The favorable outcome for patients treated with adjuvant chemotherapy in the MIOS has been sustained with follow-up approaching 5 years. This favorable result has been confirmed by experience in 88 additional patients entered on study after the randomization was closed (Figure 2B). Life tables of event-free survival for patients treated with adjuvant chemotherapy suggest that there is a plateau beyond three years, confirming results of previous trials which demonstrated that patients surviving 3 years without recurrence are likely to be cured.

The study of a large number of patients with osteosarcoma has allowed for the analysis of prognostic variables which might be used in the design of future strategies of treatment for patients with osteosarcoma. In the MIOS, elevation of serum LDH at diagnosis has emerged as the single factor most predictive of adverse outcome in patients with limb primaries presenting without metastases who received adjuvant chemotherapy (Figure 3A). Serum LDH has been found to correlate with tumor burden and with prognosis in Burkitt's lymphoma (10,11) and childhood acute lymphoblastic leukemia (12), although serum LDH did not correlate with tumor volume in the MIOS. LDH has also proven to be a useful prognostic factor in Ewing's sarcoma (13), but has not been previously reported as a prognostic factor in osteosarcoma. Patients with primary tumors in the tibia had a significantly better event-free survival than those with non-tibia primaries (Figure 3B). The association of tibia primary with favorable outcome has been noted previously (14) in the prechemotherapy era.

Refinements in therapy for patients with osteosarcoma are needed. Although the prognosis for children with osteosarcoma has improved dramatically in the past two decades, more than one-third of children presenting without metastases will relapse after receiving the therapy currently available. Recently, many investigators have recommended the use of presurgical chemotherapy to deliver systemic treatment against micrometastases earlier in the course of therapy.(15) Some investigators have utilized presurgical chemotherapy as an in vivo drug trial of drug sensitivity of the primary tumor to "customize" the postsurgical adjuvant chemotherapy. (16,17) In early trials of presurgical chemotherapy, the outcome for patients has been excellent.(17,18) Unfortunately, in multi-institutional trials utilizing presurgical chemotherapy, the overall results have not been superior to the results achieved with immediate surgery and postoperative adjuvant chemotherapy in the MIOS.(18-20) Thus, the value of presurgical chemotherapy in the treatment of osteosarcoma remains to be proven. The POG is currently studying the role of presurgical chemotherapy in an ongoing randomized trial.

REFERENCES

1. Friedman MA, Carter SK: The therapy of osteogenic sarcoma: Current status and thoughts for the future. J Surg Oncol 4:482-510, 1972.
2. Link MP: Adjuvant therapy in the treatment of osteosarcoma. In DeVita VT, Hellman S, Rosenberg S (eds.): Important Advances in Oncology, 1986. Philadelphia, JB Lippincott, pp.193-207, 1986.
3. Taylor WF, Ivins JC, Dahlin DC, Edmonson JH, Pritchard DJ: Trends and variability in survival from osteosarcoma. Mayo Clinic Proc 53:695-700, 1978.
4. Taylor WF, Ivins JC, Dahlin DC, Edmonson JH, Pritchard DJ: Trends and variability in survival among patients with osteosarcoma: A 7-year update. Mayo Clin Proc 60:91-104, 1985.
5. Edmonson J, Green S, Ivins J, et al.: A controlled pilot study of high-dose methotrexate as post surgical adjuvant treatment for primary osteosarcoma. J Clin Oncol 2:152-156, 1984.
6. Link MP, Goorin AM, Miser AW, et al.: The effect of adjuvant chemotherapy on relapse-free survival in patients with osteosarcoma of the extremity. N Engl J Med 314:1600-1606, 1986.
7. Peto R, Peto J: Asymptotically efficient rank invariant test procedures. J R Stat Soc (A) 135:185-198, 1972.
8. Kaplan EL, Meier P: Nonparametric estimation from incomplete observations. J Am Stat Assoc 53:457-481, 1958.
9. Eilber F, Giuliano A, Eckardt J, et al.: Adjuvant chemotherapy for osteosarcoma: A Randomized prospective trial. J Clin Oncol 5:21-26, 1987.
10. Magrath I, Lee YJ, Anderson T, et al.: Prognostic factors in Burkitt's lymphoma. Importance of total tumor burden. Cancer 45:1507-1515, 1980.
11. Murphy SB, Bowman WP, Abromowitch M, et al.: Results of treatment of advanced-stage Burkitt's lymphoma and B cell (SIg+) acute lymphoblastic leukemia with high dose fractionated cyclophosphamide and coordinated high-dose methotrexate and cytarabine. J Clin Oncol 4:1732-1739, 1986.
12. Pui C-H, Dodge RK, Dahl GV, et al.: Serum lactic dehydrogenase level has prognostic value in childhood acute lymphoblastic leukemia. Blood 66:778-782, 1985.
13. Glaubiger DL, Makuch RW, Schwarz J: Influence of prognostic factors on survival in Ewing's sarcoma. NCI Monogr 56:285-288, 1981.
14. Lockshin M, Higgins I: Prognosis in osteogenic sarcoma. Clin Orthop 58:85-101, 1968.
15. Rosen G, Marcove RC, Capparos B, Nirenberg A, Kosloff C, Huvos AG: Primary osteogenic sarcoma. The rationale for preoperative chemotherapy and delayed surgery. Cancer 43:2163-2177, 1979.
16. Rosen G, Capparos B, Huvos AG, et al.: Preoperative chemotherapy for osteogenic sarcoma: Selection of postoperative adjuvant chemotherapy based on the response of

the primary tumor to preoperative chemotherapy. Cancer 49:1221-1230, 1982.

17. Rosen G, Marcove RC, Huvos AG, et al.: Primary osteogenic sarcoma: Eight-year experience with adjuvant chemotherapy. J Cancer Res Clin Oncol 106(Suppl):55-67, 1983.

18. Winkler K, Beron G, Kotz R, et al.: Neoadjuvant chemotherapy for osteogenic sarcoma: Results of a Cooperative German/Austrian Study. J Clin Oncol 2:617-624, 1984.

19. Winkler K, Beron G, Delling G, et al.: Selective post-operative (pOp) adjuvant chemotherapy (CT) after aggressive vs. mild preoperative (prOp) CT in osteosarcoma. Proc ASCO 5:128, 1986.

20. Provisor A, Nachman J, Krailo M, Ettinger L, Hammond D: Treatment of non-metastatic osteogenic sarcoma of the extremities with pre- and post-operative chemotherapy. Proc Am Soc Clin Oncol 6:217, 1987.

NEOADJUVANT CHEMOTHERAPY FOR OSTEOSARCOMA - RESULTS OF A PROSPECTIVE STUDY[*]

P. Picci[1], G. Bacci[1], R. Capanna[1], E. Madon[2], G. Paolucci[3],
M. Marangolo[4], M. Avella[1], N. Baldini[1], M. Mercuri[1],
M. Campanacci[1]

In March 1983, the Bone Tumor Center of the Istituto
Ortopedico Rizzoli of Bologna, in collaboration with the
Department of Pediatric Oncology of the University of Torino,
and the 3rd Pediatric Clinic of the University of Bologna,
started a new study of preoperative chemotherapy in patients
with localized osteosarcoma of the extremities.

Design of the Study

Preoperative chemotherapy consisted of two cycles of MTX
and two cycles of CDDP. MTX was given at day 1 intravenously
at two different doses on a randomized basis: 750 mg/m2 in
half an hour vs. 7.5 g/m2 in a 1-hour infusion. In both
cases, citrovorum factor rescue was started 24 hours after
the beginning of MTX. CDDP was given intra-arterially in all
patients and at the same dose of 120-150 mg/m2 in a 72-hour
infusion starting on day 6. A second cycle of both drugs was
given starting at day 21. Surgery was usually performed after
three weeks from the end of chemotherapy.

Surgery was always performed in the same institution, by
the same surgeons with great expertise in the treatment of
bone tumors. The choice between limb salvage procedures or
ablative surgery was taken considering the size of the tumor,
the involvement of major neurovascular structures, the efficacy of preoperative treatment in delimiting the tumor, and
the residual expected functional activity. In other words,
the choice was dictated considering, on one hand, the risk of
a local recurrence, and on the other, the residual functional
activity remaining to the patient. After surgery, all the
specimens were studied by the same pathologist and the necrosis was evaluated on at least two entire sections on the two
major diameters of the tumor. Necrosis was graded as "good"
if it was greater than 90%; as "fair" if it was between 60

----

[1]Bone Tumor Center, Istituto Ortopedico Rizzoli, Bologna,
  Italy
[2]Pediatric Clinic, University of Torino, Torino, Italy
[3]3rd Pediatric Clinic, University of Bologna, Bologna, Italy
[4]Division of Clinical Oncology, Ravenna Hospital, Italy

----

[*]Supported in part by a grant from National Council for
  Research, project Oncology n. 88.02679.44, and by a grant
  from Regione Emilia Romagna, law n. 1970 of May 13th, 1986.

J. R. Ryan and L. O. Baker (eds.), Recent Concepts in Sarcoma Treatment, 291–295.
© 1988 by Kluwer Academic Publishers.

and 90%; and "poor" if it was less than 60%. Postoperatively, the treatment was chosen depending on the grade of necrosis observed:
1.   For a "good" necrosis, the same preoperative treat-
     ment at the same dose was given intravenously for
     two cycles.
2.   For a "fair" necrosis, ADM, at the dose of 90 mg/m2
     in two or three days was added to the two drugs
     employed preoperatively. The treatment started with
     ADM followed after 21 days by MTX and CDDP at the
     same doses used preoperatively for 3 complete
     cycles. Another cycle of ADM was given at the end
     of the treatment. In this way, 360 mg/m2 of ADM
     were given in about 6 months.
3.   For a "poor" necrosis, the treatment consisted of 5
     cycles of ADM with the same modalities used for
     "fair" responders, alternated to 5 cycles of BCD
     (Bleomycin 20 mg/m2, Cyclophosphamide 750 mg/m2,
     Actinomycin-D 0.6 mg/m2) for about 9 months.
     In December 1983, after four early metastases observed
in the "good" responders where ADM had not been used, this
arm was closed. After this, the "good" responders were also
treated with the same schema employed for "fair" responders.
Patients
     Until September 1986, 224 patients with osteosarcoma
were observed. Eighty patients were excluded, being considered ineligible to the study due to several reasons:
metastatic, histological varieties, previous tumor (2 retino-
blastomas and 1 leukemia), site not in an extremity, age over
45, refused the protocol.
     The remaining 144 patients entered the study and were
randomized to receive high or moderate doses of MTX. Preoperative investigations included CT scan of the lesion, and bone
scan before and after preoperative treatment. Lung tomograms
were performed after preoperative treatment before surgery.
Angiograms were performed before each infusion of CDDP.
     Of the 144 randomized patients, 18 are not evaluable for
several reasons: 10 patients, after the end of preoperative
treatment refused surgery and were, therefore, sent to other
institutions for other treatment; 3 patients, all randomized
to receive high doses of MTX developed, after the first MTX,
a severe toxicity and therefore changed their treatment; 3
patients started postoperative treatment after 50 days from
surgery due to surgical complications, and another one, for
the same reasons, was not given any postoperative treatment
other than 1 cycle of ADM. Another excluded patient suddenly
died due to unknown causes.
     The remaining 126 patients are the object of this re-
port. Sixty-six were randomized to receive high doses of MTX
and 60 to receive low doses.
Results
     Ninety-one patients (72%) were surgically treated with
limb salvage procedures and 35 (28%) with amputation or
disarticulation. In spite of this high number of limb salvage
procedures, only four local recurrences were observed (3 in

resected patients and 1 in an amputated patient). Necrosis was evaluated on all 126 specimens. Totally, 52% of the patients showed a "good" necrosis, 36 a "fair" necrosis, and 12 a "poor" necrosis. Differences were noted between the patients treated with high or moderate doses of MTX, but these were not statistically significant; in fact, "good" responders were 62% with higher doses vs. 42% with lower doses, "fair" responders were 29% and 43%, and "poor" responders 9% and 15%, respectively.

Fifteen patients, all "good" responders (9 treated with high doses of MTX and 6 with the lower doses), were postoperatively treated without ADM. Today, at a median follow-up of 48 months (range 45-54) only four (27%) are continuously disease-free (2 in each of the two groups of MTX), 10 of the remaining 11 patients developed lung metastases after 4-18 months (x=11 months), and another developed a local recurrence due to a skip metastasis erroneously not detected preoperatively, after 29 months. In December 1983, after four of these patients developed early lung metastases, this arm was closed and also the "good" responders were treated with the same postoperative schema employed for "fair" responders. The remaining 111 patients were, therefore, all treated postoperatively with ADM and will be better evaluated now. At a median follow-up of 30 months (range 12-54), 68 patients (61%) are continuously disease-free, 43 (39%) developed distant metastases. Three of these patients developed a contemporary local recurrence (3%). Regarding the doses of MTX, 70% (40/57) of the patients treated with high doses are continuously disease-free versus 52% (28/54) of the patients treated with lower doses. This difference is statistically significant (p<0.05). Evaluating the same data with Kaplan and Meier's disease-free survival curves, the figures become 68% and 51%, respectively (Figure 1).

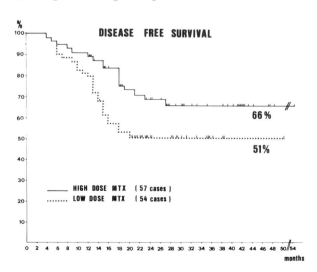

FIGURE 1.

Analyzing the results in terms of necrosis induced by preoperative chemotherapy, 82% (42/51) of "good" responders are continuously disease-free versus 47% (21/45) of the "fair" responders, and 33% (5/15) of the "poor" responders. The difference between "good" and "fair" responders is statistically highly significant (p<0.001), while the difference between "fair" and "poor" responders is not statistically significant. Evaluating the same data with Kaplan and Meier disease-free survival curves, the figures become 81% for "good" responders, 44% for "fair" responders, and 22% for "poor" responders (Figure 2).

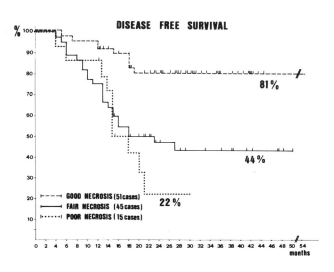

FIGURE 2.

Our study involves pediatric and adult patients and it is thus correct to evaluate the prognosis with regard to age. Fifty of our patients were 14 or younger, and 34 (58%) are continuously disease-free versus 56% (34/61) of the older patients, ranging from 15 to 45 years. Finally, again no difference in disease-free survival was observed between patients treated by amputation (64%, 21/33) and patients treated by limb salvage surgery (60%, 47/78).

Conclusions

1. In our study, with the multidrug association and doses we employed, ADM is absolutely necessary.
    Our attempt to avoid this drug for its cardiotoxicity was evaluated in 15 patients only. This attempt revealed to be prognostically negative, only 4 are disease-free, and this arm of treatment was suddenly closed.
2. Limb salvage is possible and safe. In spite of the very high percentage of limb salvage procedures (73%), only 4 experienced a local recurrence. It is to be noted

that one of these local recurrences was observed after a hindquarter amputation, and that another one was due to a skip metastasis erroneously not detected during the preoperative staging, but afterwards revealed by the careful examination of the preoperative radio- and angiograms.

3. Our study confirms that "good" responders have a very good prognosis (more than 80%).
   In our experience, to change postoperative treatment after a "poor" necrosis does not increase the disease-free survival.

4. From our experience, the "breaking point" for the choice of postoperative treatment is 90% necrosis.
   Our data, in fact, underlines that below this percentage of necrosis, postoperative treatment should be changed or increased, and these variations should not be limited to "poor" responders only.

5. The comparison between high and low doses of MTX seems to indicate a better prognosis using higher doses.
   Although our results indicate a statistically significant difference, a longer follow-up is necessary to confirm this fact.

Based on these conclusions, a new study was opened in September 1986. The aim was to increase the number of good responders, giving a more intense preoperative treatment. For this reason, in addition to the previous schema, on the third day, adriamycin, at the dose of 50-60 mg/m2, was given intravenously together with intra-arterial cisplatinum. The dose of methotrexate was established in all patients at 8 gr/m2. A second cycle was repeated on day 28.

Until June 1987, 50 patients had preoperative chemotherapy; 10 have not yet been surgically treated. Of the other 40 patients, 35 (87.5%) underwent limb saving procedures.

Necrosis was at this time evaluated in 38 cases: a "good" necrosis was obtained in 30 cases (79%), "fair" necrosis was observed in 7 (18%), and a "poor" response was seen in one case only (3%).

THE GERMAN PEDIATRIC ONCOLOGY (GPO) COOPERATIVE STUDY ON OSTEOSARCOMA

K. Winkler[1]   and H. Juergens[2]

The GPO has conducted a consecutive series of adjuvant chemotherapy trials in osteosarcoma of the extremities since 1977. Figure 1 shows the outline of the chemotherapy, and Table 1 the global outcome of the different studies.

The first trial, COSS-77, using high dose methotrexate (HDMTX), doxorubicine (DOX) and cyclosphosphamide (CP) at the same dosages as the T-4/T-5 studies of G. Rosen (1) after primary amputation resulted in a 51% calculated metastases-free survival (MFS) rate at 7 years, confirming the results of Rosen and the improved survival rate as compared to historical controls as a whole (2,3,4).

The subsequent study COSS-80 had two main objectives: 1) to further increase the MFS-rate by intensifying chemotherapy and 2) to improve the quality of survival by use of limb salvage instead of ablative surgery, if feasible.

An increased efficacy of chemotherapy was attempted by doubling the HDMTX-dosage from 6 to 12 mg/m^2, by replacing CP by either cisplatinum (CPL) or the triple drug combination bleomycin + cyclosphosphamide + dactinomycin (BCD) (5), and by additionally giving interferon (IF) after surgery to one-half of the patients. Thus, the BCD-branch without IF in schedule as well as dosage of drugs was almost identical to the T-7 study of Rosen et al (6). Actuarial MFS-rates at 40 months did not show any difference between patients receiving BCD's vs. CPL and also no difference for patients receiving IF vs. no IF. The calculated MFS-rate of the combined branches of study COSS-80 of 68% at more than five years (7) is significantly higher than that of study COSS-77 and corresponds to the results of study T-7 of Rosen (6) and compares favorably to results reported otherwise from the literature (8).

In order to gain the time necessary for preparation of limb salvage procedures, preoperative chemotherapy of 10 weeks duration was given. Patients after primary amputation from non-cooperating orthopedic clinics did no better than the study patients after delayed amputation (9). Histologic evaluation of the resected tumor revealed a close relation-

---

[1]Department of Pediatric Oncology of the University of Hamburg, Martinistr. 52, 2000 Hamburg 20.
[2]Department of Pediatric Oncology, University of Düsseldorf, W. Germany.

J. R. Ryan and L. O. Baker (eds.), Recent Concepts in Sarcoma Treatment, 296–300.
© 1988 by Kluwer Academic Publishers.

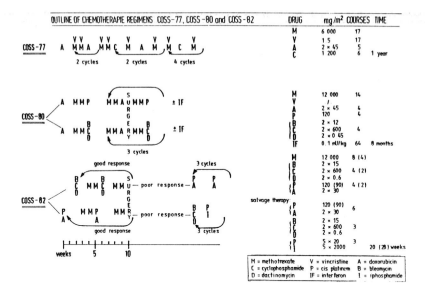

FIGURE 1: Outline of chemotherapy of the osteosarcoma stud-
-ies COSS-77, COSS-80 and COSS-82.

**TABLE 1: Global Outcome of the Osteosarcoma Studies
COSS-77, COSS-80 and COSS-82**

	COSS-77	COSS-80	COSS-82
evaluable patients	71	113	125
local failure	3	5	3
metastases	33	32	47
fatal complications	-	5	2
total fail	36	42	52
event free survival	35/71 (.49)	71/113 (.62)	73/125 (.55)
metastasis free survival	35/68 (.51)	71/103 (.68)	73/120 (.58)
median observation time	72 (57-87)mos.	54 (39-68) mos.	34 (18-52) mos.
updating	X/84	X/85	X/86

ship between the degree of tumor cell destruction (TCD) and probability of MFS (64% calculated MFS at >= 90% TCD vs. 52% at <90% TCD at 5 years). Standardized sequential digital analysis of 99m Tc-MDP scans in both early and late phases was found to be a powerful method for in vivo evaluation of tumor development, showing changes as early as within four weeks (10,11). Thirty-three patients had limb salvage procedures, 20 shank rotation plasty and the remainder ablative surgery. Local failures were not a major problem in limb salvage surgery (2 after en bloc resection vs. 2 after amputation and 1 after rotation plasty, respectively). A somewhat intriguing finding, however, was a higher rate of pulmonary metastases after en bloc resection, especially in patients with large tumors and poor response to preoperative chemotherapy (12).

The poor results for patients with tumors unresponsive to preoperative chemotherapy stimulated a trial aimed at improving their prognosis by switching to another, non cross resistant chemotherapy postoperatively. In the T-10 study, Rosen et al., using sequential chemotherapy consisting of HDMTX, DOX and BCD for preoperative chemotherapy, replaced HDMTX by CPL in patients responding poorly to the initial treatment, and claimed a disease-free survival rate approaching that of good responders for such patients (13). These encouraging results led us to question if all patients need the same aggressive DOX-containing therapy, or if it is sufficient to start with a less toxic treatment and to switch to a more aggressive therapy only in the case of poor response. Study COSS-82 followed such a strategy, and one-half of the patients received only BCD and HDMTX prior to surgery. Patients of the control arm were treated aggressively from the very beginning with a DOX/CPL combination, followed three weeks later by two HDMTX infusions weekly times two. As expected, the response rate after BCD and HDMTX was found to be significantly inferior to the DOX/CPL-HDMTX arm (26% vs. 60% > 90% TCD, p < 0.01). Salvage therapy for patients from the BCD-HDMTX branch consisted of a DOX/CPL combination, and for the DOX/CPL-HDMTX branch of BCD once every two weeks alternating with a CPL/IFO combination. However, the calculated MFS-rate of poor responders after neither the BCD-HDMTX branch nor the DOX/CPL-HDMTX branch was improved when compared to poor responders from study COSS-80 with unchanged postoperative chemotherapy (Fig. 2), indicating a failure of the employed salvage strategy in general and especially of the effort to restrict the use of the very effective but highly toxic drugs DOX and CPL to patients resistant to a less toxic initial treatment (14,15). Altogether, our results indicate that it may be difficult to markedly increase the rate of 60 to 70% long-term-metastases-free survivors in osteosarcoma if no additional and more effective drugs become available. For the time being, the most promising approach would seem to be to add an active drug like IFO as early as possible to an approved regimen of DOX, HDMTX and CPL or BCD without compromising either dosages or dose rates.

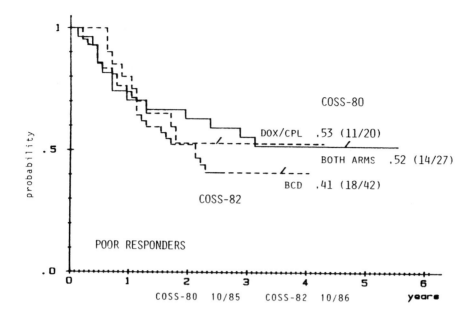

FIGURE 2: Actuarial MFS-rate of poor responders from the osteosarcoma study COSS-82 after aggressive (DOX/CPL) vs. mild (BCD) preoperative chemotherapy and postsurgical salvage chemotherapy (dashed lines) as compared to the MFS-rate of poor responders from study COSS-80 with unchanged postsurgical chemotherapy (solid line).

In the ongoing study, COSS-86 patients are stratified into a low risk and a high risk arm. High risk patients are defined by large tumors and/or insufficient decrease of bone scan activity after DOX and HDMTX and/or more than 20% chondroid groundsubstance formation in the biopsy specimen, which was found correlated to poor response after preoperative chemotherapy (16). Following DOX and HDMTX high risk patients receive the two-drug combination CPL/IFO whereas low risk patients receive CPL only. In addition, high risk patients are randomized for intra-arterial vs. intravenous CPL to increase local tumor control and to reduce the extent of surgery. A very preliminary analysis shows a $\geq$90% TCD in 9/11 low risk patients vs. 9/21 high risk patients after i. v. vs. 9/15 high risk patients after i. a. CPL treatment, indicating a higher local efficacy of i. a. CPL. The CPL content of tumor tissue, however, was not found substantially different. The impact of improved tumor response after locally intensified chemotherapy on the rate of pulmonary metastases has to be awaited.

REFERENCES

1. Rosen G et al.: Cancer 35:936-945, 1975.
2. Winkler K, Becker W, Kotz R et al.: Chemioter Oncol 2:225-228, 1978.
3. Winkler K, Beron G et al.: Klin Pädiatrie 194:251-256, 1982.
4. Purfürst C, Beron G et al.: Klin Pädiat 197:233-238, 1985.
5. Mosende C, Gutierrez M et al.: Cancer 40:2779-2786, 1977.
6. Rosen G et al.: Natl Cancer Inst Monograph 56:213-220, 1981.
7. Winkler K, Beron G et al.: J Clin Oncol 2:617-624, 1984.
8. Link MP: Important Advances in Oncology, pp.193-207, 1986.
9. Winkler K, Beron G, Kotz R et al.: Management of Soft Tissue and Bone Sarcomas, New York, Raven Press, pp.275-288, 1986.
10. Knop J, Stritzke P, Montz R et al.: Nucl Med 24:75-81, 1985.
11. Winkler K et al.: Proceedings American Society of Clin Oncol 6:220, 1987.
12. Winkler K, Beron G et al.: Verh Dtsch Krebsges 5:791-799, 1984.
13. Rosen G et al: Cancer 49:1221-1230, 1982.
14. Winkler K et al.: Proceedings American Soc of Clin Oncol 5:128, 1986.
15. Winkler K, Beron G, Delling G et al.: J Clin Oncol, submitted.
16. Delling G, Winkler K et al.: SICOT 87 Abstr. 296, 1987.

THE EXPERIENCE OF T10 PROTOCOL IN THE PEDIATRIC DEPARTMENT OF THE GUSTAVE ROUSSY INSTITUTE

C. Kalifa[1], N. Mlika[2], J. DuBousset[3], G. Contesso[4], D. Vanel[5], J. Lumbroso[6]

In 1981, the pediatric department of the Gustave Roussy Institute adopted the T10 protocol for the treatment of osteosarcomas.

I. Protocol

The schedule of the protocol is summarized in Figure 1. There are two minor differences with the original T10 design by Rosen (1): 1) The preoperative chemotherapy includes 7 perfusions of high dose methotrexate (HDMTX) instead of 8, and 2) Surgery, amputation or limb-preservation, takes place after the completion of initial chemotherapy instead of performing amputation after only 4 perfusions of methotrexate.

The modalities of the administration of HDMTX are exactly those described by Rosen. The dose of methotrexate is 8 gm/m2 before puberty and 12 gm/m2 after puberty. Intravenous sodium bicarbonate is given before and during the infusion of the methotrexate. This one is delivered for 4 hours in one liter of 5% dextrose in water. Beginning 20 hours from the start of the methotrexate infusion, calcium leucovorin is administered orally every 6 hours for 10 doses of 10 mg. Oral sodium bicarbonate is also given for 3 days following the methotrexate infusion at the dose of 2-3 meq/kg/24 hours in 4 divided doses. Patients are asked to drink enough to have a 24-hours urine output of 1.6l/m2 on day 1 and 2l/m2 on days 2 and 3 following the HDMTX infusion. Intravenous hydration is realized only in patients who are not able to drink.

The initial extension of the disease was assessed by standard x-rays and CTS of the primary tumor, standard x-rays

---

[1]Department of Pediatrics, Gustave Roussy Institute, Villejuif, France.

[2]Department of Statistics, Gustave Roussy Institute, Villejuif, France.

[3]Department of Surgery, Saint Vincent de Paul Hospital, Paris, France.

[4]Department of Pathology, Gustave Roussy Institute, Villejuif, France.

[5]Department of Radiology, Gustave Roussy Institute, Villejuif, France.

[6]Department of Nuclear Medicine, Gustave Roussy Institute, Villejuif, France

J. R. Ryan and L. O. Baker (eds.), Recent Concepts in Sarcoma Treatment, 301–305.
© 1988 by Kluwer Academic Publishers.

302

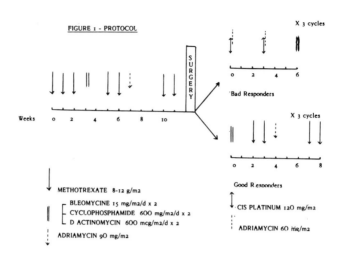

FIGURE 1 - PROTOCOL

X 3 cycles

Bad Responders

X 3 cycles

Weeks   0   2   4   6   8   10

Good Responders

METHOTREXATE 8-12 g/m2

BLEOMYCINE 15 mg/m2/d x 2
CYCLOPHOSPHAMIDE 600 mg/m2/d x 2
D ACTINOMYCIN 600 mcg/m2/d x 2

ADRIAMYCIN 90 mg/m2

CIS PLATINUM 120 mg/m2

ADRIAMYCIN 60 mg/m2

FIGURE 1

and CTS of the lungs, and bone technetium scintigraphy. Patients with a normal chest x-ray but with a suspicion of lung metastasis on CTS only, are still included in the study.

II. Materials

The 60 patients presented here received the completion of the chemotherapy in our department - except some injections of adriamycin or BCD - and had surgery performed by a single surgeon. They were treated between April 1981 and September 1986. During the same period, 32 other patients were referred to our department but are not included in this study for the following reasons: 12 had an initial amputation, 14 had metastases at diagnosis and 6 were partly treated in another institution.

There are 33 males and 27 females, aged 4 to 19 years (median 12 years).

The location of the tumor was: femur 35, tibia 19, fibula 2, humerus 4. The height of the tumor, measured on CTS, was 5 to 29 cm (median 12 cm). The delay between the biopsy and the beginning of the chemotherapy was 3 to 48 days (median 12 days).

III. Toxicity

HDMTX and citrovorum factor rescue were generally well tolerated in spite of some episodes of mucositis. Some transitory hepatic transaminase elevations were seen as usual after the perfusion of HDMTX. Benign seizures occurred during the first weeks of treatment in 3 patients, but the chemotherapy was continued. The postoperative chemotherapy was interrupted in only one patient who had hypodensity of the cerebral white matter on CTS and NMR without clinical signs. He is still in remission with normalized CTS and NMR 18 months later.

One good responder died of a pneumonitis with cardiac failure during the aplasia following the last BCD. Another patient had a pneumonitis due to pneumocystis Carinii and recovered. One patient presented a cardiac failure due to adriamycin. He is now in a good condition with medical treatment 10 months after the acute accident.

No unusual toxicity was observed in relation to Cisplatinum. One infection of an endoprosthesis of the knee occurred. It was treated by surgical washing and antibiotics.

IV. Results

During the preoperative chemotherapy, the size of the primary tumor decreased clinically in 43 patients, remained stable in 12 patients, increased in 3 patients, and was not evaluable in 2 patients. Surgical procedures were limb sparings in 49 patients, amputations in 10, and Van Ness rotation plasty in 1. The reasons to perform amputations were the progression of the tumor during chemotherapy, the young age of the patient, and the location or extension of the tumor.

The histological examination of the primary tumor after surgery was performed according to Huvos' grading (2). The distinction between bad and good responders is more or less than 5% residual viable cells. We have observed:

27 bad responders (2 Grade I and 25 Grade II)
33 good responders (16 Grade III and 17 Grade IV).

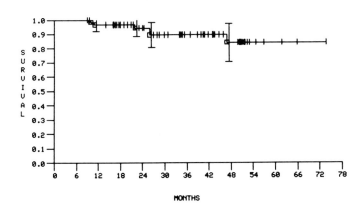

OSTEOSARCOMA (60 patients)

MONTHS

FIGURE 2

304

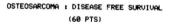

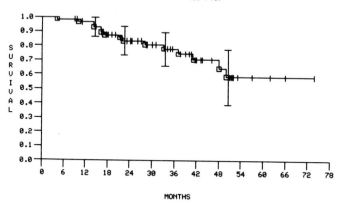

FIGURE 3

The chemotherapy was restarted between 3 and 46 days after surgery as described in the protocol, depending on the histological response.

The median follow-up of these 60 patients is 28 months.

Six patients died, 5 of disease and 1 of toxicity. The overall survival is 85% (Figure 2) and the disease-free survival is 58% (Figure 3) at 48 months. Fourteen patients have relapsed (9 bad responders and 5 good responders). The site of relapses are lungs in 9 patients, bones in 3 patients, smooth tissues in 1. After treatment of the relapses, 5 patients are in second remission since 4, 4, 4, 22, 30 months. No local relapse has been observed in this series. The disease-free survival is 75% for good responders and 32% for bad responders (Figure 4).

V. Conclusion

These results represent an important improvement of the prognosis of osteosarcomas as compared with our previous experience, but they are not as good as those obtained by Rosen. Namely, the rescue of the bad responders to HDMTX by Cis-platinum in this series was not as obvious as it was in Rosen's publication.

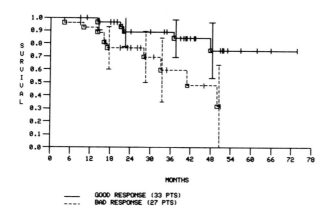

OSTEOSARCOMA : DISEASE FREE SURVIVAL

GOOD RESPONSE (33 PTS)
BAD RESPONSE (27 PTS)

FIGURE 4

REFERENCES

1. Rosen G, Caparros B, Huvos AG, et al.: Preoperative chemotherapy for osteogenic sarcoma: selection of post-operative adjuvant chemotherapy based on the response of the primary tumor to preoperative chemotherapy. Cancer 49:1221-1230, 1982.
2. Huvos AG, Rosen G, Marcove RC: Primary osteogenic sarcoma. Pathologic aspects in 20 patients after treatment with chemotherapy, en bloc resection and prosthetic bone replacement. Arch Path Lab Med 101:14-18, 1977.

ADJUVANT TREATMENT WITH RADIOTHERAPY TO THE LUNGS AND/OR CHEMOTHERAPY FOR OSTEOSARCOMA OF THE LIMBS[*]

J.M.V. Burgers, M.D. Ph.D.[1], M. van Glabbeke, Ph.D.[2],
C. Kalifa, M.D.[3], P.A. Voute, M.D. Ph.D.[4],
A. van Oosterom, M.D. Ph.D.[5], A. Busson, M.D.[6],
P. Cohen, Ph.D.[7], A. Mazabraud, M.D.[8]

Before the introduction of intensive high dose chemotherapy, adjuvant treatment did not seem feasible for osteosarcoma with the known chemotherapeutic agents. The metastatic rate for tumors in the limbs was as high as 70% in the first year after definitive surgery and practically all these metastases were situated in the lungs. In Marcove's material (8), a bone lesion as first metastasis occurred only in 6% of the total group. In Cohen's review (6) of the Dutch Bone Tumour Committee material, 24/167 = 13% of cases, developed bone metastases, but only in three patients they were not accompanied by lung lesions. It is then logical to investigate the possibilities of radiotherapy to the lungs as a locally directed adjuvant treatment.

Abbatucci (1) and Breur (2) measured growth rate and radiosensitivity of osteosarcoma lung metastases. They concluded that a tolerable dose to the lung, 20 Gy including air correction, would be able to sterilize subclinical metastases up to the size of 10^4-10^5 cells. Further, they calculated from back extrapolation of growth rates that metastases up to that size would occur in 20% of patients at the moment of treatment of the primary tumor.

On this basis, an OERTC trial was instituted in 1970, where patients with osteosarcoma of the limbs after definitive treatment of the primary with surgery or radiotherapy, were randomized to receive adjuvant radiotherapy to the lungs. A dose of 17,50 Gy without air correction was given in

----
[1]The Netherlands Cancer Institute, Dept. of Radiotherapy, Antoni van Leeuwenhoekhuis, Plesmanlaan 121, 1066 CX, Amsterdam, The Netherlands.
[2]EORTC Data Centre, Brussels
[3]Chemotherapy Committee, Institut Gustave Roussy, Villejuif
[4]Emma Kinderziekenhuis, Amsterdam
[5]Academic Hospital, Leiden
[6]Centre F. Baclesse, Caen
[7]Radiodiagnostic Committee, The Netherlands Cancer Institute, Amsterdam
[8]Pathology Committee, Institut Curie, Paris

----
[*]EORTC/SIOP Trial 20781.

J. R. Ryan and L. O. Baker (eds.), Recent Concepts in Sarcoma Treatment, 306–312.
© 1988 by Kluwer Academic Publishers.

10 fractions in 2 weeks. The trial collected 86 patients and had to be stopped in 1975 in the light of the new developments in adjuvant chemotherapy. The results were published by Breur et al. in 1978 (3), and have recently been updated. (4)

The disease-free survival at 5 years is 28% and 41%, respectively for the observed and the treated group and survival is 37% and 45%, respectively (not significant). For the 60 patients below 16 years, disease-free survival was 31% and 50%, respectively (p = 0.074).

After some discussion, a new trial, again limited to patients with osteosarcoma of the limbs below 30 years of age, was instituted in 1978 by the OERTC together with the SIOP, comparing adjuvant chemotherapy with radiotherapy to the lungs or a combination of these. The primary treatment consisted of ablative surgery or high dose radiotherapy. Adjuvant treatment had to be instituted within 4 weeks of biopsy. It consisted of either:

a) 3 months induction treatment: Vincristine (VCR) 1.5 mg/m^2 and Methotrexate (MTX) 6 g/m^2 with leucovorin rescue, were alternated every 2 weeks with Adriamycine (ADR) 70 mg/m^2, followed by a 6 months consolidation treatment: Cyclophosphamide 1.2 g/m^2 every 4 weeks alternated with either ADR or MTX -VCR - leucovorin at mid-interval (Figure 1);

b) elective irradiation to the lungs, 20 Gy including air correction over 2 weeks with megavoltage equipment;

c) induction as in a) followed by irradiation as in b).

From 1978 to 1983, 205 eligible and evaluable patients were registered by 45 European centers. The mean follow-up is now 49 months. The survival results are shown in Figures 2 and 3. At a short follow-up period of 1-2 years, there seemed

Weeks		Induction					Consolidation		
	1	3	5	7	9	11	13	15	17
CFA											
ADRIA											
VCR/MTX/CF											

Cycles of consolidation chemotherapy to be given for a total of 4 times, up to week 41.

Methotrexate	6000 mg/m^2/6 hour infusion	MTX
Citrovorum factor	15 mg/6 hour/x 12	CF
Vincristin	1.5 mg/m^2/i.v. (max. 2 mg)	VCR
Adriamycin	70 mg/m^2/i.v.	ADRIA
Cyclophophamide	1200 mg/m^2/i.v.	CFA

FIGURE 1

308

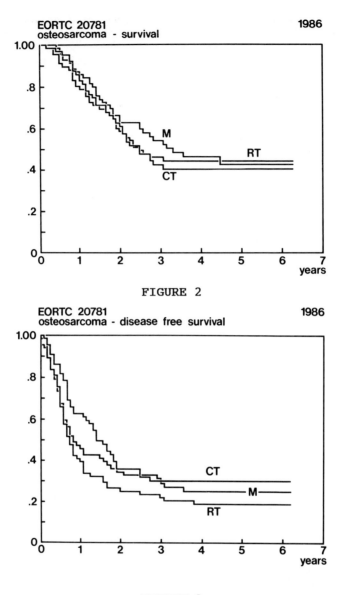

FIGURE 2

FIGURE 3

to be some disadvantage in disease-free survival for the
irradiated group, but this effect was not maintained and it
stabilized at 4 years around 24%. Survival was equal for the
3 treatment groups at 43%. In the chemotherapy arms, 3 toxic
deaths occurred. In the chemotherapy arm (a) late hematological toxicity was still reported in 31% and cardiac toxicity
in 5%, while in the combined treatment arm (c) these figures

were 4% and 1.5%, respectively. As for lung function, this
was decreased in 5% of patients of the chemotherapy arm, in
10% after adjuvant lung irradiation and in 12% after mixed
adjuvant treatment.

This trial therefore showed no advantage of the chemotherapy schedule as acceptable in 1978, over radiotherapy of
the lungs, however, with greater toxicity. Further, it seems
that treatment of metastases can be successful in a small
subgroup.

The many controversies over the best approach in the
management of osteosarcoma have been discussed by Link in
1986. (7) He points to the fact that widely differing survival figures are reported for seemingly comparable, though
relatively small patient series. We have, therefore, carefully examined the patient material of this trial in search for
prognostic factors or other aspects that might offer explana-
tions for these discrepancies.

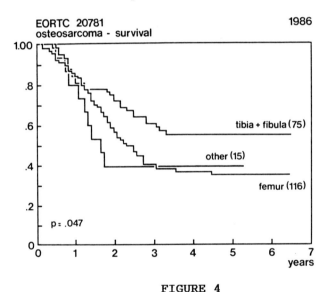

FIGURE 4

As shown in Figure 4, tibia localizations had a better
prognosis then femur lesions, survival respectively 56% and
38%, significant at p = 0.047. The same trend was also reported by Marcove (8). The influence of age was borderline
significant, with survival at 51% for patients above 15 years
and 38% for the younger patients (p = 0.055). There is,
however, a correlation between site and age, as patients with
femur localizations are significantly younger (p = 0.026).
Sex, age and localization are given in Table 1. In our material tumor size was reported by clinical measurements and by
size in the roentgenographic diagnostic films. These did not
show a correlation with prognosis, in contrast with the
German study (10), where size, reported as smaller than one-

third of the bone length, 1/3 - 1/2 or larger than 1/2, correlated to prognosis. However, 16 patients in our study had large tumors over 200 cm.^{3}, of whom 9 were over 15 years, 7 remained free of metastases and 11 survived (73%). Apparently, when such a large tumor develops without producing metastases, its course is relatively benign.

TABLE 1

Osteosarcoma 20781	AGE, SEX AND AFFECTED BONE		
	1-10 yrs.	11-15 yrs.	16+ yrs.
Male	17	52	57
Female	15	37	27
Femur	23	52	40
Tibia	7	29	31
Fibula	1	2	5
Humerus and Radius	1	6	8

The roentgenographic diagnostic films were studied for Codman's triangles: more frequent at younger age, but without significant bearing on prognosis, and for spiculae and lamellae, which were associated with a lower incidence of metastases.

Most of the pathology slides were centrally reviewed and common type osteosarcoma was seen in 150 of 178 cases. Of the 5 patients with a mixed chondro-osteoid pattern, none died, but both patients with teleangiectatic type died. Further, of the 15 patients with anaplastic features, 7 died.

The pattern of relapse was studied in relation to the type of treatment. Local failure occurred in 16%, 10% after primary amputation, and 43% after primary radiotherapy. Only 6% were isolated local recurrences without metastases. Radiotherapy of the primary tumor further led to severe dysfunction in 8/23 = 35% of cases without local recurrence. Three of these, all in the chemotherapy arms, had to be amputated.

The ratio of bone or lung metastases was not different in the 3 adjuvant treatment arms, being 24% and 62% as a first metastasis in the whole patient group. Compared to the reports by Marcove (8) and Cohen (6), the incidence of bone metastases seems to have increased with the newer treatment modalities. Also, apparently, the chemotherapy used in this trial decreases the appearance of lung metastases more effectively than the development of bone metastases.

The pattern of lung metastases has been examined by Busson (5). Up until now, not enough material has been reviewed for a definitive conclusion. There is an impression that in the radiotherapy arms, the number of metastases, when appearing, is more limited. Further, in the chemotherapy arm a) lung metastases seem to be spread out over the whole lung parenchyma, while in the radiotherapy arms, they seem to be

more frequent behind the heart, mediastinum and diaphragm. In
these areas, the dose of radiation is lower because of these
non-air containing structures.

The treatment of metastases was successful only when
further surgery was possible, as shown in Figure 5. In 50
cases, thoracotomy was undertaken and in 32 (64%) resection
was recorded as complete, divided over the adjuvant treatment
arms as follows: 8/15 after chemotherapy, 14/19 after radiotherapy, and 10/12 after mixed treatment. In 4 cases, the
result of the resection was unknown. There is no information
about second or further metastatectomies.

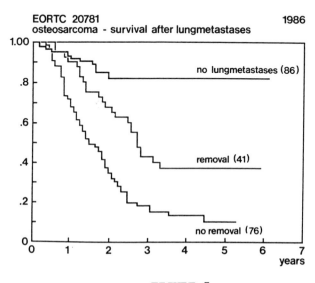

FIGURE 5

Nowadays, the treatment of osteosarcoma of the limbs has
greatly progressed and very favorable results have been
reported. Limb-saving surgery is possible in a number of
patients. At a short follow-up interval, the metastatic rate
is very low. The early toxic cost of the modern chemotherapy
schedules with Cisplatin combined with Adriamycine and/or
Methotrexate or other agents is high. Of the late morbidity,
little is known as yet.

Not all patients do well, however, with those intensive
schedules. Evaluation of the tumor viability in the surgical
specimen after neoadjuvant treatment shows that in 30-50% of
cases, a considerable amount (more than 10%) of viable tumor
tissue is still present. These patients also have a high
metastatic rate (9, 10).

The German studies try to identify presurgical characteristics of such a bad prognosis and to intensify treatment on this basis. The pathological evaluation of the specimen is indeed very time consuming and carries a high work-
load.

For these patients who are not showing a favorable response to current chemotherapy, radiotherapy to the lungs should be re-evaluated.

REFERENCES

1. Abbatucci JS, Quint R, Brune D, Fourre D, Urbajtel M: Place de la radiotherapie dans le traitement des metastases pulmonaires. Irradiation de necessite et irradiation systematiquement prevu. J Radiol Electrol 51:525-529, 1970.
2. Breur K: Growth rate and radiosensitivity of human tumours. European J Cancer 2:157-171, 1966.
3. Breur K, Cohen P, Schweisguth O, and Hart AAM: Irradiation of the lungs as an adjuvant therapy in the treatment of osteosarcoma of the limbs. An OERTC randomized study. European J Cancer 14:461-471, 1978.
4. Burgers JMV, van Glabbeke M, Busson A, et al.: Osteosarcoma of the limbs: report on the EORTC/SIOP Trial 20781, investigating the value of adjuvant treatment with chemotherapy and/or prophylactic lung irradiation (03). Cancer 1988 (in press).
5. Busson A: Personal communication.
6. Cohen P: Osteosarcoma of the long bones - clinical observations and experiences in the Netherlands. European J Cancer 14:995-1004, 1976.
7. Link MP: Adjuvant therapy in the treatment of osteosarcoma. In: Important Advances in Oncology 1986. De Vita, Hellman and Rosenberg (eds.), JB Lippincott, pp. 193-207, 1986.
8. Marcove RC, Mike V, Hajek JV, Levin AG, Hutter RVP: Osteogenic sarcoma under the age of twenty-one. J Bone Joint Surg 52A:411-423, 1970.
9. Rosen G, Marcove RC, Huvos AG, et al.: Primary osteogenic sarcoma: eight year experience with adjuvant chemotherapy. J Cancer Res Clin Oncol 2:617-624, 1984.
10. Winkler K, Bern G, Kotz R et al.: Neoadjuvant chemotherapy of osteogenic sarcoma: result of a cooperative German/Austrian study. J Clin Oncol 106 Suppl:55-67, 1984.

OSTEOSARCOMA - JAPANESE EXPERIENCE

Kiyoo Furuse, M.D.*

The incidence of osteosarcoma (OS) is 1/100,000-200,000 in the Japanese population. About 200 patients with OS are registered at the National Cancer Center Hospital (NCCH) every year.(1) Of malignant primary bone tumors, OS carries the highest percentage in incidence (ca. 43%), and is most likely to occur between the ages of 10 and 30; 60% are young adults in their 20's, with a slight predominance of males. Before 1970, therapeutic results of OS were very disappointing in Japan. Because of pulmonary metastases in more than 90% of patients within one year from ablative surgery, the 5-year survival rate was 5 to 15%, in spite of various treatment efforts.(2) In 1960, Miki (3) introduced a regional perfusion technique using anticancer agents before limb amputation, originally described by Creech et al.(4) in 1958. (Anticancer agents were circulated in the affected limb before amputation via an extra-corporeal circulation system.) Tateishi reported that the 5-year survival rate for 101 patients treated with this regimen was significantly increased to 35% from 17% over patients treated with ablative surgery alone.(5) In 1966, Akaboshi (6) introduced intra-arterial infusion of anticancer drugs with a chronometric infusor (Sullivan (7)). Five or 6 weeks after a 3- to 4-week period of infusion of drugs, ablative surgery was performed. The 5-year survival rate (31%) of 57 treated patients was significantly higher than that of patients not treated.(6)

The prognosis of OS gradually improved with adjuvant preoperative chemotherapy, and has been improving more quickly since the advent of multidisciplinary treatment in the late 70's.(2) This paper focuses on the treatment for classical OS in two large series in Japan; both were nonrandomized retrospective studies.

Treatment for OS by the Japanese Orthopedic Oncology Group (JOOG) (8)

JOOG consists of 10 Japanese orthopedic institutes. Of 176 patients with classical OS of the limbs treated by JOOG between 1973 and 1980, 117 patients received adjuvant chemotherapy after limb-ablative surgery; 59 were excluded because of distant metastasis at the start of chemotherapy. All 117 patients (70 males and 47 females, age 7 to 68 years, with a

---

*Department of Orthopedic Surgery, Tottori University School of Medicine, Yonago 683, JAPAN.

313

J. R. Ryan and L. O. Baker (eds.), Recent Concepts in Sarcoma Treatment, 313–319.
© 1988 by Kluwer Academic Publishers.

mean of 16 years) were treated with radical surgery. The sites of the primary lesions were the femur, tibia, humerus, fibula and radius, respectively in 67, 30, 14, 5 and 1 patient(s). Radiographically, the primary lesion was of the mixed type (osteolytic/sclerotic) in 64 patients, sclerotic type in 29, osteolytic type in 18, and unknown in 6. Histologically, the primary lesion was of the osteoblastic type in 84 patients, chondroblastic type in 9, fibroblastic type in 7, undifferentiated type in 3, angioblastic type in 1, and unknown in 13.

Of the 117 patients treated preoperatively, 71 had chemotherapy in the form of regional perfusion (RP), intra-arterial (IA) infusion in 52 patients, and intravenous (IV) administration in 19. Eighty were given adriamycin (ADR) alone (ADR group), and 37 ADR plus high-dose methotrexate (HDMTX) and other anticancer drugs (multi-drug group). In the latter, 75.7% of patients were treated only with ADR+HDMTX. ADR, particularly in the ADR group, was administered by the IV route at 0.6-0.8 mg/kg/day for 3 consecutive days monthly once the wound had healed. In both groups, the administration of ADR was continued until the cumulative dose totaled a level equal to 600 mg/body or 500 mg/m^2. HDMTX was generally administered by 200 mg/kg with 6-hour continuous IV infusion. Adjuvant chemotherapy was completed 18 months after radical surgery unless distant metastases were found.

As of July 1985, 53 patients were alive (follow-up period 60 to 137 months, mean 90 months): 43 of the 53 had no evidence of disease, and 10 had evidence. The remaining 64 patients were dead: 59 of the 64 died of OS, and 5 of other diseases (follow-up period 3 to 73 months, mean 20 months). The 5-year cumulative survival and continuous disease-free survival rates were 50.2% and 39.4% in the whole patients (Figure 1), 63.1% and 47.8% in the multi-drug group, and 44.4% and 35.6% in the ADR group, respectively. Both survival rates did not differ significantly between the multi-drug and

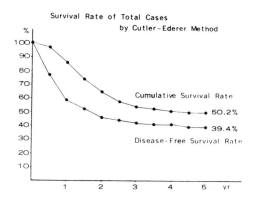

FIGURE 1.

ADR groups, although the site of primary lesions differed slightly in incidence between the groups (78% vs. 48% in the femur and 8% vs. 34% in the tibia).

The effects of preoperative adjuvant chemotherapy on the survival rate were analyzed. The 5-year cumulative survival rate for 71 patients receiving and 46 not receiving the therapy was 46.6% and 55.9%, respectively. Preoperative adjuvant chemotherapy did not influence the survival rate. The total cumulative dose of ADR was clearly correlated with the survival rate. The 5-year cumulative survival rate differed significantly between the ADR group of 500 mg and over (67 patients, 59.3%) and the ADR Group of less than 500 mg (50 patients, 36.9%) (P <0.05 by the generalized Wilcoxon test) (Figure 2). The 67 patients (ADR > 500 mg) could be subdivided into multi-drug (17 patients, 76.5%) and ADR (50 patients, 52.1%) groups. The 5-year cumulative survival rate significantly differed between the groups (P <0.01).

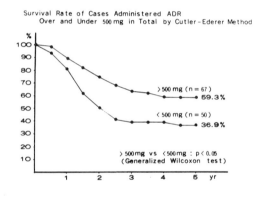

FIGURE 2.

It was difficult to find a clear correlation between the total cumulative dose of MTX and the survival rate because of the lack of complete data. The total dose was more than 20 g in 11 patients, lower than 20 g in 17, and unknown in 9. The 5-year survival rate between the groups, 72.7%, 55.7% and 66.7%, was not significant.

In follow-up studies of 66 patients who developed pulmonary metastases, their prognosis was apparently improved with thoracotomy. The 5-year survival rate differed significantly between groups treated (23 patients, 43.5%) and not treated (43 patients, 2.6%) with thoracotomy (P <0.01).

Limb-Salvage Treatment for OS by the Orthopedic Oncology Study Group (OOSG) (9)

The OOSG, consisting of 6 Japanese institutes, studied limb-salvage treatment for 225 patients with nonmetastatic and classical OS of the limbs at diagnosis. They were treated with systemic chemotherapy between 1973 and 1986: 72 (32%) received limb-salvage treatment and 153 (68%), ablative surgery. The first case of limb-salvage treatment in this study was registered in 1975. During the latest 5-year, except 1984, over 50% of evaluable patients have received limb-salvage treatment. For the purposes of analysis, the patients were subdivided into the limb-salvaged (LS) group (72 patients) and limb-amputated (LA) group (153 patients). The 5-year cumulative survival rates of the whole, LA and LS groups were 54.6%, 51.3% and 62.1%, respectively; and the 10-year cumulative survival rates were 49.3%, 46.4% and 55.6%, respectively. Statistical analysis showed no significant differences among the three groups (Figure 3).

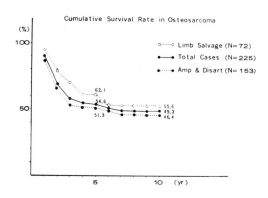

FIGURE 3.

All adjuvant chemotherapy patients were divided into 3 groups (except for 34 who were unclassifiable): 21 patients were given ADR alone (ADR group); 108 were given ADR and HDMTX (ADR+MTX group); and 62 were given carcinostatics combined with cisplatin (CDDP) (+CDDP group). The 5-year cumulative survival rates of the ADR, ADR+MTX and +CDDP groups were 15.1%, 62.4%, and 57.3%, respectively. There was a significant difference ($P < 0.001$) between the ADR group and either the ADR+MTX or +CDDP group. The 10-year cumulative survival rates of the ADR and ADR+MTX groups (10.1% and 57.5%) showed an intergroup significant difference ($P < 0.001$). There was a significant difference between the +CDDP and ADR groups in the 8-year cumulative survival rates (57.3% and 10.1%) (Figure 4) Differing from the results obtained by the JOOG, the OOSG reported significantly higher survival level for the multi-drug (ADR+MTX and +CDDP) groups than for the ADR group. The difference may be due to a greater number of patients being treated with multi-drug chemotherapy and fewer patients being treated with ADR alone in the study by the OOSG.

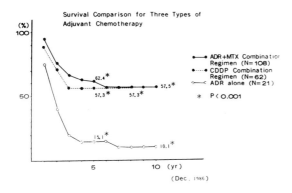

FIGURE 4.

Distant metastases appeared in 112/225 (49.5%), and the 5- and 10-year cumulative survival rates of the 112 were 21.7% and 15.8%, respectively. Of the 112, 61 (54.5%) were treated with thoracotomy, and 51 (45.5%), palliatively. The 5-year cumulative survival rates differed significantly (P <0.01) between the thoracotomy-treated (33.5%) and palliatively treated (7.6%) patients.

Complications appeared in 38/72 (52.8%) of the LS group: 14 (36.8%) of the 38 underwent further ablative surgery due to local recurrence (8 patients), infection (4) and circulatory disturbance (2). Of the whole 72, local recurrence occurred in 9 (12.5%): 6 of the 9 died of OS, 1 was alive with evidence of disease, and 2 were alive without evidence of disease. Local recurrence after limb-salvage surgery was a sign of poor prognosis. When classified according to site of the primary (fibula, humerus, femur and tibia), the incidences of complications was 75.0%, 53.0%, 51.0% and 50.0%; the incidences of secondary ablation due to complication after limb-salvage surgery were 33.0%, 38.0%, 28.0% and 56.0%; the incidence of local recurrence due to secondary ablation was 100%, 100%, 60% and 20%, respectively.

Current Status and Future Problems in Japan:

Western researchers have reported a clear correlation between the prognosis of OS and the tumor necrotic ratio. (10-13) In Japan, 32 patients with nonmetastatic classical OS of the femur and tibia, treated between 1976 and 1984, were described by Hamada and coworkers (14) in 1986: 4 patients were treated only with IA-administered ADR; 16 with Protocol A (2 preoperative IA courses of ADR in 0.6-0.8 mg/kg/day for 3 consecutive days and 2 doses of HDMTX in 100-200 mg/kg/wk); and 12 with Protocol B (2 preoperative IA courses of ADR in 1.0-1.2 mg/kg/day for 2 consecutive days, together with IV-given CDDP in 100-120 mg/m^2 and 2 doses of HDMTX in 300 mg/kg/wk).

The 5-year survival and 5-year disease-free survival rates of the 32 patients were 56% and 35%, respectively. Hamada and workers assessed the tumor necrotic ratio on the max cut surface of tumor in 29 patients receiving chemotherapy both pre- and postoperatively. In 11 patients (37.9%) with good response in tumor necrotic ration (90% or more), the 5-year disease-free survival rate was 66%; whereas in 18 patients (62.1%) with poor response (less than 90%), the survival rate was 8%. Hamada and workers also compared tumor response to preoperative chemotherapy between the 2 groups of Protocols A and B. Good responses were observed in 3/16 (19%) of Group A and 8/11 (73%) of Group B. Further, they showed a close correlation between the tumor necrotic ratio and angiographic responses.

In summarization of the results of treatment for OS in our Department since 1983 (15) (Figure 5), preoperative chemotherapy was classified by the route of drug administration into 3 groups: IA, RP and IV. The survival rate in OS exceeded 50% in Japan, irrespective of the administration route, where using multi-drug chemotherapy (mainly ADR and HDMTX). Current effort is directed toward the assessment of tumor responses to preoperative chemotherapy, with clinicopathological parameters, including imaging techniques (by radiography, computed tomography, angiography, isotope scanning and thermography), serum alkaline phosphatase and tumor necrotic ratio. The assessment of tumor responses with such parameters has correlated definitely with the prognosis of OS. However, criteria for effective tumor responses to preoperative chemotherapy using clinical parameters are not yet established.

Treatment Results of Osteosarcoma in Japan

Reporter	Radiotherapy	i.a.[1]				r.p.[2]			i.v.[3]							Prognosis	
		5FU	MTX	ADR	CDDP	ADR	MMC	CDDP	VCR	HDMTX	ADR	CYT	CDDP	PCD	MMC	Cases	Survival(%)[*]
Tateischi (1985)						○	○			○	○					41	56.2
Takata (1985)	○[a]				○[b]	○[b]			○	○	○		○	○		51	64.8
Takeuchi (1985)		○	○						○		○		○		○	46	52.1
Takeyama (1985)					○[b]	○[c]	○[c]	○[c]		○	○		○[c]			13	76.7[c]
Yamawaki (1985)									○	○	○	○				12	75.0
Furuya (1985)									○	○	○	○				25	58.4[c]
Furuse (1985)									○	○	○	○				20	55.1
Fukuma (1985)									○	○	○	○				25	56.6

1) i.a. intraarterial infusion 2) r.p. regional perfusion 3) i.v. intravenous administration

*) 5 yr cumulative survival rate
a) only for cases indicated limb salvage treatment
b) administered with i.a. and/or i.v.
c) include cases with r.p. of ADR+MMC, or with r.p. of CDDP
d) shows 3 yr cumulative survival rate
e) shows survival rate at xi months after treatment

FIGURE 5.

An attempt to apply this preoperative assessment to postoperative chemotherapy has been started. One of our future problems would be to devise a successful protocol that produces good pathological responses exceeding Grade III proposed by Rosen (12), in more than half of cases treated, and that is indicated for patients with Grade II or below. Another would be to carry out a cooperative randomized study based on the protocol.

REFERENCES

1. Bone Tumor Committee, Japanese Orthopedic Association. Bone tumor registry in Japan. National Cancer Center Hospital, Tokyo, 1985 (in Japanese).
2. Furuse K, Maeyama I, et al.: In Kimura K and Wang Y-M (eds.) Methotrexate in Cancer Therapy. New York, Raven Press, 1986.
3. Miki I, Azuma H, et al.: Seikei Geka 15:87-97, 1964 (in Japanese).
4. Creech O, Krementz JF, et al.: Ann Surg 148:616-632, 1958.
5. Tateishi T: Seikei Saigai Geka 22:675-679, 1979 (in Japanese).
6. Akaboshi Y: Rinsho Seikei Geka 1:315-319, 1969 (in Japanese).
7. Sullivan RD, Miller E, Sykes MP: Cancer 12:1248-1262, 1959.
8. Japanese Orthopedic Oncology Group. Nippon Gan Chiryo Gakkaishi 22:261, 1987 (in Japanese).
9. Orthopedic Oncology Study Group: In Interim report on study by Grant-in-Aid for cancer research. National Cancer Center, Tokyo (in Japanese) (in press).
10. Picci, P, Bacci G, et al. Cancer 56:1515-1521, 1985.
11. Winkler K, Beron G, et al.: In van Oosterom AT and van Unnik JAM (eds.) Management of Soft Tissue and Bone Sarcomas, New York, Raven Press, pp. 275-288, 1986.
12. Rosen G: Recent Results Cancer Res 103:148-157, 1986.
13. Simon MA, Nachman J: J Bone Joint Surg 68A:1458-1463, 1986.
14. Hamada H, Aoki Y, et al.: Nippon Seikei Geka Gakkai Zasshi 60:73-83, 1986.
15. Maeyama I, Furuse K: Oncologia 20:92-98, 1987 (in Japanese).

NEW THERAPEUTIC DIRECTIONS IN SARCOMAS: BIOLOGIC AND CYTOTOXIC MODALITIES*

D. Goldstein, M.D.[1], and E. C. Borden, M.D.[1]**

Although advances have occurred in the management of osteosarcomas, progress in the treatment of adult soft tissue sarcomas continues to be frustrated by a paucity of effective systemic modalities. However, the propitious data with iphosphamide has already been reviewed and two doxorubicin analogues of promise are currently being tested. Several other new approaches await Phase II assessment. Finally, preclinical data has suggested a number of potential directions for clinical evaluation. Thus, the outlook for reduction in mortality from sarcomas is brighter than at any time in the past decade.

Cytotoxics

In the case of chemotherapy, two new doxorubicin analogues which are being evaluated are epirubicin and menogaril. Epirubicin studies, in a variety of malignancies, have suggested similar efficacy to doxorubicin.(1) Recently, a study was conducted in 22 sarcoma patients in conjunction with imidazole carboximide.(2) In 19 evaluable patients there were 2 CR and 7 PR for an overall 50% response rate, which appears to confirm its comparability to doxorubicin and offer the opportunity of prolonged use in responding patients because of reduced cardiac toxicity. Menogaril is a semi-synthetic anthracycline which has good oral systemic bio-availability, comparable to IV administration.(3) It differs both structurally and biologically from doxorubicin. In comparison to doxorubicin, it inhibits cells primarily in the G1/G2 rather than the S phase of the cell cycle. Only partial cross resistance exists for the two compounds and menogaril is at least 2.5 fold less cardiotoxic in experimental models. It is currently under study by the Eastern Cooperative Oncology Group in a Phase II trial.

Cisplatinum (CDDP), at conventional doses, has had little activity in soft tissue sarcomas.(4,5,6) Hypertonic saline has allowed, however, higher doses to be given without

---

[1]Departments of Human Oncology and Medicine, University of Wisconsin Clinical Cancer Center, 600 Highland Avenue, K4/662, Madison, WI 53792.

---

*Supported in part by CA21076.
**American Cancer Society Professor of Clinical Oncology.

320

J. R. Ryan and L. O. Baker (eds.), Recent Concepts in Sarcoma Treatment, 320–327.
© 1988 by Kluwer Academic Publishers.

increasing renal toxicity. This would appear to be particularly appropriate for soft tissue sarcomas which appear to
have a steep dose response curve to most chemotherapy agents.
Two recent sarcoma studies using this approach have both
suggested improved response over standard therapy. One study
(7) used CDDP as a single agent (40 mg/m^2/dx5) in 20 patients
with previous treatment. In 19 evaluable cases there were
four partial responses including one who had failed doxorubicin and one who failed standard CDDP doses. The second was in
sarcoma of the pelvis and was CDDP combined with DTIC. This
compared 10 patients with low dose (1 mg/kg) to 10 patients
given 20 mg/m^{2}x5. In the low dose group, there were 2
responses (1 CR and 1 PR) versus 5 (3 CR and 2 PR) in the
high dose group.(8). Thus, there are indications that
sarcomas may be responsive to CDDP in a dose responsive
manner.

Sensitizers

In addition to testing new drugs, several methods of
enhancing the cytotoxicity of existing agents are in various
stages of development. These may be particularly relevant to
sarcomas because of the steep dose response curve. One
approach has been to determine whether hypoxic cell sensitizers, such as misonidazole, can augment killing of tumor
cells. The therapeutic activity of alkylating agents has been
enhanced by the nitroheterocyclic sensitizers in almost every
tumor model studied. For example, a recent study using a
mouse sarcoma model showed enhancement of the cytotoxicity of
lomustine (CCNU) by 2 fold with little increase in toxicity
using a new compound - RSU 1069, which can be used at 1/10th
the dose of misonidazole.(9) At the University of Wisconsin
Clinical Cancer Center (UWCCC), a Phase I trial of SR2508 (a
hydrophilic nitroheterocyclic sensitizer) and cyclophosphamide has begun and one could envision a similar approach with
iphosphamide.

An alternative approach for enhancing response to chemotherapy has been the use of hyperthermia. Both local and
whole body approaches have been used. In murine models,
marked synergism has been demonstrated, particularly for
alkylating agents such as cyclophosphamide, carmustine
(BCNU), phenylalanine mustard, thiotepa (10), as well as more
recently, CDDP.(11) The problem with CDDP has been enhancement not only of antitumor effects but also toxicity, particularly renal.(11) Two new strategies give some cause for
optimism about the introduction of this combination into
clinical trials. One report has shown a 2.5 fold increase in
cytotoxic effect of the combination of whole body hyperthermia (WBH) and carboplatin.(12) Since this compound is
associated with less renal toxicity, it may be preferable.
There has also been a study of a biflavinoid venoruton in a
mouse model. This compound increased the therapeutic index of
CDDP by decreasing renal toxicity without altering the
increased tumor response of the WBH/CDDP combination.(13)

These preclinical findings are now being translated into
Phase I trials. Successful heating of deep-seated sarcomatous
lesions has been reported; 89.7% of the 42 lesions studied

showed an increase in temperature of > 42°C.(14)   Three
sarcoma Phase I trials have been reported. One used WBH and
BCNU in 19 previously treated sarcoma patients; 1 CR and 4 PR
were seen, for a 26% response rate. Cumulative thrombocytopenia was dose limiting.(15)   Two other studies used local
hyperthermia. One studied 12 patients and a total of 20
lesions, half of which were radiation failures. Patients
received either CDDP, bleomycin or combination cyclophosphamide, doxorubicin and DTIC; 4 lesions responded completely
and 6 partially.(16)   Another study used hyperthermic limb
perfusion prior to surgery. This was combined with intra-
arterial doxorubicin and allowed for a 100% limb salvage in
16 patients who were Stage III or IVA and would otherwise
have had amputation.(17)
     The use of hyperthermia in combination with interferons
has been studied at the UWCCC. Preclinical work has suggested
that WBH has synergy with interferons. A Phase I trial with
alpha interferon has subsequently shown synergy of biological
response parameters.(18)   A Phase II trial is currently being
planned in soft tissue sarcomas.

Biologicals

     The impact of biological therapy is only beginning to be
explored. In vitro studies have shown sensitivity to interferons in osteogenic sarcoma cell lines (19), murine osteogenic sarcomas (20) and, more recently, human osteosarcoma
xenografts.(21,22)   The earliest clinical use of interferon
was by Strander in the mid 1970's for adjuvant therapy of
osteosarcoma.(19)   He established both concurrent and historical controls and showed a trend toward improved survival in
the adjuvant group.(19)   There have been several subsequent
trials in metastatic soft tissue sarcoma. In a trial of
interferon beta, 20 patients were treated and only one partial response was seen.(23)   In a recombinant gamma trial, 16
patients were treated and no responses were noted.(24)   Most
recently, a Phase II trial of recombinant alpha-2a in advanced bone sarcomas showed three partial responses of short
duration in 20 patients.(25)   In vitro growth arrest, but no
growth inhibition, was noted with interferon alpha as a
single agent.(22)   A more recent study showed that although
alpha or gamma interferon as single agents gave only growth
arrest, when combined they caused both tumor reduction and
even disappearance.(26)   Synergism has also been reported for
a combination of recombinant beta and gamma interferon.(27)
Clinical investigation of interferon combinations in sarcoma
would appear to be indicated.
     Two other cytokines now entering clinical use are tumor
necrosis factor (TNF) and interleukin 2 (IL-2).   TNF is a
cytokine produced by activated monocytes and may indeed have
been first used clinically for sarcoma in the 1890's by
Coley.(28)   He used bacterial cell filtrates both locally and
systemically and reported responses in 70/137 inoperable
patients.(29)   In retrospect, he was probably administering
endotoxin and stimulating TNF release.(30)   The treatment
fell out of favor because of marked toxicity and the arrival
of radiotherapy and conservative surgery. TNF has now been

produced by recombinant technology and is currently in Phase I trials at several centers including the UWCCC. Much of the preclinical data have used mouse fibrosarcoma models. While recognizing that such tumors are not directly analogous to human sarcomas, they have provided several observations about antitumor activity. Although there was no effect on cells in vitro, when transplanted into the mouse, marked regressions of fibrosarcoma were seen with TNF.(31-34) A host-mediated effect has been postulated, and there is some evidence that this is via a specific effect on tumor vascularity.(31) Phase II trials in sarcoma should be able to be commenced in the next 1-2 years.

The combination of IL-2 and LAK (lymphokine activated killer) cells has been introduced into clinical trials. All of the preclinical work used mose sarcoma models in which the combination was highly effective.(35,36) However, the six sarcoma patients reported in the most recent update failed to respond, in contrast to responses seen in both renal carcinoma and melanoma.(37) The most interesting application of IL-2/LAK for sarcomas may well be in the neoadjuvant setting. An animal model (38) has demonstrated improved regression of hepatic metastases by local infusion. This type of treatment is readily adapted to limb sarcomas as evidenced by the effectiveness of CDDP in this form.(39)

The other biological agents, which may soon impact on sarcomas, are the monoclonal antibodies (mAb). Murine mAb have been tested for diagnostic purposes both _in_ _vitro_ (40) for histopathology, and _in vivo_ in a human soft tissue sarcoma xenograft model where a tumor to blood ratio of 12:1 was reported for Mab 19-24.(41,42) There are also several therapeutic studies showing inhibition of murine sarcoma (43) and a human osteosarcoma xenograft.(44) The latter study is particularly interesting as it reports on the use of an antibody, 791T/36, which was successfully conjugated to methotrexate. The conjugate gave substantially enhanced killing over methotrexate alone. Finally, an antiganglioside antibody 3F8 has been used in a Phase I trial. Patients who had failed prior therapy, two of whom had osteosarcoma, were treated intravenously with the monoclonal. All the patients showed alteration in visible lesions consistent with an antitumor response.(45)

Summary

We may expect the following developments in therapy of sarcomas. Sensitizers and hyperthermia will lead to increased drug effectiveness in sarcomas as tumors with steep dose response curves. More effective drugs, combined with surgery and radiation techniques such as hyperfractionation, will lead to improved response rates. Biological therapy may convert these higher response rates into long-term remissions and eventually cures.

REFERENCES

1. Cerosimi RJ and Hong WK: Epirubicin: A review of the pharmacology, clinical activity, and adverse effects of

an adriamycin analogue. J Clin Oncol 4:425-439, 1986.

2. Lopez M, Carpano S, Vici P, Di Laurol L, Papaldo P: Epirubicin and DTIC (EDIC) in the treatment of advanced soft tissue sarcomas in adults (abstr.) Proc Am Soc Clin Oncol 6:256, 1987.

3. Adams WJ, Brewer JE, Hosley JD, Earhart RH, Kuhn J, Weiss G, Brown T: Systemic Bioavailability and Pharmacokinetics of orally administered Menogaril. Proc Am Assoc Cancer Res 28:195, 1987.

4. Sordillo PP, Magill GB, Brenner J, Cheng EW, Dosik M, Yagoda A: Cisplatin. A Phase II evaluation in previously untreated patients with soft tissue sarcoma. Cancer 59:884-886, 1987.

5. Brenner J, Magill GB, Sordillo PP, Cheng EW, Yagoda A: A Phase II trial of cisplatin (CDDP) in previously treated patients with advanced soft tissue sarcoma. Cancer 50:2031-2033, 1982.

6. Samson MK, Baker LH, Benjamin RS, Lane M, Plager C: CisDichlorodiammineplatinum (II) in advanced soft tissue sarcoma: A Southwest Oncology Group study. Cancer Treat Rep 63:2027-2029, 1979.

7. Budd GT, Balcerzak S, Mortimer J, Fletcher W: SWOG 8465: High-dose cisplatin (CDDP) for advanced sarcomas. Proc Am Soc Clin Oncol 6:137, 1987.

8. Piver MD, Lele SB, Patsner B: Cis-Diamminedichloroplatinum plus Dimethyltriazenoimidazol Carboxamide as second and third line chemotherapy for sarcomas of the female pelvis. Gynecol Oncol 23:371-375, 1986.

9. Siemann DW, Alliet K, Maddison K, Wolf K: Enhancement of the antitumor efficacy of lomustine by the radiosensitizer RSU 1069. Cancer Treat Rep 69:1409-1414, 1985.

10. Hiramoto RN, Ghanta VK, Lilly MB: Reduction of tumor burden in a murine osteosarcoma following hyperthermia combined with cyclophosphamide. Cancer Res 44:1405-1408, 1984.

11. Bull JM, Strebel FR, Khokar AR, Bulger R, Newman RA: A synergistic combination of two platinum chemotherapy agents with hyperthermia in a fibrosarcoma. Proc Am Assoc Cancer Res (abstr.) 27:400, 1986.

12. Cohen JD, Robins HI: Hyperthermic enhancement of Cis-Diammine-1,1-cyclobutane Dicarboxylate Platinum(II) cytotoxicity in human leukemia cells in vitro. Cancer Res 47:4335-4337, 1987.

13. Bull JM, Strebel FR, Dobyan D, Sunderland B, Bulger R: Increased therapeutic index (TI) using Venoruton (V) combined with Cisplatin (CDDP) and whole body hyperthermia (WBH). Proc Am Assoc Cancer Res 28:447, 1987.

14. Jabboury K, Corry P, Plager C, Benjamin R: Hyperthermia induction in sarcoma. Proc Am Assoc Cancer Res 28:222, 1987.

15. Bull JMC, Mansfield B, Jabboury K, et al.: An update of whole body hyperthermia + BCNU in advanced sarcoma. Proc Am Assoc Clin Oncol 5:144, 1986.

16. Jabboury K, Duffin H, Bartley D, Corry P: Local hyperthermia for resistant soft tissue sarcoma. 34th Annual

Meeting of the Radiation Research Society, April 12-17, 1986, Las Vegas NV, (abstr.) p.18, 1986.

17. Cavaliere R, Di Fillipo F, Cavallari A, Calabro A, Carlini S, Piarulli L, Cerulli P: Hyperthermic perfusion as a first step of a multimodality approach to limb protocol for soft tissue sarcoma. 3rd European Conference on Clinical Oncology and Cancer Nursing, June 16-20, 1985, Stockholm, p.66, 1985.

18. Robins HI, Storer B, Longo WL, Sauserig J, Jendre R, Scacterle LM, Hugander AH, Hawkins MJ, Sielaff KC, Borden EC: Interferon alpha and whole body hyperthermia: a Phase I trial. Proc Am Assoc Cancer Res 27:205, 1986.

19. Strander H, Aparisi T, Brostom LA, Einhorn S, Ingimarson S: Nilsonne U, Soderborg G: Adjuvant interferon therapy of primary osteosarcoma. In Current Concepts of Diagnosis and Treatment of Bone Tissue and Soft Tissue Tumors, Berlin, Springer-Verlag, pp. 119-127, 1984.

20. Crane JL, Glasgow LA, Kern ER, Younger JS: Inhibition of murine osteogenic sarcomas by treatment with Type I or Type II interferons. J Natl Cancer Inst 61:871-874, 1978.

21. Hoffman V, Groscurth P, Morant R, Cserhati M, Honegger H, VonHochstetter A: Effects of leukocyte interferon (E. Coli) on human bone sarcoma growth in vitro and in the nude mouse. Eur J Cancer Clin Oncol 21:859-863, 1985.

22. Brosjo, O, Bauer HEF, Brostrom LA, Nillson OS, Reiholt FP, Tribukati B, et al.: Growth inhibition of human osteosarcomas in nude mice by human interferon - alpha: Significance of dose and tumor differentiation. Cancer Res 47:258-262, 1987.

23. Harris J, Das Gupta T, Vogelzang N, Badrinath K, Bonomi P, Dresser R, Locker G, Blough R, Johnson C, et al.: Treatment of soft tissue sarcoma with fibroblast interferon (beta-interferon): An American Cancer Society/ Illinois Cancer Council Study. Cancer Treat Rep 70:293-294, 1986.

24. Edmonson JH, Long HJ, Creagan ET, Frytak S, Sherwin S, Chang MN: Phase II study of recombinant gamma - interferon in patients with advanced nonosseous sarcomas. Cancer Treat Rep 71(2):211-213, 1987.

25. Edmonson JH, Long HJ, Frytak S, Smithson WA, Itri IM: Phase II study of recombinant Alfa-2a interferon in patients with advanced bone sarcomas. Cancer Treat Rep 71(7-8):747-748, 1987.

26. Brosjo O, Bauer HC, Brostrom LA, Nillson OS, Reinholt FP, Strander H, Tribuklati B, et al.: IFN-gamma inhibits osteosarcoma xenografts in nude mice. J Interferon Res (abstr.) 6(suppl.1):27, 1986.

27. Gonic K, Oka T, Morimoto M: Antitumor effect of human recombinant interferon gamma and beta against human osteosarcoma transplanted into nude mice. J Pharmacobiodyn 9:879-888, 1986.

28. Coley WB: The treatment of malignant tumors by repeated inoculations of erysipelas. The Am J of the Med Sciences 105: May 1883.

29. Nauts HC: Beneficial effects of immunotherapy (bacterial toxins) on sarcoma of soft tissues, other than lymphosarcoma. NY Cancer Res Inst (monogr.) 16:1-219, 1975.

30. Old LJ: Tumor necrosis factor (TNF). Science 230:630-632, 1985.

31. Palladino MA, Shalaby MR, Kramer SM, Ferraiolo BL, Baughman RA, Deleo AB, Crase D, Marafino B, Aggarawal BB, Figari IS, Liggit D, Patton JS: Characterization of the antitumor activities of human tumor necrosis factor alpha and the comparison with other cytokines: induction of tumor specific immunity. J Immunol 138(11):4023-4032, 1987.

32. Tomazic VJ, Farha M, Loftus A, Elias GE: Therapeutic effects of recombinant tumor necrosis factor on growth of mouse fibrosarcoma. Proc Am Assoc Cancer Res 28:398, 1987.

33. Bloksma N, Hofhuis FMA: Synergistic action of human recombinant tumor necrosis factor with endotoxins or nontoxic poly A:U against solid Meth a tumors in mice. Cancer Immunol Immunother 24(2):165-171, 1987.

34. Regenass U, Muller M, Curschellas E, Matter A: Antitumor effects of tumor necrosis factor in combination with chemotherapeutic agents. Intl J Cancer 39:266-273, 1987.

35. Mule JJ, Yang JC, Lafreniere R, Shu S, Rosenberg SA: Identification of cellular mechanisms operational in vivo during the regression of established pulmonary metastases by the systemic administration of high dose recombinant interleukin 2. J Immunol 139:285-294, 1987.

36. Mule JJ, Shu S, Rosenberg SA: The antitumor efficacy of lymphokine activated killer cells and recombinant interleukin-2 in vivo. J Immunol 135:646-652, 1985.

37. Rosenberg SA, Lotze MT, Chang AE, Avis FP, Leitman S, Linehan WM, Robertson CN, Lee RE, Rubin JT, Seipp CA, Simpson CG, White DE: A progress report on the treatment of 157 patients with advanced cancer using lymphokine activated killer cells and interleukin-2 or high dose interleukin-2 alone. New Engl J Med 316:889-897, 1987.

38. Lafraniere R and Rosenberg SA: Adoptive immunotherapy of murine hepatic metastases with lymphokine activated killer cells and recombinant interleukin 2 can mediate the regression of both immunogenic and non-immunogenic sarcomas and an adenocarcinoma. J Immunol 135:4273-4280, 1985.

39. Benjamin RS: Limb salvage surgery for sarcomas: A good idea receives formal blessing (editorial). JAMA 254:1795-1796, 1985.

40. Feit C, Bartal AH, Fass B, Bushkin Y, Cardo CC, Hirshaut Y: Monoclonal antibodies to human sarcoma and connective tissue differentiation antigens. Cancer Res 44:5752, 1984.

41. Brown JM, Greager JA, Pavel DG, Das Gupta TK: Localization of radiolabelled monoclonal antibody in a human soft tissue sarcoma xenograft. J.N.C.I. 75:637-644, 1985.

42. Greager JA, Atcher RW, Blend M, Brechbiel MW, Gansow OA, Das Gupta TK: Evaluation of ^{111}In-1-(p-Isothiocyanato-benzyl) - DTPA labelling of an anti-sarcoma monoclonal antibody for sarcoma Radioimmunodetection. Proc Am Assoc Cancer Res 28:356, 1986.
43. Lamon EW, Powell TJ, Walia AS, Lidin BIM, Srinivas RV, Baskin JG, Kearney JF: Monoclonal IgM antibodies that inhibit primary moloney murine sarcoma growth. J.N.C.I. 78:547-556, 1987.
44. Baldwin RW, Embleton MJ, Garnett MC, Pimm MV: Conjugates of monoclonal antibody 791T/36 with methotrexate in cancer therapy: NCI Monograph 3:95-99, 1987.
45. Cheung NK, Berger N, Coccia P, Kallick S, Lazarus H, Miraldi F, Saringen U, Strandjord S: Murine monoclonal antibody specific for GD2 ganglioside: A Phase I trial in patients with neuroblastoma, melanoma and osteogenic sarcoma. Proc Am Assoc Cancer Res 27:318, 1986.